As a neonatal nurse and educator for more than 30 years I have seen firsthand the impact our neonatal intensive care units (NICUs) have on infants and their families. While not a new concept, few health professionals understand or necessarily like the term "trauma-informed care," yet that is what our neonates and families need. This book addresses the most important issues that impact neonatal care. Using evidence to support the interventions may lead more health professionals to support the implementation. Use of a competency model will assist supervisors in measuring outcomes for both the health professional's own performance and the care provided. Trauma-informed care supports family-centered integrative, transdisciplinary care, which is vital to the provision of safe, high-quality neonatal care.

Carole Kenner, PhD, NNP, RN, FAAN
Carol Kuser Loser Dean and Professor
School of Nursing, Health, and Exercise Science
The College of New Jersey

Mary Coughlin's new book, *Trauma-Informed Care in the NICU: Evidence-Based Practice Guidelines for Neonatal Clinicians*, draws on the growing evidence regarding the effectiveness of strength-based, individualized, developmentally supportive and relationship-based care delivery in the neonatal intensive care unit (NICU) setting. Much of this evidence has accumulated over the last three decades due to the international Newborn Individualized Developmental Care and Assessment Program (NIDCAP) research trials, which demonstrate, enduring into school age, improved brain development and overall health and developmental outcomes, as well as enhanced parent competence and lowered stress. Ms. Coughlin's sensitive and thoughtful work emphasizes the significant trauma that parents and infants, as well as staff, experience in the face of intensive newborn medical care. It will give pause to even the most hardened intensivists, who may attempt to wall off the feelings that come from recognizing the traumatizing events they must deliver repeatedly in the course of a NICU day, thus denying the humanity of infants and families, as well as their own. Coughlin's text supports clinicians in recapturing their true caring personhoods and reenergizes their emotional attunement to caring with compassion *and* technical excellence for the infants and families entrusted to them. This book is a must for every clinician and caregiver in newborn intensive care nurseries everywhere.

Heidelise Als, PhD
Professor of Psychology (Department of Psychiatry)
Harvard Medical School
Director, Neurobehavioral Infant and Child Studies
Boston Children's Hospital
Founder, NIDCAP Federation International

Ms. Coughlin's work on trauma-informed care in the neonatal intensive care unit (NICU) provides the neonatal (and health care) community with a sound and reliable resource for providing excellent age-appropriate care. She articulates and substantiates the necessity for improved and consistent practices to positively affect both short- and long-term outcomes for premature infants. Because of the innate link between neonatal therapy and trauma-informed care, Ms. Coughlin has delivered the keynote speech on this topic at our national conference and I have personally recommended her first book time and time again—to our membership, to health care leaders, and to parents of premature infants.

Sue Ludwig, OTR/L
President and Founder
National Association of Neonatal Therapists (NANT)

This important new book by an experienced and knowledgeable neonatal clinician provides a practical and evidence-based approach to apply the Institute of Medicine's six aims for health care improvement to the care of medically fragile neonatal intensive care unit (NICU) patients. A clear message is the central role of the neonatal nurse as a member of the transdisciplinary team in providing the optimal environment for age-appropriate care and family engagement to ensure the best possible outcomes.

Ann R. Stark, MD, FAAP
Professor of Pediatrics
Division of Neonatology
Vanderbilt University School of Medicine

Trauma-Informed Care in the NICU

Mary E. Coughlin, MS, NNP, RNC-E, is an inspirational speaker, motivational coach, and transformational consultant. With a clinical background that spans more than 30 years, Ms. Coughlin is the internationally recognized expert in the field of trauma-informed, age-appropriate care in the neonatal intensive care unit (NICU).

Ms. Coughlin is a graduate of Northeastern University, Boston, Massachusetts, where she received her baccalaureate and master's degrees in nursing. Following 7 years of active duty service in the U.S. Air Force Nurses Corps, Ms. Coughlin transitioned to civilian practice at the Brigham and Women's Hospital NICU in Boston, assuming roles as staff nurse, charge nurse, and neonatal nurse practitioner. After a 1-year interim faculty position, Ms. Coughlin realized her passion for education and currently provides multimodal continuing professional education for interdisciplinary neonatal clinicians aimed at translating evidence-based research into clinical practice for measurable results. She is a published author and keynote speaker for national and international conferences.

Trauma-Informed Care in the NICU

Evidence-Based Practice Guidelines
for Neonatal Clinicians

Mary E. Coughlin, MS, NNP, RNC-E

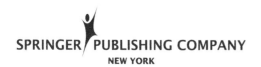

SPRINGER PUBLISHING COMPANY
NEW YORK

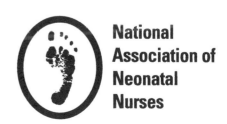

**National
Association of
Neonatal
Nurses**

Springer Publishing Company, LLC
11 West 42nd Street
New York, NY 10036
www.springerpub.com

Acquisitions Editor: Elizabeth Nieginski
Senior Production Editor: Kris Parrish
Composition: Newgen KnowledgeWorks

ISBN: 978-0-8261-3196-6
e-book ISBN: 978-0-8261-3197-3
Professional Practice Resources ISBN: 978-0-8261-3149-2

A Professional Practice Resources ancillary is available at springerpub.com/coughlin.

16 17 18 19 20 / 5 4 3 2 1

The author and the publisher of this Work have made every effort to use sources believed to be reliable to provide information that is accurate and compatible with the standards generally accepted at the time of publication. Because medical science is continually advancing, our knowledge base continues to expand. Therefore, as new information becomes available, changes in procedures become necessary. We recommend that the reader always consult current research and specific institutional policies before performing any clinical procedure. The author and publisher shall not be liable for any special, consequential, or exemplary damages resulting, in whole or in part, from the readers' use of, or reliance on, the information contained in this book. The publisher has no responsibility for the persistence or accuracy of URLs for external or third-party Internet websites referred to in this publication and does not guarantee that any content on such websites is, or will remain, accurate or appropriate.

Library of Congress Cataloging-in-Publication Data
Names: Coughlin, Mary, author. | Sequel to (work): Coughlin, Mary. Transformative nursing in the NICU.
Title: Trauma-informed care in the NICU: evidence-based practice guidelines for neonatal clinicians/ Mary E. Coughlin.
Description: New York, NY: Springer Publishing Company, LLC, [2017] | "Follow-up to Transformative nursing in the NICU: trauma-informed, age-appropriate care. This book is the direct result of my experience working with the amazing and dedicated neonatal intensive care unit (NICU) team at Children's Healthcare of Atlanta, Egleston campus"—Preface. | Includes bibliographical references and index.
Identifiers: LCCN 2016035326| ISBN 9780826131966 | ISBN 9780826131973 (e-book) | ISBN 9780826131492
Subjects: | MESH: Intensive Care, Neonatal—psychology | Infant, Newborn—psychology | Family Health | Evidence-Based Practice | Practice Guideline
Classification: LCC RJ253.5 | NLM WS 421 | DDC 618.92/01—dc23
LC record available at https://lccn.loc.gov/2016035326

Printed in the United States of America by Bradford & Bigelow.

Contents

Foreword

Neonatal care has gotten increasingly complex over the past decade. The concept of trauma to describe the neonatal intensive care unit (NICU) journey for the infant, family, and care providers has brought a new and different understanding to care practices in the NICU. Trauma-informed care speaks to the impact of the NICU environment and needed medical treatments and procedures for the infant who is often premature and critically ill, and the impact on his or her family who is dealing with the unexpected NICU admission after the birth of their infant.

The concept of trauma, as it relates to neonates and families, is clinically relevant to all neonatal care providers. Understanding the impact the NICU environment and treatment plans have on the developing infant and new family will have long-term implications in improving outcomes in this fragile population. Combining the core measures for age-appropriate care in the NICU and the principles of trauma-informed care within evidence-based clinical practice guidelines will lead to a standardization of practice, with the goal of improving neonatal and family outcomes.

Within this text, Mary Coughlin discusses clinically relevant, transdisciplinary practice guidelines within the five core measures, which include the importance of a healing environment, protection from pain and stress, time for protected sleep for the infant while continuing to provide for the daily care and treatment for the infant, and the integration of the family throughout the course of treatment in the NICU. Use of current scientific research along with explanations of the clinical rationale and the association with both short- and long-term outcomes make this an important resource for all involved in neonatal care. The guidelines include implementation strategies to support practice improvement, as well as sample competencies and teaching tools to support the changes that may be needed within the NICU.

Integration of families at the very beginning of the NICU journey is vital to improve positive family outcomes. It is recognized that the families require assistance in dealing with this difficult situation and the NICU environment. They need to identify their roles as parents, when others are often providing the daily hands-on care for their infant. The understanding of parent–clinical partnerships is important in the improvement of positive family outcomes.

But it is not only infants and their families that deal with the trauma of the NICU. Care providers need to understand issues within their work environment and workplace dynamics in addition to how the NICU environment and caring for critically ill infants can affect them individually, and what resources may be available for self-care and making healthy choices.

This text is a crucial resource for all neonatal care providers as a way to improve quality care to infants and families when faced with starting family life in the NICU. I would encourage all neonatal care providers to have this as a resource as we continue to develop new care technologies for the very smallest and critically ill infants who are in the NICU.

Cheryl Ann Carlson, PhD, APRN, NNP-BC
National Association of Neonatal Nurses President, 2012–2015

Preface

It was with great gratitude and excitement that I wrote this book as a follow-up to *Transformative Nursing in the NICU: Trauma-Informed, Age-Appropriate Care.* This book is the direct result of my experience working with the amazing and dedicated neonatal intensive care unit (NICU) team at Children's Healthcare of Atlanta, Egleston campus. The team and I embarked on a 3-year cultural transformation to adopt and integrate the National Association of Neonatal Nurses (NANN) Clinical Practice Guidelines for Age-Appropriate Care of the Premature and Critically Ill Hospitalized Infant. The vehicle for transformation was the Quantum Caring program from Caring Essentials, which combines the latest evidence-based research in trauma-informed, developmentally supportive, age-appropriate care with best practices in andragogy and uses proven implementation strategies and improvement methodologies to achieve measurable results. Launched in February 2013, the team has presented their progressive and statistically significant results at 10 international conferences to include the Gravens Conference on the Physical and Developmental Environment of the High Risk Infant (three times), the NANN Annual Educational Conference (twice), and the International Association for the Study of Pain Conference, as well as several local conferences.

As we approached the halfway point of the program (approximately 18 months in), the project leader, NICU nurse manager, and division director asked if I could put together a "core curriculum" handbook for them to use as a resource and reference once the program was completed. Knowing that cultural transformation isn't a destination but a journey, this sounded like a great idea. Since I am only as successful as my clients, I began compiling the latest and greatest evidence and best practice strategies for trauma-informed, age-appropriate care. I wanted a user-friendly format for the guidelines and so adopted the format used by the Agency for Healthcare Research and Quality—National Guideline Clearinghouse. As the work progressed I wondered if other folks might be interested in this type of resource and I contacted Elizabeth Nieginski at Springer Publishing (the amazing editor responsible for the first book) and ran the idea by her. She was very positive, asked me to put together a formal proposal, and, well, here we are!

Given how the first book resonated so profoundly with the global neonatal community, I am convinced that the concept of trauma-informed care in the NICU aligns with the mission, goals, and objectives of my transdisciplinary neonatal colleagues around the world. This book expands on the content from its predecessor and provides the reader with the next steps to adopt and implement a trauma-informed paradigm in their NICU.

A review of trauma and trauma-informed care and evidence-based updates to the core measures for age-appropriate care is presented in Part I. Part II dives deeper into each core measure set, providing updated evidence-based research to substantiate the practice recommendations, and includes practical implementation strategies and resources to support success. As a result of many invites to present on the topic of trauma and the clinician's experience, I have included a separate part addressing this critical challenge with guidelines and recommendations to support and promote self-care for my frontline colleagues.

Companion resources to this book are available at the Quality Caring Institute of Caring Essentials Collaborative, LLC, an online virtual learning environment. To begin, go to http://moodle.caringessentials.org, select login, and then register. (Guest login will not give you access to the learning materials and resources; you must register.) Once you have registered, select the course category titled Trauma-Informed Age-Appropriate Care and enroll using the enrollment key TAC2016. Please share your feedback and constructive comments regarding this web-based learning experience at contact@caringessentials.org. *A Professional Practice Resources ancillary is available from springerpub.com/coughlin.*

Mary E. Coughlin

Acknowledgments

As I mentioned in the Preface, this book is a direct result of my work with the wonderful team at Children's Healthcare of Atlanta (CHOA), Egleston NICU, and as such, I would like to formally express my profound gratitude to Myra Rolfes, Clinical Nurse Leader, for her passion, persistence, and capacity to engage, mentor, and inspire her colleagues. It has been a privilege to work with you; I am energized and inspired by our journey and I look forward to our next collaboration—just keep swimming, Myra!

I would also like to recognize and thank Deb LaPorte, Director of Critical Care at CHOA, for believing in and supporting the program and the work and your enthusiastic encouragement for this book—there are no words to express my gratitude!

In addition, I would like to acknowledge each and every staff member at the Egleston NICU—thank you for inspiring me, and giving me the chance to walk with you on your journey to provide trauma-informed, age-appropriate care to the infants and families you serve at Egleston's NICU! I hope this book helps others on that same journey!

Thanks to Dr. Ann Stark, my former colleague and dear friend from the Brigham and Women's NICU, currently Professor of Pediatrics, Division of Neonatology at Vanderbilt University School of Medicine; Sue Ludwig, President and Founder of the National Association of Neonatal Therapists; Dr. Carole Kenner, scholar and "mother of neonatal nursing"; and Dr. Heidelise Als, creator of the Newborn Individualized Developmental Care and Assessment Program (NIDCAP) and a prolific researcher who proposed the Synactive Theory, which forms the basis of developmentally supportive care. I want you all to know how honored and humbled I am that you each took time out of your busy lives to write your recommendations for this new book; I am truly grateful.

Last, but never least, I want to thank my husband, Dan McNeil, whose critical eye and attention to detail have been invaluable in editing, proofreading, and revising the manuscript—I know my writing style sometimes made you twitch (Dan was an English major), but I appreciate you balancing your passion for grammar with my need to express myself with as many "-ing" words as I choose. Although after the first book, I had vowed I would never write another one, I am very happy that I went back on my word and completed this manuscript. I hope you find it helpful and clinically relevant.

Take care and always care well.

PART I

Introduction to Trauma-Informed Care in the NICU

CHAPTER 1

Trauma and the NICU Experience

*There are wounds that never show on the body that are deeper and
more hurtful than anything that bleeds.*
         —Laurell K. Hamilton, *Mistral's Kiss*

■ WHAT IS TRAUMA?

The *Merriam-Webster Dictionary* defines trauma as both "an injury to living tissue
caused by an extrinsic agent and/or a disordered psychic or behavioral state resulting from severe mental or emotional stress or physical injury" (Merriam-Webster
Dictionary, 2016). The National Child Traumatic Stress Network (NCTSN) describes
pediatric medical trauma as a life-threatening situation that induces intense fear
activating a traumatic stress response comprised of physiological and psychological
phenomena. Adverse early-life experiences play a formative role in lifelong health
mediated by chronic fear, dysregulation of the hypothalamic–pituitary–adrenal
(HPA) axis, activation of the vagus nerve, and epigenetic factors that disrupt the
developmental trajectory of the individual physically, emotionally, and behaviorally.

For many, the word trauma conjures up visions of gunshot wounds, motor
vehicle accidents, domestic violence, sexual and/or physical abuse, war and other
forms of violence, or natural disasters such as hurricanes, floods, and earthquakes.
Hospitalization for a life-threatening illness is synonymous with trauma.

> Trauma is the unique individual experience of an event or enduring conditions
> in which the individual's ability to integrate his or her emotional experience is
> overwhelmed and the individual experiences a threat to his or her life, bodily
> integrity, or that of a caregiver or family. (Saakvitne, Gamble, Pearlman, & Tabor
> Lev, 2000)

The perception of trauma varies by age and stage of development and this may
be where there is a disconnect in understanding that an infant or neonate may experience and perceive trauma. As the brain's most primitive and essential role is to
ensure survival of the organism, experiences that pose a *perceived or actual* threat to
survival will trigger chemical, behavioral, and structural modifications within the
individual. Extreme fear and even terror develop in response to an aggressive world
of pain and isolation detected at a subcortical level, regardless of the intention or

medical necessity (Callaghan & Richardson, 2012). Early interpersonal trauma coupled with a paucity of loving care and confounded by excessive, repeated exposure to pain-related stress alters the psychoemotional development of the hospitalized infant and is associated with a decrease in white brain matter in critical brain regions when compared to healthy controls (Bick et al., 2015; Engelhardt et al., 2015; Montirosso & Provenzi, 2015; Smith et al., 2011).

The neural correlates of consciousness are capable of integrating exteroceptive and interoceptive inputs with emotions, feelings, and memories as early as 24 weeks gestation (Lagercrantz, 2014; Lagercrantz & Changeux, 2010). At the cortical level, a neonate's somatosensory awareness of peripheral noxious stimulation is intact at approximately 23 to 24 weeks gestation (Lagercrantz & Changeux, 2010; McGlone, Wessberg, & Olausson, 2014). How this relates to the infant's perception of trauma involves the role of the amygdala or the brain's emotional processor located in the temporal subcortex, which is functionally competent by the second trimester with continued pruning of regional connections influenced by experience throughout adolescence (Bock, Rether, Gröger, Xie, & Braun, 2014; Kiernan, 2012; Phelps & LeDoux, 2005; Saygin et al., 2015). The amygdala receives sensory information from the external world; rapidly assigns emotional significance to the event (i.e., what is the level of danger or threat); regulates physiological and behavioral responses to these external stimuli; and, when these events are repeated, reinforces the response sequence to create Pavlovian associations (LeDoux, 2010; McEwen & Gianaros, 2011). These threats underlie learning of fear and are associated with reduced hippocampal volume and function in adulthood, elevated amygdala reactivity to threats, attention bias or hypervigilance, reduced prefrontal cortex volume, and compromised attachment and interpersonal relationships as infant behavior is shaped to match the environment and his or her experiences (Landers & Sullivan, 2012; National Scientific Council on the Developing Child, 2010; Sheridan & McLaughlin, 2014). When combined with socioemotional deprivation or the absence of maternal care, the neural and genetic consequences associated with this early-life adversity are compounded (Montirosso & Provenzi, 2015; Sheridan & McLaughlin, 2014).

Neonatal intensive care is an adverse early-life experience that includes experiences of threat and deprivation. Figure 1.1 highlights institutionalization (e.g., hospitalization) as an experience associated with high deprivation and high threat (Sheridan & McLaughlin, 2014).

Neglect or unresponsive care overshadows the experience in an institutional setting and can be manifested at varying levels as described by the Center on the Developing Child (Table 1.1), which acknowledges that although the term *neglect* has a specific meaning with regard to the social welfare system, for researchers, neglect is synonymous with deprivation and refers to "the absence of attention, responsiveness, and protection that are appropriate to the age and needs of a child" (National Scientific Council on the Developing Child, 2012).

Neglect, deprivation, or unresponsive care initiates a toxic stress response that disrupts homeostasis, undermines attachment learning, alters gene expression, and derails healthy development (Chen & Baram 2016; Johnson, Riley, Granger, & Riis,

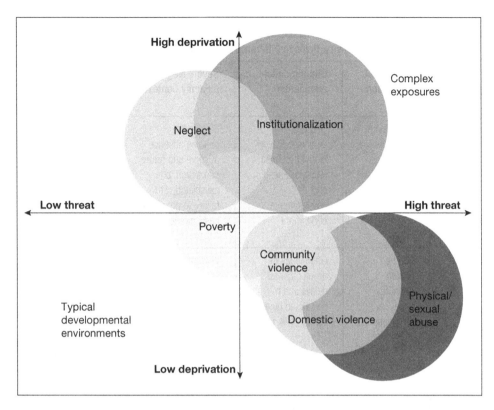

FIGURE 1.1   Threat and deprivation are dimensions of experiences associated with early-life adversity.
Reprinted with permission from Sheridan and McLaughlin (2014) and Elsevier.

2013; Moriceau, Shionoya, Jakubs, & Sullivan, 2009; National Scientific Council on the Developing Child, 2005/2014; Provenzi & Santoro, 2015; Shonkoff & Garner, 2012; Sullivan & Perry, 2015). The biologic mechanism of the trauma experience is exemplified by the allostatic-load model (Figure 1.2) put forth by Moore, Berger, and Wilson (2014).

Repeated activation of the stress response system superimposed on the structurally and functionally immature body systems of the hospitalized neonate creates a unique constellation of maladaptive physiologic patterns that compromises and exaggerates immune function, overwhelms the antioxidant system, and alters cortisol and catecholamine levels (Ganzel & Morris, 2011; Moore et al., 2014). It is important to note that all stress is not bad (Figure 1.3). However, excessive stress, also known as toxic stress, referring to intense, frequent, protracted activation of the stress response system, alters the very architecture of the brain impacting the developmental trajectory of the individual physically, emotionally, and behaviorally (National Scientific Council on the Developing Child, 2005/2014).

TABLE 1.1   Four Types of Unresponsive Care

| | Science Helps to Differentiate Four Types of Unresponsive Case | | | |
	Occasional Inattention	Chronic Under-stimulation	Severe Neglect in a Family Context	Severe Neglect in an Institutional Setting
Features	Intermittent, diminished attention in an otherwise responsive environment	Ongoing, diminished level of child-focused responsiveness and developmental enrichment	Significant, ongoing absence of serve and return interaction, often associated with failure to provide for basic needs	"Warehouse-like" conditions with many children, few caregivers, and no individualized adult–child relationships that are reliably responsive
Effects	Can be growth promoting under caring conditions	Often leads to developmental delays and may be caused by a variety of factors	Wide range of adverse impacts, from significant developmental impairments to immediate threat to health or survival	Basic survival needs may be met, but lack of individualized adult responsiveness can lead to severe impairments in cognitive, physical, and psychosocial development
Action	No intervention needed	Interventions that address the needs of caregivers combined with access to high-quality early care and education for children can be effective	Intervention to ensure caregiver responsiveness and address the developmental needs of the child required as soon as possible	Intervention and removal to a stable, caring, and socially responsive environment required as soon as possible

Source: National Scientific Council on the Developing Child (2012).

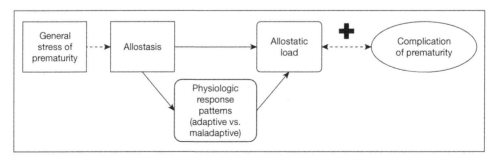

FIGURE 1.2   General stress of prematurity (or neonatal critical illness) has a direct relationship with allostasis (the stress response), which over time becomes an allostatic load on the individual mediated by adaptive or maladaptive physiological responses.

Moore, Berger, and Wilson (2014) adapted this model from the work of McEwen (1998). Reprinted with permission of SAGE Publications, Inc.

Positive stress

- Stress associated with everyday life, for example, immunization
- Short episode of autonomic reactivity, supported by a caring adult
- Positive adaption

Tolerable stress

- Stress associated with a more significant event and has the potential to be harmful (i.e., surgery–with appropriate or inappropriate pain management)
- The presence of absence of a supportive adult can ease or exacerbate the stress

Toxic stress

- Strong, frequent, prolonged periods of unmanaged/unrecognized stress
- Maternal separation
- Unresponsive care/caring from an adult

FIGURE 1.3 Types of stress.
Adapted from National Scientific Council on the Developing Child (2005/2014).

The trauma experience of the neonatal intensive care unit (NICU) transcends the infant's life-threatening admission diagnosis and associated medical/surgical invasive procedures, and includes the infant's postural orientation, feeding encounters, sleep requirements, sensual experiences, and other age-appropriate core needs of the developing human being, but most significantly, the primary trauma experienced by the hospitalized infant is separation from mother, from family, from a secure, constant, loving relationship that is completely devoted to protecting, reassuring, and validating the infant's existence and personhood (Coughlin, 2014).

Trauma by definition is unbearable and intolerable with lifelong physiological and psychological implications; it is a very personal, individualized experience. Regardless of the diagnosis, infants requiring neonatal intensive care are at higher risk of psychological, behavioral, cognitive, relational, and emotional pathology then their term counterparts as a result of their trauma experience (Coughlin, 2014). The physiological, developmental, and psychological implications of pain-related stress (a component of the NICU trauma experience) have been well studied and report alterations in brain microstructure and function, changes in biological set-point circuitry (i.e., HPA axis), aberrations in stress responsivity and stress-sensitive behaviors, alterations in brain oscillations that negatively impact visual perceptual capabilities at school-age, and a predisposition to a number of neuropsychiatric and behavioral disorders that severely limits the infant's quality of life (Anand & Scalzo, 2000; Coughlin, 2014; Doesburg et al., 2013; Grunau, 2013; Vinall & Grunau, 2014).

▪ THE CONTEXT OF TRAUMA

It's often said that a traumatic experience early in life marks a person
forever, pulls her out of line, saying, "Stay there. Don't move."
     —Jeffrey Eugenides

Contextual factors influence an infant's response to the trauma of life-threatening illness and intensive care hospitalization and modulates long-term plasticity framed by the infant's neurobiological susceptibility to the environment (Boyce, 2016). The social ecology or environment of the infant requires dynamic engaging and responsive "serve and return" interactions with adults (parents and professionals) to support healthy development and cultivate resilience in the developing human (National Scientific Council on the Developing Child, 2012). Biobehavioral synchrony between parent and infant is requisite for social growth, shaping oxytocin functionality, building capacity for empathy and self-regulatory capabilities (Figure 1.4; Feldman, 2015a).

Establishing zero parent–infant separation as the context for care in the NICU enables the parent to accept and embrace the traumatic reality of the newborn infant's critical illness and begin the neurobiological and behavioral transformation to parenthood (Bergman, 2014; Blomqvist, Rubertsson, Kylberg, Jöreskog, & Nyqvist, 2012; Cleveland, 2008; Feldman, 2016). Fragmented and unpredictable parent–infant interactions, especially within the context of trauma, exert profound deleterious effects on both infants and parents (Baram et al., 2012; Feldman, 2015b). In a systematic review of qualitative studies, fathers of preterm infants identify five main themes describing the paternal experience within the context of the NICU: the experience of an emotional roller coaster, the need to be informed and treated respectfully, feelings of helplessness and out of control, an emerging sense of parenthood restricted by the critical nature of the environment, and the desire to provide care juxtaposed with the fear of hurting the fragile infant (Provenzi & Santoro, 2015).

Research confirms parental expectations to participate in the care of the hospitalized infant, attitudes and behaviors of health care professionals, as well as other contextual factors of the NICU (e.g., rituals, routines, culture) can prohibit or facilitate parental involvement (Power & Franck, 2008). Recognizing the impact of trauma and toxic stress on the hospitalized infant–family dyad necessitates consistently reliable experiences that mitigate the trauma—that is, responsive, relation-based care encounters that not only address the medical or surgical needs of the individual but the infant's age-appropriate, experience-expected needs (Coughlin, 2014).

The context of trauma in the NICU can be rewarding and fulfilling or overwhelming and morally distressing for the health care professional. Caring for profoundly fragile individuals with diverse cultural backgrounds in a technologically oriented environment, the caring professional can lose sight of the shared humanity with the families they serve. The trauma experience of the professional is shaped by the professional's own unique personal history, views on family, past and present

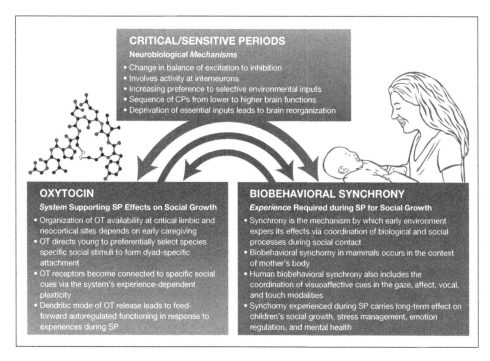

FIGURE 1.4   Critical/sensitive periods.

CP, critical period; OT, oxytocin; SP, sensitive period.
Feldman (2015a). Reproduced with permission from Cambridge University Press.

relationships, and experiences with illness, dying, and death. All of this is brought to bear on the service they provide within the context of trauma. Clinical expertise and technical proficiency may serve as a shield to the ever-present suffering we bear witness to every day, but a price is paid.

The context of trauma for the professional is presented in more detail in Part III.

■ REFERENCES

Anand, K. J., & Scalzo, F. M. (2000). Can adverse neonatal experiences alter brain development and subsequent behavior? *Biology of the Neonate, 77*(2), 69–82.

Baram, T. Z., Davis, E. P., Obenaus, A., Sandman, C. A., Small, S. L., Solodkin, A., & Stern, H. (2012). Fragmentation and unpredictability of early-life experience in mental disorders. *The American Journal of Psychiatry, 169*(9), 907–915.

Bergman, N. J. (2014). The neuroscience of birth—and the case for Zero Separation. *Curationis, 37*(2, Art. #1440), 4. Retrieved from http://dx.doi.org/10.4102/curationis.v37i2.1440

Bick, J., Zhu, T., Stamoulis, C., Fox, N. A., Zeanah, C., & Nelson, C. A. (2015). Effect of early institutionalization and foster care on long-term white matter development: A randomized clinical trial. *JAMA Pediatrics, 169*(3), 211–219.

Blomqvist, Y. T., Rubertsson, C., Kylberg, E., Jöreskog, K., & Nyqvist, K. H. (2012). Kangaroo mother care helps fathers of preterm infants gain confidence in the paternal role. *Journal of Advanced Nursing, 68*(9), 1988–1996.

Bock, J., Rether, K., Gröger, N., Xie, L., & Braun, K. (2014). Perinatal programming of emotional brain circuits: An integrative view from systems to molecules. *Frontiers in Neuroscience, 8*, 11.

Boyce, W. T. (2016). Differential susceptibility of the developing brain to contextual adversity and stress. *Neuropsychopharmacology, 41*(1), 142–162.

Callaghan, B. L., & Richardson, R. (2012). The effect of adverse rearing environments on persistent memories in young rats: Removing the brakes on infant fear memories. *Translational Psychiatry, 2*, e138.

Chen, Y., & Baram, T. Z. (2016). Toward understanding how early-life stress reprograms cognitive and emotional brain networks. *Neuropsychopharmacology, 41*(1), 197–206.

Cleveland, L. M. (2008). Parenting in the neonatal intensive care unit. *Journal of Obstetric, Gynecologic, and Neonatal Nursing, 37*(6), 666–691.

Coughlin, M. (2014). *Transformative nursing in the NICU: Trauma-informed, age-appropriate care*. New York, NY: Springer Publishing.

Doesburg, S. M., Chau, C. M., Cheung, T. P., Moiseev, A., Ribary, U., Herdman, A. T.,… Grunau, R. E. (2013). Neonatal pain-related stress, functional cortical activity and visual-perceptual abilities in school-age children born at extremely low gestational age. *Pain, 154*(10), 1946–1952.

Engelhardt, E., Inder, T. E., Alexopoulos, D., Dierker, D. L., Hill, J., Van Essen, D., & Neil, J. J. (2015). Regional impairments of cortical folding in premature infants. *Annals of Neurology, 77*(1), 154–162.

Feldman, R. (2015a). Sensitive periods in human social development: New insights from research on oxytocin, synchrony, and high-risk parenting. *Development and Psychopathology, 27*(2), 369–395.

Feldman, R. (2015b). The adaptive human parental brain: Implications for children's social development. *Trends in Neurosciences, 38*(6), 387–399.

Feldman, R. (2016). The neurobiology of mammalian parenting and the biosocial context of human caregiving. *Hormones and Behavior, 77*, 3–17.

Ganzel, B. L., & Morris, P. A. (2011). Allostasis and the developing human brain: Explicit consideration of implicit models. *Development and Psychopathology, 23*(4), 955–974.

Grunau, R. E. (2013). Neonatal pain in very preterm infants: Long-term effects on brain, neurodevelopment and pain reactivity. *Rambam Maimonides Medical Journal, 4*(4), e0025.

Johnson, S. B., Riley, A. W., Granger, D. A., & Riis, J. (2013). The science of early life toxic stress for pediatric practice and advocacy. *Pediatrics, 131*(2), 319–327.

Kiernan, J. A. (2012). Anatomy of the temporal lobe. *Epilepsy Research and Treatment, 2012*, 1–12. doi:10.1155/2012/176157

Lagercrantz, H. (2014). The emergence of consciousness: Science and ethics. *Seminars in Fetal & Neonatal Medicine, 19*(5), 300–305.

Lagercrantz, H., & Changeux, J. P. (2010). Basic consciousness of the newborn. *Seminars in Perinatology, 34*(3), 201–206.

Landers, M. S., & Sullivan, R. M. (2012). The development and neurobiology of infant attachment and fear. *Developmental Neuroscience, 34*(2–3), 101–114.

LeDoux, J. (2010). *The amygdala in 5 minutes.* Retrieved from http://bigthink.com/videos/the-amygdala-in-5-minutes

McEwen, B. S. (1998). Stress, adaptation, and disease. Allostasis and allostatic load. *Annals of the New York Academy of Sciences, 840,* 33–44.

McEwen, B. S., & Gianaros, P. J. (2011). Stress- and allostasis-induced brain plasticity. *Annual Review of Medicine, 62,* 431–445.

McGlone, F., Wessberg, J., & Olausson, H. (2014). Discriminative and affective touch: Sensing and feeling. *Neuron, 82*(4), 737–755.

Merriam-Webster Dictionary. Retrieved from http://www.merriam-webster.com/dictionary/trauma

Montirosso, R., & Provenzi, L. (2015). Implications of epigenetics and stress regulation on research and developmental care of preterm infants. *Journal of Obstetric, Gynecologic, and Neonatal Nursing: JOGNN/NAACOG, 44*(2), 174–182.

Moore, T. A., Berger, A. M., & Wilson, M. E. (2014). A new way of thinking about complications of prematurity. *Biological Research for Nursing, 16*(1), 72–82.

Moriceau, S., Shionoya, K., Jakubs, K., & Sullivan, R. M. (2009). Early-life stress disrupts attachment learning: The role of amygdala corticosterone, locus ceruleus corticotropin releasing hormone, and olfactory bulb norepinephrine. *The Journal of Neuroscience, 29*(50), 15745–15755.

National Scientific Council on the Developing Child. (2005/2014). *Excessive stress disrupts the architecture of the developing brain: Working paper 3* (updated edition). Retrieved from http://www.developingchild.harvard.edu

National Scientific Council on the Developing Child. (2010). *Persistent fear and anxiety can affect young children's learning and development: Working paper no. 9.* Retrieved from http://www.developingchild.net

National Scientific Council on the Developing Child. (2012). *The science of neglect: The persistent absence of responsive care disrupts the developing brain: Working paper 12.* Retrieved from http://www.developingchild.harvard.edu

Phelps, E. A., & LeDoux, J. E. (2005). Contributions of the amygdala to emotion processing: From animal models to human behavior. *Neuron, 48*(2), 175–187.

Power, N., & Franck, L. (2008). Parent participation in the care of hospitalized children: A systematic review. *Journal of Advanced Nursing, 62*(6), 622–641.

Provenzi, L., & Santoro, E. (2015). The lived experience of fathers of preterm infants in the neonatal intensive care unit: A systematic review of qualitative studies. *Journal of Clinical Nursing, 24*(13–14), 1784–1794.

Saakvitne, K., Gamble, S., Pearlman, L., & Tabor Lev, B. (2000). *Risking connection: A training curriculum for working with survivors of childhood abuse.* Baltimore, MD: Sidran Press.

Saygin, Z. M., Osher, D. E., Koldewyn, K., Martin, R. E., Finn, A., Saxe, R.,...Sheridan, M. (2015). Structural connectivity of the developing human amygdala. *PloS One, 10*(4), e0125170.

Sheridan, M. A., & McLaughlin, K. A. (2014). Dimensions of early experience and neural development: Deprivation and threat. *Trends in Cognitive Sciences, 18*(11), 580–585.

Shonkoff, J. P., & Garner, A. S.; Committee on Psychosocial Aspects of Child and Family Health; Committee on Early Childhood, Adoption, and Dependent Care; Section on Developmental and Behavioral Pediatrics. (2012). The lifelong effects of early childhood adversity and toxic stress. *Pediatrics, 129*(1), e232–e246.

Smith, G. C., Gutovich, J., Smyser, C., Pineda, R., Newnham, C., Tjoeng, T. H.,…Inder, T. (2011). Neonatal intensive care unit stress is associated with brain development in preterm infants. *Annals of Neurology, 70*(4), 541–549.

Sullivan, R. M., & Perry, R. E. (2015). Mechanisms and functional implications of social buffering in infants: Lessons from animal models. *Social Neuroscience, 10*(5), 500–511.

Van der Kolk, B. (2014). *The body keeps the score: Brain, mind, and body in the healing of trauma.* New York, NY: Penguin.

Vinall, J., & Grunau, R. E. (2014). Impact of repeated procedural pain-related stress in infants born very preterm. *Pediatric Research, 75*(5), 584–587.

CHAPTER 2

Core Measures for Age-Appropriate Care

Core measures for age-appropriate care in the neonatal intensive care unit (NICU), framed by the Universe of Developmental Care (UDC) model, define measurable, evidence-based best practices in developmentally supportive, whole-person care (Coughlin, 2011; Coughlin, Gibbins, & Hoath, 2009; Gibbins, Hoath, Coughlin, Gibbins, & Franck, 2008). This concept, adapted from The Joint Commission (TJC) to quantify disease-independent evidence-based practices, was introduced by Coughlin et al. (2009), reviewed and published by the National Association of Neonatal Nurses (Coughlin, 2011), and has been successfully implemented and adapted as both a standard to assess existing practices and a vehicle to guide practice improvement in NICUs across the globe (Coughlin, 2014; Coughlin & Rolfes, 2016; Goudarzi et al., 2015; Montirosso et al., 2012; Soleimani, Torkzahrani, Rafiey, Salavati, & Nasiri, 2016; Valizadeh, Asadollahi, Mostafa Gharebaghi, & Gholami, 2013).

Integrating the concept of trauma-informed care operationalized by the core measures for age-appropriate care in the NICU meets the developmentally sensitive and critical needs of the hospitalized infant and aims to restore health through healing relationships and integrative care. The concept of health is complex and multifaceted. The World Health Organization defines health as "a state of complete physical, mental, and social well-being and not merely the absence of disease or infirmity" (WHO, 2016; p. 100). Accordingly, the presence of disease should not diminish an individual's need for physical and psycho-emotional comfort and supportive social interactions; however, in today's technologically driven, task-oriented health care system, patients are often reduced to their diagnostic circumstances, stripped of their personhood and humanity. In the eloquent plenary speech at the 2009 International Forum on Quality and Safety in Healthcare, former president of the Institute for Healthcare Improvement Dr. Don Berwick speaks about his fear of becoming a patient:

> What chills my bones is indignity...homogenized, anonymous, powerless....It scares me to be made helpless before my time, to be made ignorant when I want to know...or to be alone when I need to hold my wife's hand....You can call it patient-centeredness if you choose, but I suggest to you, this is the core, it is that property of care that welcomes me to assert my humanity and my individuality and my uniqueness. And if we be healers, that is not a root to the point, it *is* the point (Berwick, 2009, July 4).
>
> —Reprinted from www.IHI.org with permission of the
> Institute for Healthcare Improvement (IHI), © 2011

Healing is "a holistic, transformative process of repair and recovery in mind, body, and spirit resulting in positive change, finding meaning, and movement toward self-realization of wholeness, regardless of the presence or absence of disease" (Sakallaris, MacAllister, Voss, Smith, & Jonas, 2015, p. 1). Ignoring a healing, trauma-informed approach to care in the NICU places the hospitalized individual at risk of healthcare–acquired conditions mediated and exacerbated by stress and distress with lifelong implications both physiologically and psychologically (Coughlin, 2014; Feldman, 2015; Moore, Berger, & Wilson, 2014).

■ THE HEALING ENVIRONMENT

We are now approaching a day when the best medical care and
nurturing are not mutually exclusive concepts, and where the mother's
arms are considered the optimal locus of care.
       —White (2011)

The importance of the physical environment in health, healing, and recovery has been acknowledged as early as 400 BCE by Hippocrates in ancient Greece. Florence Nightingale in the 19th century reiterated the importance of the physical environment and added the relevance of the human and organizational dimensions of the environment on quality patient outcomes. Nurse theorist Myra Levine in her Conservation model describes the importance of congruence between person and environment to restore health. Levine's concept is echoed in the work of Aaron Antonovsky, who proposed a *salutogenic* model to guide health promotion and promote a paradigm shift from a dualistic perspective of illness and wellness to a holistic and integrated view of health as a movement on a continuum between disease and "ease" or wellness (Antonovsky, 1996; Jonas, Chez, Smith, & Sakallaris, 2014; Lindström & Eriksson, 2005).

An individual's health continuum is dynamic and influenced by the environment—healing or otherwise. The attributes associated with the healing environment of the NICU include the physical, human, and organizational dimensions (Coughlin, 2011, 2014; Coughlin et al., 2009). These attributes are integrated yet distinct from each other and are supported by a substantial body of evidence demonstrating relevance across clinical, psycho-emotional, and economic domains. Optimal healing environments acknowledge the complex needs of the hospitalized individual as an integrated organism with psychic, social, and somatic dimensions (Jonas et al., 2014; Sakallaris et al., 2015; Schweitzer, Gilpin, & Frampton, 2004).

In 2004, a research team from Texas A&M University and Georgia Tech identified more than 600 studies that established how hospital design impacts clinical outcomes (Ulrich, Quan, Zimring, Joseph, & Choudhary, 2004). They discovered not only a large body of evidence to guide hospital design but found rigorous studies linking the physical environment to patient and staff outcomes, specifically:

- Decreased levels of stress and fatigue among staff members
- Increased effectiveness in delivering care
- Improved patient safety
- Decreased patient stress and improved patient outcomes
- Improved overall health care quality

Just as medicine has moved toward an evidence-based framework, health care design is increasingly guided by research that links the physical environment to patient and staff outcomes. As defined by the core measures for age-appropriate care in the NICU, the physical environment includes the sensory milieu, the physical layout, and spatial dimensions, as well as the aesthetics. The combination of these attributes demonstrates a respect for human dignity, supports the socioemotional gestation of the infant through continuous family presence, and provides neuroprotection for the developing somatosensory and interoceptive systems. Integrating these dimensions of the healing environment consistently and reliably into the culture of care has far-reaching implications when viewed through the lens of human behavioral epigenetics. Provenzi and Montirosso (2015) define prematurity as an example of early-life adversity. Our understanding of the epigenetic vulnerability of this unique patient population to the caregiving environment and caregiving experiences poses an intriguing ethical and moral conundrum. As NICU clinicians, do we have an *epigenethical* responsibility to manage the environmental and early-life stressors inherent to a stay in the NICU (Provenzi & Montirosso, 2015)?

The professional's internal and interpersonal environments (the human environment) mediate this ethical and moral dilemma and impact quality and patient safety, job satisfaction, and professional fulfillment. Healing intention and healing relationships are the foundation for conscious transpersonal caring—the therapeutic use of self (Barba, Stump, & Fitzsimmons, 2014; Roley et al., 2008; Sakallaris et al., 2015; Taylor, Lee, Kielhofner, & Ketkar, 2009; Watson, 2002). Insight into our own personal journey with suffering and our experience with bearing witness to the suffering of others must be continuously assessed to ensure that we are able to be fully present in the caring moment, that critical turning point when we touch and are touched by another's humanity (Watson, 2002, 2006).

> Often we hear about burnout, but increasingly we learn that the burnout is not because we care too much. It's because we wall ourselves off and close off our heart, and close off our very source of love, and the human connectedness that gives us the life-generating force for that work. (Watson, 2006)

Presence, mindfulness, and empathy underpin our ability to consistently and reliably provide trauma-informed, age-appropriate care with regard to managing and mitigating pain and stress, promoting and protecting sleep, providing optimal postural alignment, ensuring infant-guided feeding experiences, preserving skin integrity, and securing collaborative partnerships with parents and families.

The assurance of optimal healing environments requires leadership and organizational commitment to an ethic of trauma-informed, age-appropriate care. Transformational and relational leadership, grounded by a strong moral compass, ensures that resources are sufficient to deliver the desired standards of care, support, and role-model professionalism and accountability, and endorse zero tolerance for substandard care or unethical behavior (Cummings et al., 2010; Gustafsson & Stenberg, 2015; Mannix, Wilkes, & Daly, 2015).

◼ PAIN AND STRESS

It seems unbelievable how long it took the medical community to
realize that newborns also feel pain.
    —Krishnan (2013)

Pain prevention, assessment, and management are complex health challenges across all patient populations and pose a unique challenge in the NICU. Infants rely on their adult caregivers to interpret and respond to their pain experience by "reading" physiological and behavioral cues and employing a high index of suspicion, presuming that pain is present in all situations to be considered painful for an adult, even if the biobehavioral signs are not present (Walden & Gibbins, 2012).

Pain relief is a basic right of every human being, regardless of age or size, and yet it is ubiquitous in the NICU (Krishnan, 2013). Carbajal et al. (2008b) completed a prospective epidemiological study on procedural pain management on a cohort of 430 infants ranging from 24 to 42 weeks gestational age at birth during the first 2 weeks following NICU admission. Of the greater than 42,000 painful procedures performed during this 2-week period, 79.2% were performed without any type of specific analgesia (Carbajal et al., 2008b). Cruz, Fernandes, and Oliveira (2016) confirm that painful procedures in the NICU are performed frequently and, more often than not, with inadequate pain management. Neonatal pain and pain-related stress are associated with compromised postnatal growth, poor early neurodevelopment, high cortical activation, altered brain development, negative affective temperament, cognitive and motor impairments, decreased pain tolerance, changes in cortical thickness, and increased incidence of internalizing behaviors (anxiety/depression) negatively correlated with visual-perceptual abilities at school age (Hatfield, Meyers, & Messing, 2013; Valeri, Holsti, & Linhares, 2015; Vinall & Grunau, 2014).

Therefore, the big question is: Why? Why is the treatment of neonatal pain so inconsistent? Despite an expansive body of evidence on the efficacy of various pharmacological and nonpharmacological pain-relief strategies as well as national and international evidence-based guidelines for preventing and treating neonatal pain, the translation of published research into routine clinical practice is inconsistent at best (Carbajal, Nguyen-Bourgain, & Armengaud, 2008a). Nurse–physician collaboration, parental presence, written pain-management protocols, and integrated approaches that include education, the use of validated assessment tools, and audit and feedback processes have been associated with more consistent translation of evidence-based pain care strategies into clinical practice (Allegaert, Tibboel, & van den Anker, 2013; Guedj et al., 2014; Latimer, Johnston, Ritchie, Clarke, & Gilin, 2009; Walker, 2014).

The prevention of pain and pain-related stress in neonates is a moral and ethical priority for pediatric and neonatal health care professionals. All health care settings that provide care for neonates must adopt comprehensive pain-prevention programs, as well as pain assessment and management care plans that use pharmacological and nonpharmacological strategies to prevent pain and pain-related stress associated with invasive procedures, surgical interventions, and hospitalization (Table 2.1; American Academy of Pediatrics [AAP] Committee on Fetus and Newborn & Section on Anesthesiology and Pain Medicine, 2016).

Undermanaged and/or unmanaged pain and pain-related stress must become a *never event* in the NICU and requires a commitment of organizational leadership, the transdisciplinary team, and the individual professional to ensure the consistently reliable provision of evidence-based, humane pain care to this profoundly vulnerable population.

TABLE 2.1   The 2016 Updated Recommendations From the American Academy of Pediatrics on Neonatal Procedural Pain Prevention and Management

1	Preventing and minimizing neonatal pain must be an expressed, measured, and monitored goal for facilities that serve the neonatal and infant patient population.
2	A validated neonatal pain assessment tool must be consistently and reliably used before, during, and after all painful procedures monitoring the effectiveness (or lack of effectiveness) of various pain-relief strategies; pain and stress must be continuously assessed throughout the infant's hospital course to ensure pain prevention and pain management.
3	Nonpharmacological interventions (e.g., facilitated tuck, nonnutritive sucking with or without sucrose/glucose/expressed breast milk, breastfeeding, and skin-to-skin care) must be an integral part of the pain prevention and procedural pain management plan of care.
4	Sucrose and/or glucose use for procedural pain management should be prescribed and tracked and should be part of an evidence-based pain prevention policy.
5	Caution and prudence should be taken when using pharmacological agents for neonatal pain, particularly when there is limited or nonexistent research for use in neonates.
6	Neonatal and pediatric clinicians as well as family members must receive continuing education on recognizing, assessing, and managing pain in neonates.
7	Continued research on pain assessment and pharmacological/nonpharmacological strategies must be ongoing and include studies on the pharmacokinetics and dynamics of newer medications to ensure safety and efficacy.

Adapted from American Academy of Pediatrics (AAP) Committee on Fetus and Newborn & Section on Anesthesiology and Pain Medicine (2016).

Educating parents and family members on the context of pain and pain-related stress in the NICU, as well as the biobehavioral indicators of pain and pain-related stress, is a first step to minimize unnecessary suffering in the NICU. In addition to education, however, parents must be empowered to advocate for their infant's pain care needs in partnership with the health care team. Parents should be informed of scheduled painful and stressful procedures to facilitate their presence in supporting and comforting their infant during these all too frequent, medically necessary events.

■ PROTECTED SLEEP

Sleep solves everything.
        —Unknown

Sleep plays a critical role in early cortical development. Sleep disturbances early in life are associated with alterations in cognitive, attentional, and psychosocial development (Kurth, Olini, Huber, & LeBourgeois, 2015). Sleep deprivation is associated with obesity and poor cognitive performance, and sleep fragmentation has been linked to asthma (Kurth et al., 2015). Qureshi, Malkar, Splaingard, Khuhro, and Jadcherla (2015) report a decrease in episodes of gastroesophageal reflux during sleep, and Scher et al. (2009) report that sleep, facilitated by skin-to-skin care, improves autonomic stability. Rapid eye movement (REM) sleep exerts a higher degree of importance during early cortical development for synaptic plasticity of the visual cortex and transitions to an emphasis on non-REM slow-wave activity for learning and developmental refinements of neural networks (Frank, Issa, & Stryker, 2001; Kurth et al., 2015).

The structure and quality of infant sleep in the NICU are impacted by frequent handling during caregiving routines, environmental factors (noise and light), underlying disease processes that are the source of pain and stress, and the use of various pharmacological substances that are known to interfere with sleep dynamics (Allen, 2012; Axelin, Cilio, Asunis, Peloquin, & Franck, 2013; Kudchadkar, Aljohani, & Punjabi, 2014). Mahmoodi, Arbabisarjou, Rezaeipoor, and Pishkar Mofrad (2015) report that nurses' knowledge of infant sleep and sleep–wake states is limited and may compromise neonatal brain development in the NICU. Providing evidence-based interventions in the NICU to support and protect sleep in partnership with parents improves infant and parent short- and long-term outcomes (Allen, 2012; Craig et al., 2015; Gerstein, Poehlmann-Tynan, & Clark, 2015).

Infant sleep goes through significant changes over the first year of life and is influenced by parent/caregiver behaviors. Empowering parents during the NICU stay to take an active role in parenting their infant and cultivating sleep routines and rituals facilitates the transition to home and supports ongoing healthy sleep patterns for the NICU graduate (Mindell, Sadeh, Kohyama, & How, 2010; Sadeh, Tikotzky, & Scher, 2010). Healthy sleep patterns include both daytime and nighttime sleeping over the first 2 years of life. Cultivating early regulatory behaviors (e.g., sleep patterns and rituals) and optimal interpersonal interactions during the NICU enriches parenting behaviors, supports parenting confidence postdischarge, and promotes infant brain development, which improves the developmental trajectory (Raines & Brustad, 2012; Schwichtenberg et al., 2011).

Preparation for discharge to home includes transitioning the infant and parents for supine sleep ("Back to Sleep"); however, inconsistencies in practice and significant knowledge gaps place the NICU infant–family dyad in grave danger of sudden, unexplained infant death (Patton, Stiltner, Wright, & Kautz, 2015). The AAP issued an expansion of its recommendations for a safe infant sleeping environment and includes a call to action for neonatal professionals to be vigilant in adopting, role-modeling, and endorsing safe sleep practices in the NICU (AAP, 2011). Translating these recommendations into practice requires a commitment to evidence-based practice at the organizational, unit, and individual levels as well as a clearly designed implementation strategy to achieve statistically significant improvements in knowledge and practice compliance (Hwang et al., 2015; McMullen, Fioravanti, Brown, & Carey, 2016).

ACTIVITIES OF DAILY LIVING

Ensuring postural alignment for comfort and optimal neuromotor development, employing cue-based and infant-directed oral feeding experiences, and maintaining skin and mucous membrane integrity through the adoption of evidence-based best practices form the triumvirate of infant care practices in the NICU. The essential nature of these basic human needs (even in the NICU), however, goes beyond the physical aspects of these care activities and presents the clinician with a unique opportunity to build a trusting relationship with the infant through attunement and authentic presence with each caring moment (Watson, 2002).

Humanizing perfunctory nursing care practices requires a fully engaged professional with healing intention; going beyond the checklist of activities that need to be completed before the end of the shift, nursing is a human endeavor that is transpersonal and transformative (Warelow, Edward, & Vinek, 2008; Watson, 2005). With each infant encounter we communicate to the infant his or her worth as an individual and he or she (the infant) derives self-meaning and worth in relationship to other (Stone, DeKoeyer-Laros, & Fogel, 2012; Trevarthen & Aitken, 2001; Tronick & Beeghly, 2011).

Truth be told, these care activities of positioning, feeding, and bathing are best described as parenting activities and promote parent–infant attachment, validate parent role identity, build parental competence and confidence, and reduce infant stress behaviors (Baylis et al., 2014; Craig et al., 2015; Flacking et al., 2012).

Best practices in the provision of activities of daily living require a transdisciplinary and collaborative approach to ensure that the infant's care encounters consistently convey trust and trustworthiness during this very sensitive period of human psychosocial development (Coughlin, 2014). It is the art of consistency that conveys trust, not inconsistency; evidence-based practice is not a "flavor of the month" phenomenon but a fundamental component of safe, quality-driven health care (Golec, 2009). Proper body alignment impacts physiologic function and comfort. Take, for example, the intubated infant whose head is positioned and repositioned at a greater than 60° angle from midline, impeding cerebral perfusion and venous drainage—you try and put your chin on either shoulder and see if you can hold it there for 3 hours (Malusky & Donze, 2011). Breast is best, and yet NICUs struggle with adopting practices, routines, and resources to fully support direct breastfeeding in the NICU. (I know we have a million "plausible" reasons—but it can and has been done for even the most complex surgical situations; Briere, McGrath, Cong, Brownell, & Cusson, 2015; Edwards & Spatz, 2010.) Then there are bathing issues: An infant is either bathed excessively or not at all (outside of spot baths). We rationalize that there are infection control considerations, yet we seldom consider adopting even the simplest hygiene practice of washing the infant's hands and face with each care encounter to minimize his or her risk of hospital-acquired infection (Landers, Abusalem, Coty, & Bingham, 2012).

Providing age-appropriate postural support, identifying breastfeeding as the preferred feeding method while adopting oral feeding practices that place the infant at the helm of the experience, and protecting skin and mucous membrane integrity using sensory sensitive strategies that also preserve a healthy microbiome are quintessential for physiologic and psychoemotional health of the developing human!

FAMILY COLLABORATIVE CARE

Family, where life begins and love never ends.
   —Unknown

Parental presence, emotional well-being, and confidence and competence in parenting comprise the attributes of the family collaborative care core measure that are fundamental to the recovery of the hospitalized infant and the integrity of the family in crisis (Coughlin, 2014; Lee, Carter, Stevenson, & Harrison, 2014). Antiquated and restrictive policies that limit parent and family access to their hospitalized infant have no place in 21st-century health care and significantly undermine quality and patient safety. That being said, even NICUs that advertise 24-hour unrestricted access to families do not guarantee that parents and families will feel welcome within this highly specialized environment by way of a thousand small gestures that accumulate over time. These small gestures welcome or alienate the NICU family in crisis and include the simplest of things such as a pleasant greeting, adequate seating, a welcoming attitude, and even nonverbal communication through facial expression that can make or break a family's perception of reception in the NICU (Cleveland, 2008).

Organizations committed to family-centered, collaborative care must "walk the talk" and ensure that these values are internalized by the organization at every level from administration to frontline, and shape attitudes, behaviors, and priorities that reflect the tenets of family-centered care (Table 2.2; Meek, 2010).

Translating these tenets into clinical practice at the bedside can be challenging for the nurse due to a myriad of factors that include competing priorities in patient care, getting to know the parents and their readiness to participate in their infant's care, and finding a happy medium between completing clinical priorities and involving novice and sometimes even frightened parents into the caregiving routine (Trajkovski, Schmied, Vickers, & Jackson, 2012). For the parents, however, needing to negotiate with a nurse who controls parent access to and participation in the care of their own infant compounded by poor communication and information sharing disempowers and disengages parents (Corlett & Twycross, 2006).

TABLE 2.2   The Tenets of Family-Centered Care

Principle of Family-Centered Care	American Academy of Pediatrics and the Institute for Patient- and Family-Centered Care Joint Statement
Information sharing	Sharing honest and unbiased information in useful and affirming ways
Respecting and honoring differences	Respecting each child and his or her family; honoring racial, ethnic, cultural, and socioeconomic diversity, and the effect on families' experience and perception of care. Recognizing and building on strengths of the child in the family
Partnership and collaboration	Collaborating with families at all levels of health care, in the care of the child, professional education, policy making, and program development. Supporting and facilitating choice on approaches to care. Providing/ensuring formal and informal support for patient and family of all ages
Negotiation	Empowering families to discover their own strengths, build confidence, and make choices and decisions about their health and the health of their child
Care in context of the family and community	Flexibility in organization policies, procedures, and practices so that services can be tailored to the unique needs, beliefs, and cultural values of the child and family

Source: Kuo et al. (2012).

Building effective, authentic, person-centered communication strategies to cultivate healing relationships and partnerships can successfully overcome many of these existing barriers (Weis, Zoffmann, & Egerod, 2014; Wigert, Dellenmark, & Bry, 2013).

In addition to communication challenges, parents experience profound emotional distress following admission to the NICU and clinicians must be competent in recognizing signs and symptoms of emotional distress, postpartum depression, and acute stress disorder in order to make appropriate referrals and effectively support families through the trauma of NICU hospitalization (Greene et al., 2015; Hynan & Hall, 2015). Peer-to-peer parent support programs are an integral and effective component of family-centered care grounded in the self-help philosophy with proven positive results that span four decades (Hall, Ryan, Beatty, & Grubbs, 2015; Levick, Quinn, & Vennema, 2014). In addition to alleviating and/or validating the emotional upheaval of the NICU experience, peer support also helps with parent role development, particularly maternal identity, which is crucial to the short- and long-term health and well-being of the infant–family dyad (Rossman, Greene, & Meier, 2015).

Honoring the lived reality of the families we serve in the NICU requires authentic presence and empathy as we touch lives and impact lifetimes! Our presence is not only heard, but felt through our nonverbal communication. Reiss and Kraft-Todd (2014) developed a novel teaching tool to build clinician skill and awareness in projecting empathy during clinical encounters using a simple acronym: E.M.P.A.T.H.Y.—E, eye contact; M, muscles of facial expression; P, posture; A, affect; T, tone of voice; H, hearing the whole patient/parent; Y, your (the clinician's) response.

*I've learned that people will forget what you said, people will forget
what you did, but people will never forget how you made them feel.*
        —Maya Angelou

Complete the following developmental care practice self-assessment form. This will provide you with some insight into the latest evidence-based best practices associated with the provision of trauma-informed, age-appropriate care (Quantum Caring) in the NICU (this resource is also available for download at www.springerpub.com).

Quantum Caring Self-Assessment

The Healing Environment

This self-assessment will provide you with insight into the evidence-based best practices associated with the provision of trauma-informed age-appropriate care (Quantum Caring) in the neonatal care unit (NICU).

*1. Please indicate the frequency in which you or your unit provides the following as part of the healing environment

	Never	Occasionally	Sometimes	Often	Always	Don't know OR N/A
Sound levels in the patient care area are maintained within the recommended range (< 45 decibels = sound of a library)	○	○	○	○	○	○

Comment

[   ]

	Never	Occasionally	Sometimes	Often	Always	Don't know OR N/A
Light levels are maintained within the recommended range (1–60 foot candles or no brighter than your living room)	○	○	○	○	○	○

Comment

[   ]

	Never	Occasionally	Sometimes	Often	Always	Don't know OR N/A
You provide cycled lighting (lighting during the night is in the lower recommended range and daytime lighting is at the higher end)	○	○	○	○	○	○

Comment

[   ]

Quantum Caring Self-Assessment					
The Healing Environment					
	Never	Occasionally	Sometimes	Often	Always	Don't know OR N/A

	Never	Occasionally	Sometimes	Often	Always	Don't know OR N/A
You shield the infant's eyes from direct light	○	○	○	○	○	○

Comment

Infant exposure to noxious odors is managed (such as skin prep pads are opened outside the infant's microenvironment)	○	○	○	○	○	○

Comment

Infants are provided positive olfactory and gustatory experiences (i.e., through kangaroo care, holding, breast-milk for oralcare, parent scented materials are placed within the infant's microenvironment)	○	○	○	○	○	○

Comment

Quantum Caring Self-Assessment					
The Healing Environment					
	Never	Occasionally	Sometimes	Often	Always	Don't know OR N/A
When moving an infant, you proceed slowly and provide containment (e.g., when transferring the infant from one location to another, the infant is brought close to youa nd supported versus "flying")	○	○	○	○	○	○

Comment

| Parent privacy is protected at the bed-side (either through the use of a screen or single family room) | ○ | ○ | ○ | ○ | ○ | ○ |

Comment

| The patient care environment is aesthetically pleasing, welcoming, and displays a respect for human dignity (e.g., there is artwork, maybe the walls are painted muted pastels, there is a warm feeling to the space you work in) | ○ | ○ | ○ | ○ | ○ | ○ |

Comment

Quantum Caring Self-Assessment					
The Healing Environment					
	Never	Occasionally	Sometimes	Often	Always	Don't know OR N/A
Collaboration, shared decision making, and interprofessional rounding occurs daily	○	○	○	○	○	○
Comment						
Age-appropriate or developmentally supportive care is provided	○	○	○	○	○	○
Comment						
Staff comply with hand hygiene protocol	○	○	○	○	○	○
Comment						
Staff respond to infant's alarms or infant crying promptly, regardless of patient assignment status	○	○	○	○	○	○
Comment						

Quantum Caring Self-Assessment					
The Healing Environment					
	Never	Occasionally	Sometimes	Often	Always	Don't know OR N/A
Addressing practice that is not in the best service to the patient (i.e., when watching a colleague perform a painful procedure without a pain management intervention, how frequently do staff intervene on behalf of the infant?)	○	○	○	○	○	○
Comment						
Staff are held accountable to the provision of age-appropriate (developmentally supportive) care (i.e., annual performance appraisal includes evidence of age-appropriate care practices)	○	○	○	○	○	○
Comment						

Quantum Caring Self-Assessment
Pain and Stress: Prevention, Assessment, Management

*2. Please indicate the frequency in which you or your unit provides the following as part of pain and stress prevention, assessment, and management.

	Never	Occasionally	Sometimes	Often	Always	Don't know/NA
Routine painful or stressful activities are reviewed, revised, and modified based on the individual needs of each patient (i.e.,r outine lab draws are based on the infant's needs not the rituals of the unit)	○	○	○	○	○	○

Comment

ALL painful and stressful proce-dures are managed effectively (i.e., when performing a feeding tube insertion or needle stick procedure, the infant receives sucrose with nonnutritive sucking prior to the procedure)	○	○	○	○	○	○

Comment

Quantum Caring Self-Assessment					
Pain and Stress: Prevention, Assessment, Management					
	Never	Occasionally	Sometimes	Often	Always	Don't know/ NA
When parents are present they are invited and encouraged to support their infant during procedures (i.e., through skin-to-skin care, breastfeeding, containment etc.)	◯	◯	◯	◯	◯	◯
Comment						
Pain and stress are managed and assessed continuously throughout the procedure and the post-procedure period until the infant reaches baseline status	◯	◯	◯	◯	◯	◯
Comment						
All nonpharmacologic pain/stress interventions are recorded accurately in the medical record (to include time of administration and infant response)	◯	◯	◯	◯	◯	◯
Comment						

Quantum Caring Self-Assessment					
Pain and Stress: Prevention, Assessment, Management					
	Never	Occasionally	Sometimes	Often	Always	Don't know/ NA
Skin-to-skin (or kangaroo care) is used as a non-pharmaco-logic intervention to manage procedural pain	○	○	○	○	○	○
Comment					
Caregiving activities are modified based on the infant's behavioral stress cues	○	○	○	○	○	○
Comment					
A validated, age-appropriate pain assessment tool is used	○	○	○	○	○	○
Comment					
Staff are competent in the proper use of the pain assessment tool	○	○	○	○	○	○
Comment					

Quantum Caring Self-Assessment

Pain and Stress: Prevention, Assessment, Management

	Never	Occasionally	Sometimes	Often	Always	Don't know/ NA
Pain and stress prevention is an expressed goal on daily rounds	○	○	○	○	○	○

Comment

Quantum Caring Self-Assessment

Protected Sleep

*3. Please indicate the frequency in which you and/or your unit provides the following as part of protecting sleep.

	Never	Occasionally	Sometimes	Often	Always	Don't know/ N/A
Infant sleep-wake state is assessed prior to nonemergent caregiving	○	○	○	○	○	○

Comment

| | | | | | | |

	Never	Occasionally	Sometimes	Often	Always	Don't know/ N/A
Nonemergent caregiving is provided during wakeful states	○	○	○	○	○	○

Comment

	Never	Occasionally	Sometimes	Often	Always	Don't know/ N/A
Skin-to-skin care is an integral part of the daily care of eligible infants	○	○	○	○	○	○

Comment

Quantum Caring Self-Assessment					
Protected Sleep					
	Never	Occasionally	Sometimes	Often	Always	Don't know/ N/A
Skin-to-skin care is documented to capture the dose-dependent effect (i.e., start and stop time for each session)	○	○	○	○	○	○

Comment

| Parents maintain a sleep diary for their convalescing infant | ○ | ○ | ○ | ○ | ○ | ○ |

Comment

| Parents of convalescing infants provide bedtime routines for their infants in the hospital | ○ | ○ | ○ | ○ | ○ | ○ |

Comment

| Staff participate in annual "back to sleep" or safe sleep competency-based education | ○ | ○ | ○ | ○ | ○ | ○ |

Comment

Quantum Caring Self-Assessment					
Protected Sleep					
	Never	Occasionally	Sometimes	Often	Always	Don't know/ N/A
Eligible infants are transitioned to "back to sleep" (i.e., medically stable, anticipating discharge, term corrected gestational age)	○	○	○	○	○	○
Comment						
Staff role model "back to sleep" practices for parents (i.e., eligible infants are sleeping supine, without additional bedding, with head of bed flat)	○	○	○	○	○	○
Comment						
Parents are educated on the importance of safe sleep in the hospital and at home	○	○	○	○	○	○
Comment						

Quantum Caring Self-Assessment

Activities of Daily Living: Positioning, Feeding, and Skin Care Practices

*4. Please indicate the frequency in which you or your unit provides the following as part of age-appropriate activities of daily living (positioning, feeding, skin care).

	Never	Occasionally	Sometimes	Often	Always	Don't know OR N/A
Infants are positioned in flexion, with containment and postural alignment	○	○	○	○	○	○

Other (please specify)

Staff receive competency-based education in positioning infants in the NICU	○	○	○	○	○	○

Other (please specify)

When infants are handled, they are supported in flexion and postural alignment throughout the caregiving experience	○	○	○	○	○	○

Other (please specify)

Head and neck orientation is maintained in midline with head rotation no greater than 45 degrees to either side	○	○	○	○	○	○

Other (please specify)

Quantum Caring Self-Assessment					
Activities of Daily Living: Positioning, Feeding, and Skin Care Practices					
	Never	Occasionally	Sometimes	Often	Always	Don't know OR N/A
Infants are swaddled for weighing	○	○	○	○	○	○
Other (please specify)						
Infants are swaddled for bathing	○	○	○	○	○	○
Other (please specify)						
Infant eligibility for skin-to-skin care is discussed daily on rounds	○	○	○	○	○	○
Other (please specify)						
Staff receive competency-based education in skin-to-skin care including there commended infant transfer method	○	○	○	○	○	○
Other (please specify)						
Staff employ the standing infant transfer method for skin-to-skin care	○	○	○	○	○	○
Other (please specify)						
Staff employ the seated infant transfer method for skin-to-skin care	○	○	○	○	○	○
Other (please specify)						

Quantum Caring Self-Assessment						
Activities of Daily Living: Positioning, Feeding, and Skin Care Practices						
	Never	Occasionally	Sometimes	Often	Always	Don't know OR N/A
Neonatal therapy is consulted on admission (OT/PT/SLP)	○	○	○	○	○	○
Other (please specify)						
Breastmilk is actively recommended for all infants in your NICU	○	○	○	○	○	○
Other (please specify)						
Intubated and non-intubated infants begin skin-to-skin care when medically stable	○	○	○	○	○	○
Other (please specify)						
Staff receive competency-based education on breastfeeding support in the NICU	○	○	○	○	○	○
Other (please specify)						
Lactation consultants are readily available resources in your NICU	○	○	○	○	○	○
Other (please specify)						
The first oral feed is at the breast for breastfeeding mothers	○	○	○	○	○	○
Other (please specify)						

	Never	Occasionally	Sometimes	Often	Always	Don't know OR N/A
Quantum Caring Self-Assessment						
Activities of Daily Living: Positioning, Feeding, and Skin Care Practices						
Staff receive competency-basede ducation on infant feeding readiness cues	○	○	○	○	○	○
Other (please specify)						
Infant feeding readiness cues drive the initiation of oral feedings	○	○	○	○	○	○
Other (please specify)						
A bottle feeding is discontinued when the infant is no longer able to be safely engaged in the activity (e.g., shows signs of stress, leakage at the lips, eyes are closed, breathing is erratic) regardless of the volume taken	○	○	○	○	○	○
Other (please specify)						
Skin and mucous membrane integrity is assessed at least daily using a validated, age-appropriate assessment tool	○	○	○	○	○	○
Other (please specify)						

Quantum Caring Self-Assessment						
Activities of Daily Living: Positioning, Feeding, and Skin Care Practices						
	Never	Occasionally	Sometimes	Often	Always	Don't know OR N/A
Colostrum and/or mother's own milk isused for mouth care in infants who are not receiving oral feedings	◯	◯	◯	◯	◯	◯
Other (please specify)						
Bathing mode and frequency is individualized for each infant	◯	◯	◯	◯	◯	◯
Other (please specify)						
Infant's hands and face are gently wiped with each care encounter or a minimum of once per shift	◯	◯	◯	◯	◯	◯
Other (please specify)						
Skin barrier films are used as an interface when applying medical devices or adhesives to infant's skin	◯	◯	◯	◯	◯	◯
Other (please specify)						
Adhesives are removed gently to minimize skin injury; solutions with toxic chemicals are not employed	◯	◯	◯	◯	◯	◯
Other (please specify)						

Quantum Caring Self-Assessment

Family Collaborative Care

*5. Please indicate the frequency in which you provide the following as part of family collaborative care.

	Never	Occasionally	Sometimes	Often	Always	Don't know OR N/A
Parents have 24-hour unrestricted access to their infant in the NICU	○	○	○	○	○	○
Parents are invited and encouraged to be present during procedures	○	○	○	○	○	○
Parents are expected to provide care for their infant in the NICU	○	○	○	○	○	○
Parents receive competency-based education on infant caregiving in the NICU (to include skin-to-skin, bathing, feeding, comforting, etc.)	○	○	○	○	○	○
Parents are never referred to as visitors	○	○	○	○	○	○
Parents participate in clinical bedside rounds	○	○	○	○	○	○
Parents participate in change of shift report	○	○	○	○	○	○
Parent presence in the NICU is recorded in the medical record	○	○	○	○	○	○

Quantum Caring Self-Assessment						
Family Collaborative Care						
	Never	Occasionally	Sometimes	Often	Always	Don't know OR N/A
Parents have adequate space to be at their infant's bedspace	○	○	○	○	○	○
Parents are assessed routinely for their emotional well-being	○	○	○	○	○	○
Mental health professionals are readily available to support parents	○	○	○	○	○	○
Mental health professionals are readily available to support staff	○	○	○	○	○	○
Parents have access to family support group or peer-to-peer support resources	○	○	○	○	○	○
Culturally sensitive parenting resoucres are available in your NICU	○	○	○	○	○	○
Staff receive competency-based cultural sensitivity education to meet the needs of the patient demographics served in your NICU	○	○	○	○	○	○

Comment

■ REFERENCES

Allegaert, K., Tibboel, D., & van den Anker, J. (2013). Pharmacological treatment of neonatal pain: In search of a new equipoise. *Seminars in Fetal & Neonatal Medicine, 18*(1), 42–47.

Allen, K. A. (2012). Promoting and protecting infant sleep. *Advances in Neonatal Care, 12*(5), 288–291.

American Academy of Pediatrics (AAP) Committee on Fetus and Newborn & Section on Anesthesiology and Pain Medicine. (2016). Prevention and management of procedural pain in the neonate: An update. *Pediatrics, 137*(2), e20154271.

American Academy of Pediatrics Task Force on Sudden Infant Death Syndrome. (2011). SIDS and other sleep-related infant deaths: Expansion of recommendations for a safe sleeping environment. *Pediatrics, 128*(5), 1030–1039.

Antonovsky, A. (1996). A salutogenic model as a theory to guide health promotion. *Health Promotion International, 11*(1), 11–18.

Axelin, A., Cilio, M. R., Asunis, M., Peloquin, S., & Franck, L. S. (2013). Sleep-wake cycling in a neonate admitted to the NICU: A video-EEG case study during hypothermia treatment. *The Journal of Perinatal & Neonatal Nursing, 27*(3), 263–273.

Barba, B., Stump, M., & Fitzsimmons, S. (2014). The role of therapeutic use of self in the application of nonpharmacological interventions. *Journal of Gerontological Nursing, 40*(8), 9–12.

Baylis, R., Ewald, U., Gradin, M., Hedberg Nyqvist, K., Rubertsson, C., & Thernström Blomqvist, Y. (2014). First-time events between parents and preterm infants are affected by the designs and routines of neonatal intensive care units. *Acta Paediatrica, 103*(10), 1045–1052.

Berwick, D. (2009, July 4). Don *What patient centred care really means* [Video File]. Retrieved from https://www.youtube.com/watch?v=SSauhroFTpk

Briere, C. E., McGrath, J. M., Cong, X., Brownell, E., & Cusson, R. (2015). Direct-breastfeeding premature infants in the neonatal intensive care unit. *Journal of Human Lactation, 31*(3), 386–392.

Carbajal, R., Nguyen-Bourgain, C., & Armengaud, J. B. (2008a). How can we improve pain relief in neonates? *Expert Review of Neurotherapeutics, 8*(11), 1617–1620.

Carbajal, R., Rousset, A., Danan, C., Coquery, S., Nolent, P., Ducrocq, S., . . . Bréart, G. (2008b). Epidemiology and treatment of painful procedures in neonates in intensive care units. *Journal of the American Medical Association, 300*(1), 60–70.

Cleveland, L. M. (2008). Parenting in the neonatal intensive care unit. *Journal of Obstetric, Gynecologic, & Neonatal Nursing, 37*, 666–691.

Corlett, J., & Twycross, A. (2006). Negotiation of parental roles within family-centred care: A review of the research. *Journal of Clinical Nursing, 15*(10), 1308–1316.

Coughlin, M. (2011). *Age-appropriate care of the premature and critically ill hospitalized infant: Guideline for practice.* Glenview, IL: National Association of Neonatal Nurses.

Coughlin, M. (2014). *Transformative nursing in the NICU: Trauma-informed, age-appropriate care.* New York, NY: Springer Publishing.

Coughlin, M., Gibbins, S., & Hoath, S. (2009). Core measures for developmentally supportive care in neonatal intensive care units: Theory, precedence and practice. *Journal of Advanced Nursing, 65*(10), 2239–2248.

Coughlin, M., & Rolfes, M. (2016). *Quantum caring: A systematic approach to cultural transformation in the NICU.* Paper presented at the International Forum on Quality and Safety in Healthcare Asia, Singapore.

Craig, J. W., Glick, C., Phillips, R., Hall, S. L., Smith, J., & Browne, J. (2015). Recommendations for involving the family in developmental care of the NICU baby. *Journal of Perinatology, 35*(Suppl. 1), S5–S8.

Cruz, M. D., Fernandes, A. M., & Oliveira, C. R. (2016). Epidemiology of painful procedures performed in neonates: A systematic review of observational studies. *European Journal of Pain, 20*(4), 489–498.

Cummings, G. G., MacGregor, T., Davey, M., Lee, H., Wong, C. A., Lo, E.,…Stafford, E. (2010). Leadership styles and outcome patterns for the nursing workforce and work environment: A systematic review. *International Journal of Nursing Studies, 47*(3), 363–385.

Edwards, T. M., & Spatz, D. L. (2010). An innovative model for achieving breast-feeding success in infants with complex surgical anomalies. *The Journal of Perinatal & Neonatal Nursing, 24*(3), 246–253; quiz 254.

Feldman, R. (2015). Sensitive periods in human social development: New insights from research on oxytocin, synchrony, and high-risk parenting. *Development and Psychopathology, 27*(2), 369–395.

Flacking, R., Lehtonen, L., Thomson, G., Axelin, A., Ahlqvist, S., Moran, V. H.,…Dykes, F.; Separation and Closeness Experiences in the Neonatal Environment (SCENE) group. (2012). Closeness and separation in neonatal intensive care. *Acta Paediatrica, 101*(10), 1032–1037.

Frank, M. G., Issa, N. P., & Stryker, M. P. (2001). Sleep enhances plasticity in the developing visual cortex. *Neuron, 30*(1), 275–287.

Gerstein, E. D., Poehlmann-Tynan, J., & Clark, R. (2015). Mother-child interactions in the NICU: Relevance and implications for later parenting. *Journal of Pediatric Psychology, 40*(1), 33–44.

Gibbins, S., Hoath, S. B., Coughlin, M., Gibbins, A., & Franck, L. (2008). The universe of developmental care: A new conceptual model for application in the neonatal intensive care unit. *Advances in Neonatal Care, 8*(3), 141–147.

Golec, L. (2009). The art of inconsistency: Evidence-based practice my way. *Journal of Perinatology, 29*(9), 600–602.

Goudarzi, Z., Rahimi, O., Khalessi, N., Soleimani, F., Mohammadi, N., & Shamshiri, A. (2015). The rate of developmental care delivery in neonatal intensive care unit. *Iran Journal of Critical Care Nursing, 8*(2), 117–124.

Greene, M. M., Rossman, B., Patra, K., Kratovil, A. L., Janes, J. E., & Meier, P. P. (2015). Depression, anxiety, and perinatal-specific posttraumatic distress in mothers of very low birth weight infants in the neonatal intensive care unit. *Journal of Developmental and Behavioral Pediatrics, 36*(5), 362–370.

Guedj, R., Danan, C., Daoud, P., Zupan, V., Renolleau, S., Zana, E.,…Carbajal, R. (2014). Does neonatal pain management in intensive care units differ between night and day? An observational study. *BMJ Open, 4*(2), e004086.

Gustafsson, L. K., & Stenberg, M. (2015). Crucial contextual attributes of nursing leadership toward an ethic of care. *Nursing Ethics*, pii: 0969733015614879. [Epub ahead of print].

Hall, S. L., Ryan, D. J., Beatty, J., & Grubbs, L. (2015). Recommendations for peer-to-peer support for NICU parents. *Journal of Perinatology, 35*(Suppl. 1), S9–13.

Hatfield, L. A., Meyers, M. A., & Messing, T. M. (2013). A systematic review of the effects of repeated painful procedures in infants: Is there a potential to mitigate future pain responsivity? *Journal of Nursing Education and Practice, 3*(8), 99–112.

Hwang, S. S., O'Sullivan, A., Fitzgerald, E., Melvin, P., Gorman, T., & Fiascone, J. M. (2015). Implementation of safe sleep practices in the neonatal intensive care unit. *Journal of Perinatology, 35*(10), 862–866.

Hynan, M. T., & Hall, S. L. (2015). Psychosocial program standards for NICU parents. *Journal of Perinatology, 35*(Suppl. 1), S1–S4.

Jonas, W. B., Chez, R. A., Smith, K., & Sakallaris, B. (2014). Salutogenesis: The defining concept for a new healthcare system. *Global Advances in Health and Medicine, 3*(3), 82–91.

Krishnan, L. (2013). Pain relief in neonates. *Journal of Neonatal Surgery, 2*(2), 19.

Kudchadkar, S. R., Aljohani, O. A., & Punjabi, N. M. (2014). Sleep of critically ill children in the pediatric intensive care unit: A systematic review. *Sleep Medicine Reviews, 18*(2), 103–110.

Kuo, D. Z., Houtrow, A. J., Arango, P., Kuhlthau, K. A., Simmons, J. M., & Neff, J. M. (2012). Family-centered care: Current applications and future directions in pediatrics health care. *Maternal Child Health Journal, 16*(2), 297–305.

Kurth, S., Olini, N., Huber, R., & LeBourgeois, M. (2015). Sleep and early cortical development. *Current Sleep Medicine Reports, 1*(1), 64–73.

Landers, T., Abusalem, S., Coty, M. B., & Bingham, J. (2012). Patient-centered hand hygiene: The next step in infection prevention. *American Journal of Infection Control, 40*(4, Suppl. 1), S11–S17.

Latimer, M. A., Johnston, C. C., Ritchie, J. A., Clarke, S. P., & Gilin, D. (2009). Factors affecting delivery of evidence-based procedural pain care in hospitalized neonates. *Journal of Obstetric, Gynecologic, and Neonatal Nursing, 38*(2), 182–194.

Lee, L. A., Carter, M., Stevenson, S. B., & Harrison, H. A. (2014). Improving family-centered care practices in the NICU. *Neonatal Network, 33*(3), 125–132.

Levick, J., Quinn, M., & Vennema, C. (2014). NICU parent-to-parent partnerships: A comprehensive approach. *Neonatal Network, 33*(2), 66–73.

Lindström, B., & Eriksson, M. (2005). Salutogenesis. *Journal of Epidemiology and Community Health, 59*(6), 440–442.

Mahmoodi, N., Arbabisarjou, A., Rezaeipoor, M., & Pishkar Mofrad, Z. (2015). Nurses' awareness of preterm neonates' sleep in the NICU. *Global Journal of Health Science, 8*(5), 54945.

Malusky, S., & Donze, A. (2011). Neutral head positioning in premature infants for intraventricular hemorrhage prevention: An evidence-based review. *Neonatal Network, 30*(6), 381–396.

Mannix, J., Wilkes, L., & Daly, J. (2015). "Good ethics and moral standing": A qualitative study of aesthetic leadership in clinical nursing practice. *Journal of Clinical Nursing, 24*(11–12), 1603–1610.

McMullen, S. L., Fioravanti, I. D., Brown, K., & Carey, M. G. (2016). Safe sleep for hospitalized infants. *MCN. The American Journal of Maternal Child Nursing, 41*(1), 43–50.

Meek, K. (2010). Customer service in healthcare: Optimizing your patients' experience. *Bulletin, 89*(6), 1–5.

Mindell, J. A., Sadeh, A., Kohyama, J., & How, T. H. (2010). Parental behaviors and sleep outcomes in infants and toddlers: A cross-cultural comparison. *Sleep Medicine, 11*(4), 393–399.

Montirosso, R., Del Prete, A., Bellù, R., Tronick, E., & Borgatti, R.; Neonatal Adequate Care for Quality of Life (NEO-ACQUA) Study Group. (2012). Level of NICU quality of developmental care and neurobehavioral performance in very preterm infants. *Pediatrics, 129*(5), e1129–e1137.

Moore, T. A., Berger, A. M., & Wilson, M. E. (2014). A new way of thinking about complications of prematurity. *Biological Research for Nursing, 16*(1), 72–82.

Patton, C., Stiltner, D., Wright, K. B., & Kautz, D. D. (2015). Do nurses provide a safe sleep environment for infants in the hospital setting? An integrative review. *Advances in Neonatal Care, 15*(1), 8–22.

Provenzi, L., & Montirosso, R. (2015). "Epigenethics" in the neonatal intensive care unit: Conveying complexity in health care for preterm children. *JAMA Pediatrics, 169*(7), 617–618.

Qureshi, A., Malkar, M., Splaingard, M., Khuhro, A., & Jadcherla, S. (2015). The role of sleep in the modulation of gastroesophageal reflux and symptoms in NICU neonates. *Pediatric Neurology, 53*(3), 226–232.

Raines, D. A., & Brustad, J. (2012). Parent's confidence as a caregiver. *Advances in Neonatal Care, 12*(3), 183–188.

Riess, H., & Kraft-Todd, G. (2014). E.M.P.A.T.H.Y.: A tool to enhance nonverbal communication between clinicians and their patients. *Academic Medicine, 89*(8), 1108–1112.

Roley, S. S., DeLany, J. V., Barrows, C. J., Brownrigg, S., Honaker, D., Sava, D. I., … Youngstrom, M. J.; American Occupational Therapy Association Commission on Practice. (2008). Occupational therapy practice framework: Domain and practice, 2nd edition. *The American Journal of Occupational Therapy, 62*(6), 625–683.

Rossman, B., Greene, M. M., & Meier, P. P. (2015). The role of peer support in the development of maternal identity for "NICU moms." *Journal of Obstetric, Gynecologic, and Neonatal Nursing, 44*(1), 3–16.

Sadeh, A., Tikotzky, L., & Scher, A. (2010). Parenting and infant sleep. *Sleep Medicine Reviews, 14*(2), 89–96.

Sakallaris, B. R., MacAllister, L., Voss, M., Smith, K., & Jonas, W. B. (2015). Optimal healing environments. *Global Advances in Health and Medicine, 4*(3), 40–45.

Scher, M. S., Ludington-Hoe, S., Kaffashi, F., Johnson, M. W., Holditch-Davis, D., & Loparo, K. A. (2009). Neurophysiologic assessment of brain maturation after an 8-week trial of skin-to-skin contact on preterm infants. *Clinical Neurophysiology, 120*(10), 1812–1818.

Schweitzer, M., Gilpin, L., & Frampton, S. (2004). Healing spaces: Elements of environmental design that make an impact on health. *Journal of Alternative and Complementary Medicine, 10*(Suppl. 1), S71–S83.

Schwichtenberg, A. J., Shah, P. E., & Poehlmann, J. (2013). Sleep and attachment in preterm infants. *Infant Mental Health, 34*(1), 37–46.

Soleimani, F., Torkzahrani, S., Rafiey, H., Salavati, M., & Nasiri, M. (2016). Development and psychometric testing of a scale for the assessment of the quality of developmental care in neonatal intensive care units in Iran. *Electronic Physician, 8*(1), 1686–1692.

Stone, S. A., DeKoeyer-Laros, I., & Fogel, A. (2012). Self and other dialogue in infancy: Normal versus compromised developmental pathways. In H. J. M. Hermans (Ed.),

Applications of dialogical self theory: New directions for child and adolescent development (Vol. 137, pp. 23–38). Hoboken, NJ: John Wiley & Sons, Inc.

Taylor, R. R., Lee, S. W., Kielhofner, G., & Ketkar, M. (2009). Therapeutic use of self: A nationwide survey of practitioners' attitudes and experiences. *The American Journal of Occupational Therapy, 63*(2), 198–207.

Trajkovski, S., Schmied, V., Vickers, M., & Jackson, D. (2012). Neonatal nurses' perspectives of family-centred care: A qualitative study. *Journal of Clinical Nursing, 21*(17–18), 2477–2487.

Trevarthen, C., & Aitken, K. J. (2001). Infant intersubjectivity: Research, theory, and clinical applications. *Journal of Child Psychology and Psychiatry, and Allied Disciplines, 42*(1), 3–48.

Tronick, E., & Beeghly, M. (2011). Infants' meaning-making and the development of mental health problems. *The American Psychologist, 66*(2), 107–119.

Ulrich, R., Quan, X., Zimring, C., Joseph, A., & Choudhary, R. (2004). *The role of the physical environment in the hospital of the 21st century: A once-in-a-lifetime opportunity.* The Center for Health Design. Retrieved from https://www.healthdesign.org/sites/default/files/Role%20Physical%20Environ%20in%20the%2021st%20Century%20Hospital_0.pdf

Valeri, B. O., Holsti, L., & Linhares, M. B. (2015). Neonatal pain and developmental outcomes in children born preterm: A systematic review. *The Clinical Journal of Pain, 31*(4), 355–362.

Valizadeh, L., Asadollahi, M., Mostafa Gharebaghi, M., & Gholami, F. (2013). The congruence of nurses' performance with developmental care standards in neonatal intensive care units. *Journal of Caring Sciences, 2*(1), 61–71.

Vinall, J., & Grunau, R. E. (2014). Impact of repeated procedural pain-related stress in infants born very preterm. *Pediatric Research, 75*(5), 584–587.

Walden, M., & Gibbins, S. (2012). *Newborn pain assessment and management: Guideline for practice.* Glenview, IL: National Association of Neonatal Nurses.

Walker, S. M. (2014). Neonatal pain. *Paediatric Anaesthesia, 24*(1), 39–48.

Warelow, P., Edward, K. L., & Vinek, J. (2008). Care: What nurses say and what nurses do. *Holistic Nursing Practice, 22*(3), 146–153.

Watson, J. (2002). Intentionality and caring-healing consciousness: A practice of transpersonal nursing. *Holistic Nursing Practice, 16*(4), 12–19.

Watson, J. (2005). *Caring science as sacred science.* Philadelphia, PA: F. A. Davis.

Watson, J. (2006). The caring moment. In G. Malkin & M. Stilwater (Producers), *Care for the journey: Music and messages for sustaining the heart of healthcare.* Companion Arts in Association with Wisdom of the World Inc. Retrieved from http://watsoncaringscience.org/images/features/library/Caring%20Moment_WatsonTranscript.pdf

Weis, J., Zoffmann, V., & Egerod, I. (2014). Improved nurse-parent communication in neonatal intensive care unit: Evaluation and adjustment of an implementation strategy. *Journal of Clinical Nursing, 23*(23–24), 3478–3489.

White, R. D. (2011). The newborn intensive care unit environment of care: How we got here, where we're headed, and why. *Seminars in Perinatology, 35*(1), 2–7.

World Health Organization (WHO). (2016). *WHO definition of Health.* Retrieved from http://www.who.int/about/definition/en/print.html

Wigert, H., Dellenmark, M. B., & Bry, K. (2013). Strengths and weaknesses of parent-staff communication in the NICU: A survey assessment. *BMC Pediatrics, 13*, 71.

CHAPTER 3

Trauma-Informed, Age-Appropriate Care in the NICU

The concept of trauma-informed care in the neonatal intensive care unit (NICU) has been gaining global acceptance. The relevance of this paradigm for the hospitalized infant is grounded in an understanding of the impact of toxic, traumatic stress on the physiologic, genetic, and psychic dimensions of the developing human. Insight into the scientific and professional organizations that support this paradigm will facilitate transformation of the neonatal patient's experience of intensive care through the adoption of evidence-based best practices in age-appropriate care.

▪ SCIENTIFIC SUPPORT

Polyvagal Theory

The polyvagal theory brings new acumen into the reactivity of the stress response system mediated by evolutionary changes to the autonomic nervous system (Porges, 2007, 2009). Building on earlier work linking the autonomic nervous system with emotion and social behavior, Dr. Stephen Porges, a renowned neuroscientist, describes the phylogeny of the vagus nerve from its unmyelinated form to its more sophisticated myelinated counterpart, thus giving rise to the term *polyvagal*—describing the vagus as not a single nerve but several nerves originating in unique areas of the brainstem (Sanders, 2013). Physiologic defense strategies (stress response mechanisms) are associated with both myelinated and unmyelinated vagal activity mediating parasympathetic inhibitory responses, the hypothalamic–pituitary–adrenal (HPA) axis, and the social engagement system (Porges, 2009). This theory

> explains why a kind face or a soothing tone of voice can dramatically alter the way we feel...look[ing] beyond the effects of fight or flight and put[ing] social relationships front and center in our understanding of trauma. (van der Kolk, 2014, p. 78)

Human beings across the age continuum process information from the environment through sensory perception to assess risk and threat. The term *neuroception* describes how neural circuits, on a subconscious level, distinguish between situations or people that are safe, dangerous, or life-threatening (Porges, 2004). In response to perceived threats, the polyvagal theory describes how our adaptive behavioral strategies balance defensive and prosocial behaviors via neural circuitry involving the myelinated and unmyelinated vagus nerves of the autonomic nervous system (Porges, 2004).

The three neural circuits that regulate reactivity are as follows:

1. Immobilization (feigning death or playing possum) is the most primitive defense behavior mediated by the unmyelinated portion of the vagus nerve originating from the dorsal motor nucleus of the brainstem and is observed when your patient passes out and/or decompensates when you override his or her stress communication behaviors.

2. Mobilization (also referred to as fight or flight behaviors) increases cardiac output and metabolic activity, contingent on the individual's sympathetic nervous system capabilities and is observed when your patient is swatting you away with his or her arms and/or legs and crying—if these defense behaviors are unsuccessful, he or she may revert to immobilization as a defense or disengagement strategy.

3. Social engagement, comprised of facial expressions, vocalizations, and attentiveness, is mediated by the myelinated vagus originating in the nucleus ambiguus of the brainstem and supports a sense of calm, inhibiting sympathetic activity and is observed when you introduce yourself before a care encounter and the patient exhibits engagement or readiness cues; you proceed with caregiving contingent on the infant's continuous display of engagement behaviors and modify the interaction should the infant show signs of distress).

We know that stress during fetal, neonatal, and early life has a negative impact on neurodevelopmental and neuropsychiatric outcomes and the polyvagal theory describes a grounded, neurobiological mechanism to better understand these outcomes. This biologically based theory guides our understanding about the vulnerability and neuroceptive capabilities of the hospitalized infant to the physical environment, relationships, and interpersonal experiences.

Epigenetics

Epigenetics is the study of cellular and physiological variations to the genome by environmental factors affecting gene expression (Figure 3.1). These environmental or external factors create reversible genetic modifications that shape an individual's phenotype along with the phenotype of subsequent generations and demonstrates critical and sensitive periods of vulnerability that have specific relevance for the neonatal patient population (Tammen, Friso, & Choi, 2013).

Epigenetic effects begin at conception influencing the development and function of neuronal networks (Samra, McGrath, Wehbe, & Clapper, 2012). Infants born prematurely or infants who require the NICU endure maternal separation, repeated

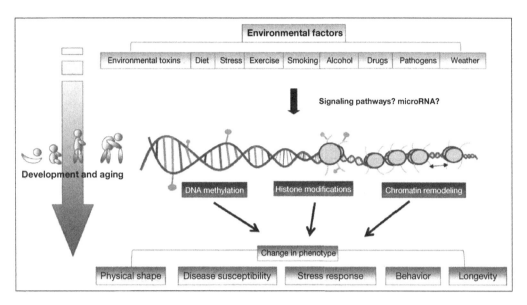

FIGURE 3.1   Epigenetic mechanisms.

Source: Tammen, Friso, and Choi (2013). Reprinted with permission from Elsevier.

noxious experiences, alterations in nutrition and exposure to various pharmaco-logic agents that exert an epigenetic influence that alters an individual's develop-mental trajectory at the molecular level (Samra et al., 2012).

The epigenetic impact of early-life adversity results in striking modifications to HPA axis function, and stress responsivity and regulation (Figure 3.2; Brummelte et al., 2015; Chau, Cepeda, Devlin, Weinberg, & Grunau, 2015; Kundakovic & Champagne, 2015; Montirosso & Provenzi, 2015). Grunau et al. (2013) report gen-der-specific persistent alterations of stress/inflammatory mechanisms in HPA axis programming at the genomic level in preterm boys at school age mediated by neo-natal pain-related stress.

Early-life stress alters neural, hormonal, and behavioral systems and is a path-way linking the individual's experience of early-life adversity and severe illness to altered brain development influencing lifelong risks of psychopathology and other morbidities (Boyce & Kobor, 2015; Heim & Nemeroff, 2002; Richards & Wadsworth, 2004; Smith et al., 2011). These dynamic gene–environment interactions are bidirec-tional and can also play a positive and enriching role in human development when optimal nurturing experiences are available for the individual during critical and sensitive periods of development (Boyce & Kobor, 2015).

The quality of early caregiving environments influences biobehavioral devel-opment to include epigenetic alterations that program the individual for stress reactivity or resilience as seen through the protective influence of skin-to-skin care mediated by epigenetic mechanisms (Boyce & Kobor, 2015; Hane & Fox, 2016; Provenzi & Montirosso, 2015).

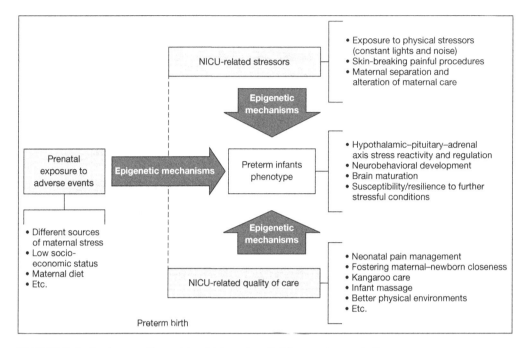

FIGURE 3.2   A prospective model explaining epigenetic influences in prematurity.

NICU, neonatal intensive care unit.

Source: Montirosso and Provenzi (2015).

Understanding the interplay among genes, early-life experiences, and early-life stress creates an ethical framework to inform and guide clinical practice in the provision of evidence-based age-appropriate care to support healthy development and later life health outcomes (Boyce & Kobor, 2015; Provenzi & Montirosso, 2015; Vaiserman, 2015).

Caring Science

Caring science, guided by scientific knowledge, affirms a deep, relational ethic that recognizes the integral role of the clinician to the clinician–patient encounter at the shared interface of care—being with other in a reciprocal caring moment (Cowling, Smith, & Watson, 2008; Gibbins, Hoath, Coughlin, Gibbins, & Franck, 2008; Jarrín, 2012; Watson, 2005). The deeply human dimensions of caring (Table 3.1), realized in clinical practice, has the power to transform and transcend the suffering of other at spiritual, physiologic, and genomic levels (Watson, 2007).

Loving, caring, kind, and sensitively meaningful personal connections underpin a trauma-informed paradigm poised to mitigate the adversity associated with the NICU (Watson, 2009). Relationship-based care grounded by human caring science reunites the ethos of health care and is crucial for human development biologically, psychoemotionally, and spiritually (Faber, 2013; Lachman, 2012).

TABLE 3.1   Watson's 10 Caritas Processes

1. Practicing loving-kindness and equanimity for self and other within the context of caring consciousness
2. Being authentically present to and enabling, sustaining, and honoring the belief system and subjective world of self and other
3. Cultivating one's own spiritual practices, deepening self-awareness, and going beyond self
4. Developing and sustaining a helping–trusting authentic, caring relationship
5. Being present to and supportive of the expression of positive and negative feelings as a connection with a deeper spirit of self and other
6. Creatively using self and all ways of knowing and being a part of the caring process
7. Engaging in genuine teaching–learning experiences attending to the whole person and their meaning
8. Creating healing environments at all levels to potentiate the wholeness, beauty, comfort, and dignity of other
9. Assisting other with his or her basic needs with an intentional caring consciousness that potentiates alignment of mind–body–spirit wholeness in all aspects of care
10. Being open and attending to the spiritual allowing miracles to happen; attending to soul care for self and other

Source: Watson (2007).

The neural circuits of emotional saliency (the amygdala, insula, and anterior cingulate cortex), the central executive network (the prefrontal and posterior parietal cortex), and caregiving circuitry (the brainstem, hypothalamus, basal ganglia, ventromedial prefrontal cortex) are modulated by neuroendocrine mechanisms, specifically oxytocin, and are responsible for our cognitive empathy and empathic concern for other (Decety & Fotopoulou, 2014). We operationalize our empathic concern for other through authentic transpersonal caring and nonverbal communication of compassion to reduce autonomic reactivity, cultivate healing relationships and meet the experience expectant needs of the developing human in the NICU (Kemper & Shaltout, 2011; Pickler et al., 2010; Porges, 2004; Watson, 2002).

Nature alone heals and it is the clinician's responsibility to create and maintain an environment conducive to the healing process (Dossey, 2000). Open-minded caring, intentionality, unconditional acceptance and awareness of our shared humanity, empathy, and authentic healing presence allow us to see the subtle and perceive the wholeness of other in the caring encounter (Koerner, 2011; Willis, Grace, & Roy, 2008).

The purpose of healthcare is not occupational status, or the fulfillment
of the individual clinician, it is the patient.
        —Adapted from Bradshaw, 1999

■ SOCIETAL SUPPORT

The American Academy of Pediatrics

Advances in the basic sciences of human development are now exposing the biological mechanisms that underlie the fetal and neonatal origins of adult disease framed by an ecobiodevelopmental framework whereby the ecology or the environment and experiences of the developing individual impact his or her biology (Block, 2016; Garner, Forkey, & Szilagyi, 2015; Odgers & Jaffee, 2013; Shonkoff & Garner, 2012). Exposure to toxic stress during early life accelerates the wear and tear on the infant's body and restructures the developing architecture of the brain (Odgers & Jaffee, 2013). AAP addresses the consequences of early childhood adversity and toxic stress in its 2012 policy statement, "Early Childhood Adversity, Toxic Stress, and the Role of the Pediatrician," and entreats pediatricians and pediatric professionals to advocate for and catalyze change in policy, practice, and clinical care across all service lines (Garner & Shonkoff, 2012). Pediatric service lines encompass a wide range of medical and surgical specialties and subspecialties serving individuals and their families from birth to 18 years of age. As trusted guardians of child health, pediatric and neonatal professionals in partnership with parents are poised to improve the future health of society by understanding the power of prevention and of very early intervention to build resilience in the infant–family dyad combatting the effects of toxic stress in early life and cultivating nurturing parent–infant relationships and capabilities (Block, 2016; Garner & Shonkoff, 2012).

Prevention and early-intervention strategies that form the foundation of healthy development and physical and mental well-being include: (a) a stable responsive environment of relationships, which provide consistent nurturing and protective interactions within the infant–family dyad facilitating the development of an adaptive, well-regulated stress response systems; (b) safe and supportive physical environments that are free from noxious and injurious elements supporting family interactions that nurture child rearing; and finally (c) appropriate nutrition, healthy eating habits, and age-appropriate eating behaviors and experiences (Shonkoff & Garner, 2012).

Looking at the NICU patient's lived experience of critical illness, requiring life-saving interventions, undergoing various medically necessary stressful and painful procedures, one can see why the NICU experience, with its inherent toxic stress, can readily be classified as early-life adversity (Odgers & Jaffee, 2013). Applying an ecobiodevelopmental framework to neonatology provides an opportunity to shift the paradigm to embrace and integrate age-appropriate care to mitigate toxic stress, enhance infant and family outcomes, and improve quality and patient safety (Shonkoff & Garner, 2012).

Efforts to reduce toxic stress and cultivate infant and family resilience in the NICU require a comprehensive and coordinated approach to care that offers continuity and is culturally effective, family centered, and compassionate (AAP, 2004).

Building clinician competence in anticipatory guidance to support age-appropriate socioemotional skills and language development in the hospitalized infant through parental presence and positive parenting; consistently and reliably resolving stressful and/or painful experiences; creatively adapting and innovating on existing practice routines to reduce infant–parent separation; and advocating for necessary resources and practice improvements will mitigate toxic stress in the NICU and, in partnership with parents, promote secure attachment and resilience (Coughlin, 2014; Garner & Shonkoff, 2012; Odgers & Jaffee, 2013).

It is easier to build strong children than to repair broken men.
    —Frederick Douglass

National Scientific Council on the Developing Child

Established in 2003, the National Scientific Council on the Developing Child is a multidisciplinary academic and scientific community of professionals dedicated to translating the science of human development to inform and engage society at local, national, and international levels to promote child health and well-being. The council has published numerous white papers presenting the science of early childhood development to include the following key concepts:

- *Brain architecture*—built over time and from the bottom up (subcortex to cortex) with approximately 1,000 new neural connections forming every second over the first year of life, this critical developing structure is highly sensitive to experiences and interactions with the world
- *Serve and return*—responsive relationships and interactions are expected and essential for child development; the child serves and the adult returns (e.g., when a child cries and an adult responds, neural connections that support communication and social skills are strengthened)
- *Toxic stress*—the prolonged activation of stress response systems disrupts brain development and increases the individual's risk for stress-related disease into adulthood
- *Executive function and self-regulation*—mental processes that allow us to focus, remember, and multitask, but are impaired when the system is exposed to toxic stress
- *Resilience*—the ability to overcome adversity that can be cultivated when a child has at least one stable, caring relationship with an adult: "Age-appropriate, health-promoting activities can significantly improve the odds that an individual will recover from stress-inducing experiences" (Center on the Developing Child)

In addition, the council has drilled down on critical content (deep dives) presenting evidence-based research that informs the public, policy decision makers, and professionals about early childhood mental health; why early health matters for lifelong health; how the absence of responsive relationships (neglect) threatens development; and gene–environment interactions that shape health and development (Center on the Developing Child).

The Council has embarked on a series of innovative projects to address some of the root causes of compromised infant/child development in community and outpatient settings, primarily focused on the adult caregiver. These effective strategies can easily be adapted for the inpatient setting, specifically the FIND project (Filming Interactions to Nurture Development). Coaching clinicians in "serve and return" interactions with the hospitalized infant is an effective, simple, evidence-based prevention strategy to mitigate toxic stress mediated by unresponsive caregiving. In addition, clinicians can then mentor parents in "serve and return" during the hospital stay, building parental confidence and competence and preparing them for positive parenting postdischarge.

The Institute for Healthcare Improvement Triple Aim Initiative

The Institute for Healthcare Improvement (IHI), founded in 1991, is a recognized global innovator and leader that focuses on improving health and health care worldwide. The organization began by building capacity for change through education and then, moving beyond best practice to innovate health care design, to unify industry to rally around health care improvement, transform mainstream practice standards, and ultimately improve the health of populations. Improving the health of populations is the goal of the IHI Triple Aim initiative. The Triple Aim Initiative proposes that improving the patient's experience of care will improve population health and reduce per capita health care costs. The five components of a system that would achieve the Triple Aim include (a) a focus on the individual and family; (b) a redesign of services and structures; (c) population health management; (d) cost-control platform; and (e) system integration and execution (Figure 3.3).

Focusing on the individual and family is at the heart of trauma-informed age-appropriate care. Redesigning workflows, practice routines, and the environment requires clinicians to ask the critical question, "How does our current approach to care serve the whole patient and family—is there a different way that may be better?" The foundation of population health management includes information-powered clinical decision making—for example, using big data to validate adoption and measure the impact of best practices, embracing a "primary-care" clinical

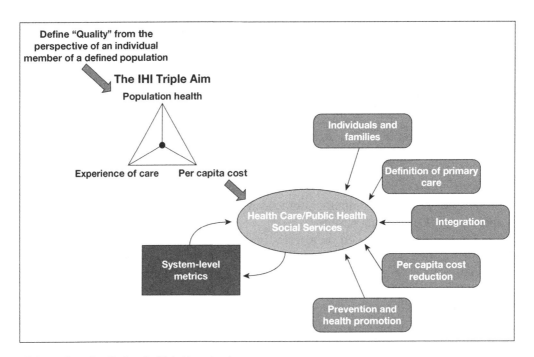

FIGURE 3.3   Design of a Triple Aim enterprise.

IHI, Institute for Healthcare Improvement.

Source: Institute of Healthcare Improvement (2012).

model—to ensure consistency in care and the cultivation of healing relationships, and engaging and integrating the patient–family dyad into care planning (The Advisory Board, 2013). The cost-control platform gives us an opportunity to measure success in a quantifiable way—for example, looking at decreasing hospital-acquired conditions, increasing breastfeeding rates, and decreasing length of hospital stay— to allow us to select appropriate economic goals and objectives that can guide and drive the practice improvement project. And lastly system integration focuses on the individual's experience of care and how your existing system resources support this key driver—for example, if your goal is to increase direct breastfeeding rates, do you have adequate lactation support to achieve that objective.

The IHI advocates for a systematic approach to change that includes identification of the target population, defining system aims and success metrics, developing a project plan that is realistic and actionable, and undergoing rapid cycles to test, evaluate, revise, and subsequently implement the change.

When you come upon a wall, throw your hat over it, and then go get your hat.
        —Anonymous Irish proverb

The "wall" in this proverb is your current way of doing things in the NICU; maybe it is the way you have been doing things for 30 years, it is your culture. Evidence-based best practice is not a wall or a static process, and neither is the journey to excellence. Throw your hat over the wall and go get it—the journey will be well worth it for your patient, the family, your organization, society at large, and *you*!

■ REFERENCES

The Advisory Board. (2013). *Three key elements for successful population management*. Retrieved from https://www.advisory.com/-/media/Advisory-com/Research/HCAB/Research -Study/2013/Three-Elements-for-Successful-Population-Health-Management/Three -Key-Elements-for-Successful-Population-Health-Management.pdf?la=en

American Academy of Pediatrics (AAP). (2004). Policy statement: Organizational principles to guide and defined the child healthcare system and or improve the health of all children. *Pediatrics, 113*(5), 1545–1547.

Block, R. W. (2016). All adults once were children. *Journal of Pediatric Surgery, 51*(1), 23–27.

Boyce, W. T., & Kobor, M. S. (2015). Development and the epigenome: The "synapse" of gene–environment interplay. *Developmental Science, 18*(1), 1–23.

Bradshaw, A. (1999). The virtue of nursing: The covenant of care. *Journal of Medical Ethics, 25*(6), 477–481.

Brummelte, S., Chau, C. M., Cepeda, I. L., Degenhardt, A., Weinberg, J., Synnes, A. R., & Grunau, R. E. (2015). Cortisol levels in former preterm children at school age are predicted by neonatal procedural pain-related stress. *Psychoneuroendocrinology, 51,* 151–163.

Center on the Developing Child. Harvard University. *Resilience*. Retrieved from http://developingchild.harvard.edu/science/key-concepts/resilience

Center on the Developing Child. Harvard University. *Science*. Retrieved from http://developingchild.harvard.edu/science

Chau, C. M., Cepeda, I. L., Devlin, A. M., Weinberg, J., & Grunau, R. E. (2015). The Val66Met brain-derived neurotrophic factor gene variant interacts with early pain exposure to predict cortisol dysregulation in 7-year-old children born very preterm: Implications for cognition. *Neuroscience*, Aug 28, pii: S0306–4522(15)00776–9. doi:10.1016/j.neuroscience.2015.08.044

Coughlin, M. (2014). *Transformative nursing in the NICU: Trauma-informed, age-appropriate care*. New York, NY: Springer Publishing.

Cowling, W. R., Smith, M. C., & Watson, J. (2008). The power of wholeness, consciousness, and caring: A dialogue on nursing science, art, and healing. *Advances in Nursing Science, 31*(1), E41–E51.

Decety, J., & Fotopoulou, A. (2014). Why empathy has a beneficial impact on others in medicine: Unifying theories. *Frontiers in Behavioral Neuroscience, 8*, 457.

Dossey, B. (2000). *Florence Nightingale: Mystic, visionary, healer*. Springhouse, PA: Springhouse.

Faber, K. (2013). Relationship-based care in the neonatal intensive care unit. *Creative Nursing, 19*(4), 214–218.

Garner, A. S., Forkey, H., & Szilagyi, M. (2015). Translating developmental science to address childhood adversity. *Academic Pediatrics, 15*(5), 493–502.

Garner, A. S., & Shonkoff, J. P.; Committee on Psychosocial Aspects of Child and Family Health; Committee on Early Childhood, Adoption, and Dependent Care; Section on Developmental and Behavioral Pediatrics. (2012). Early childhood adversity, toxic stress, and the role of the pediatrician: Translating developmental science into lifelong health. *Pediatrics, 129*(1), e224–e231.

Gibbins, S., Hoath, S. B., Coughlin, M., Gibbins, A., & Franck, L. (2008). The universe of developmental care: A new conceptual model for application in the neonatal intensive care unit. *Advances in Neonatal Care, 8*(3), 141–147.

Grunau, R. E., Cepeda, I. L., Chau, C. M., Brummelte, S., Weinberg, J., Lavoie, P. M.,… Turvey, S. E. (2013). Neonatal pain-related stress and NFKBIA genotype are associated with altered cortisol levels in preterm boys at school age. *PloS One, 8*(9), e73926.

Hane, A. A., & Fox, N. A. (2016). Early caregiving and human biobehavioral development: A comparative physiology approach. *Current Opinion in Behavioral Sciences, 7*, 82–90.

Heim, C., & Nemeroff, C. B. (2002). Neurobiology of early life stress: Clinical studies. *Seminars in Clinical Neuropsychiatry, 7*(2), 147–159.

Jarrín, O. F. (2012). The integrality of situated caring in nursing and the environment. *Advances in Nursing Science, 35*(1), 14–24.

Kemper, K. J., & Shaltout, H. A. (2011). Non-verbal communication of compassion: Measuring psychophysiological effects. *BMC Complementary and Alternative Medicine, 11*(132), 1–9. Retrieved from http://www.biomedcentral.com/1472–6882/11/132

Koerner, J. (2011). *Healing presence: The essence of nursing.* New York, NY: Springer Publishing.

Kundakovic, M., & Champagne, F. A. (2015). Early-life experience, epigenetics, and the developing brain. *Neuropsychopharmacology, 40*(1), 141–153.

Lachman, V. D. (2012). Applying the ethics of care to your nursing practice. *MEDSURG Nursing, 21*(2), 112–4, 116.

Montirosso, R., & Provenzi, L. (2015). Implications of epigenetics and stress regulation on research and developmental care of preterm infants. *Journal of Obstetric, Gynecologic, and Neonatal Nursing: JOGNN/NAACOG, 44*(2), 174–182.

Odgers, C. L., & Jaffee, S. R. (2013). Routine versus catastrophic influences on the developing child. *Annual Review of Public Health, 34*, 29–48.

Pickler, R. H., McGrath, J. M., Reyna, B. A., McCain, N., Lewis, M., Cone, S.,...Best, A. (2010). A model of neurodevelopmental risk and protection for preterm infants. *The Journal of Perinatal & Neonatal Nursing, 24*(4), 356–365.

Porges, S. W. (2004). Neuroception: A subconscious system for detecting threats and safety. *Zero to Three, 24*(5), 19–24.

Porges, S. W. (2007). The polyvagal perspective. *Biological Psychology, 74*(2), 116–143.

Porges, S. W. (2009). The polyvagal theory: New insights into adaptive reactions of the autonomic nervous system. *Cleveland Clinic Journal of Medicine, 76*(Suppl. 2), S86–S90.

Provenzi, L., & Montirosso, R. (2015). "Epigenethics" in the neonatal intensive care unit: Conveying complexity in health care for preterm children. *JAMA Pediatrics, 169*(7), 617–618.

Richards, M., & Wadsworth, M. E. (2004). Long-term effects of early adversity on cognitive function. *Archives of Disease in Childhood, 89*(10), 922–927.

Samra, H. A., McGrath, J. M., Wehbe, M., & Clapper, J. (2012). Epigenetics and family-centered developmental care for the preterm infant. *Advances in Neonatal Care, 12*(Suppl. 5), S2–S9.

Sanders, M. R. (2013). Rich, dense, and not for the faint of heart. The polyvagal theory: Neurophysiological foundations of emotions, attachment, communication, and self-regulation by Stephen W. Porges. *Journal of Unified Psychotherapy and Clinical Science, 2*(1), 98–103.

Shonkoff, J. P., & Garner, A. S.; Committee on Psychosocial Aspects of Child and Family Health; Committee on Early Childhood, Adoption, and Dependent Care; Section on Developmental and Behavioral Pediatrics. (2012). The lifelong effects of early childhood adversity and toxic stress. *Pediatrics, 129*(1), e232–e246.

Smith, G. C., Gutovich, J., Smyser, C., Pineda, R., Newnham, C., Tjoeng, T. H.,...Inder, T. (2011). Neonatal intensive care unit stress is associated with brain development in preterm infants. *Annals of Neurology, 70*(4), 541–549.

Tammen, S. A., Friso, S., & Choi, S. W. (2013). Epigenetics: The link between nature and nurture. *Molecular Aspects of Medicine, 34*(4), 753–764.

Vaiserman, A. M. (2015). Epigenetic programming by early-life stress: Evidence from human populations. *Developmental Dynamics, 244*(3), 254–265.

van der Kolk, B. (2014). Body-brain connections. In B. van der Kolk (Ed.), *The body keeps the score: Brain, mind, and body in the healing of trauma* (p. 78). New York, NY: The Penguin Group.

Watson, J. (2002). Intentionality and caring-healing consciousness: A practice of transpersonal nursing. *Holistic Nursing Practice, 16*(4), 12–19.

Watson, J. (2005). *Caring science as sacred science*. Philadelphia, PA: F. A. Davis.

Watson, J. (2007). Watson's theory of human caring and subjected living experiences: Keratin factors/care test processes as a disciplinary guide to the professional nursing practice. *Texto Contexto Enfermagem, Florianopolis, 16*(1), 129–135.

Watson, J. (2009). Caring science and human caring theory: Transforming personal and professional practices of nursing and health care. *Journal of Health and Human Services Administration, 31*(4), 466–482.

Willis, D. G., Grace, P. J., & Roy, C. (2008). A central unifying focus for the discipline: Facilitating humanization, meaning, choice, quality of life, and healing in living and dying. *Advances in Nursing Science, 31*(1), E28–E40.

CHAPTER 4

Summary: The Need for Standardization of Trauma-Informed, Age-Appropriate Care in the NICU

Adopting a trauma-informed paradigm for neonatal intensive care acknowledges and honors the lived experience of the infant–family dyad in crisis. Neonatal clinicians must integrate evidence-based best practices in age-appropriate care to manage and mitigate the trauma and adversity associated with neonatal intensive care unit (NICU) hospitalization to cultivate resilience through authentic healing relationships with the infant and his or her family. Nursing plays a key role in transforming culture but cannot achieve the desired results alone—it takes a village! This first section aspired to engage the hearts and minds of my transdisciplinary colleagues grounded by science and guided by our moral compass to lead and be the necessary change-makers that positively impact the families we serve today and tomorrow (Coughlin, 2014; Small & Small, 2011). Standardizing developmentally supportive, age-appropriate care, framed by a trauma-informed paradigm, is at the heart of safe, patient-centered quality care in the NICU and is a global health imperative (Coughlin, 2014).

The patient's experience is the sum of all interactions, shaped by an organization's culture, that influence patient perceptions across the continuum of care.
          —The Beryl Institute

This section presented both an overview and an update on the concept and the science behind trauma-informed, age-appropriate care in the NICU, expanding on this author's first book, *Transformative Nursing in the NICU*. In addition, Chapter 2 delineated the core measure categories and introduced new knowledge, insights, and better practices in the healing environment; pain and stress prevention, assessment and management; the constituents of protected sleep; activities of daily living, and family collaborative care. The dynamic nature of health care embraces the continual pursuit of excellence and the discovery of new and potentially better practices; however, knowledge alone is not sufficient to transform culture (Coughlin, 2014).

The adoption of evidence-based best practices, often formulated into guidelines, has proven to reduce morbidity and mortality in all areas of health care; however, translation and implementation of best practices continue to be a challenge. Implementation science explores methodologies and barriers to the translation of research into clinical practice acknowledging a greater demand for accountability in research (Kelly, 2013). To that end, collaborative quality networks and quality organizations, such as the Institute for Healthcare Improvement, are at the forefront of the quality movement tackling quality improvement initiatives using proven improvement methodologies (Profit & Soll, 2015). Figure 4.1 provides an overview and comparison of the two phases associated with the Plan-Do-Study-Act (PDSA)

Pilot Phase	Implementation Phase
PEOPLE: **FEW** The number of people affected by a pilot test is relatively small. Thus, the resistance to the change is often relatively low.	PEOPLE: **MANY** The number of people affected during implementation is relatively large. There may be stronger resistance to the change that improvement teams must overcome.
SUPPORT NEEDED: **LOW** Testers do not yet intend changes to be permanent and therefore do not need processes to maintain changes beyond the test period.	SUPPORT NEEDED: **HIGH** Testers expect the change to become part of the routine operations of the system; supporting processes to maintain the change—feedback and measurement systems, job descriptions, training, etc.—must be in place.
TIME: **SHORTER** Cycles for testing changes can be rapid.	TIME: **LONGER** Test cycles, which are larger in scale and more diverse in scope, generally require more time than in the pilot.
TOLERANCE FOR FAILURE: **HIGH** It's OK (in fact it is encouraged!) for testers to learn from mistakes. Between 25% and 50% of tests may not produce the desired results; these "failures" are important opportunities to learn.	TOLERANCE FOR FAILURE: **LOW** Due to all of the above (i.e., the people, resources, and time involved) the tolerance for failure is relatively low during implementation. Testers should have a high degree of confidence that the changes they are implementing will result in improvement.

FIGURE 4.1   Plan-Do-Study-Act (PDSA) comparison of the pilot phase and the implementation phase of improvement work.

Source: © 2014 Institute for Healthcare Improvement.

model for improvement, a framework for accelerating the translation of evidence into practice. The model asks three fundamental questions:

1. What are you trying to accomplish or what is the aim of your improvement project?
2. How will you know that a change is an improvement? Not all change is better than what you are doing now, so, what will tell you that the new practice is an improvement?
3. What changes will you make to achieve your desired results? What ideas will you test in the pilot phase, then tweak (or throw out) to arrive at the practice that works best, in your environment, for your patients? (This will determine what you implement; Langley et al., 2009.)

The purpose of guidelines is to tell clinicians the right things to do; however, most guidelines fail to tell clinicians how to do these things—how to implement evidence-based best practices (Vander Schaaf, Seashore, & Randolph, 2015). This book presents the latest evidence, best practice recommendations, and suggested implementation strategies and resources to facilitate adoption and integration of trauma-informed, age-appropriate care and best practices in your NICU.

I have been impressed with the urgency of doing. Knowing is not
enough; we must apply. Being willing is not enough; we must do.
        —Leonardo da Vinci

▪ REFERENCES

Coughlin, M. (2014). *Transformative nursing in the NICU: Trauma-informed, age-appropriate care.* New York, NY: Springer Publishing.

Kelly, B. (2013). Implementing implementation science: Reviewing the quest to develop methods and frameworks for effective implementation. *Journal of Neurology and Psychology, 1*(1), 5.

Langley, G. L., Moen, R., Nolan, K. M., Nolan, T. W., Norman, C. L., & Provost, L. P. (2009). *The improvement guide: A practical approach to enhancing organizational performance* (2nd ed.). San Francisco, CA: Jossey-Bass.

Profit, J., & Soll, R. F. (2015). Neonatal networks: Clinical research and quality improvement. *Seminars in Fetal & Neonatal Medicine, 20*(6), 410–415.

Small, D. C., & Small, R. M. (2011). Patients first! Engaging the hearts and minds of nurses with a patient-centered practice model. *Online Journal of Issues in Nursing, 16*(2), 2.

Vander Schaaf, E. B., Seashore, C. J., & Randolph, G. D. (2015). Translating clinical guidelines into practice: Challenges and opportunities in a dynamic health care environment. *North Carolina Medical Journal, 76*(4), 230–234.

PART II

Clinical Practice Guidelines for Trauma-Informed, Age-Appropriate Care in the NICU: The Core Measures

■ OVERVIEW

The scope and purpose of these practice guidelines is to standardize the experience of care for the hospitalized infant to reflect adoption of evidence-based best practices in the provision of trauma-informed, age-appropriate care in the neonatal intensive care unit (NICU). The intended users of these practice guidelines include all health care professionals who interface with hospitalized newborns and infants.

The target population includes all hospitalized newborns (both preterm and term) in the NICU. These guidelines may also have implications for newborns and infants hospitalized in other settings to include mother–baby units, postpartum wards, special care or other intensive care settings (surgical, medical, and cardiothoracic), as well as infants requiring neonatal transport.

Evidence to support practice recommendations was collected via electronically accessible, peer-reviewed studies from MEDLINE, Neonatal Cochrane Collaboration, and the Cumulative Index to Nursing and Allied Health Literature published between 1982 and 2015. Search words correlated with the specific attributes and criteria associated with each core measure for age-appropriate care set. Systematic reviews and randomized controlled trials were considered the strongest level of evidence. When unavailable, cohort, case control, consensus statements, and qualitative methods were considered the strongest level of evidence for a particular practice strategy.

CHAPTER 5

Guidelines for the Healing Environment

Embracing a caring–healing framework incorporates attending to the wholeness of humans in their everyday creation and sustenance of a meaningful life.
      —Swanson and Wojnar (2004)

This guideline presents the latest evidence-based research, along with clinical practice recommendations and implementation strategies related to the healing environment in the neonatal intensive care unit (NICU) across the physical, the human, and the organizational domains (as detailed in Table 5.1).

TABLE 5.1   Attributes and Criteria of the Healing Environment

Attributes	Criteria
The physical environment is a soothing, spacious, and aesthetically pleasing space that is conducive to rest, healing, and establishing therapeutic relationships.	1. Sensory input is age-appropriate; dose and duration of sensory input is guided by infant's behavioral and physiologic responses. 2. Space safely accommodates the provision of quality clinical care, 24-hr parental presence, and privacy. 3. The design honors the holistic and human dimensions of those that inhabit the space, integrates stress-reducing strategies (e.g., art, music), and facilitates social and therapeutic interactions for patients, families, and professionals.
The human environment emanates teamwork, mindfulness, and caring.	1. The interprofessional team exhibits shared responsibility in problem solving and decision making to formulate holistic plans for patient care; team members assume complementary roles that facilitate cooperation. 2. Team members support each other in "always doing the right thing" for the patient, family, and staff. 3. All verbal, written, and behavioral communication is respectful, complete, and patient centered; there is zero tolerance for behaviors that compromises safety and/or undermines respectful relationships.

(continued)

TABLE 5.1 Attributes and Criteria of the Healing Environment *(continued)*

Attributes	Criteria
The organizational environment reflects a just culture committed to safety.	1. Core measures for age-appropriate care provide the standard of care for all patient care encounters and are reviewed/revised annually to reflect the latest evidence-based best practices. 2. Practice standards are integrated into the annual performance evaluation across all the disciplines and professionals who interface with the neonatal/infant population. 3. A just culture framework ensures balanced accountability at the individual and organizational level for continuous learning, quality improvement, and patient safety.

GUIDELINE OBJECTIVES

- To define the properties associated with a healing environment
- To present the evidence that supports this definition
- To present evidence-based recommendations
- To present clinical practice strategies to integrate this definition into the culture of neonatal intensive care

MAJOR OUTCOMES CONSIDERED

The impact of the healing environmental dimensions on the NICU patient, family, and staff includes:

- Physiologic, psychosocial, and psychoemotional outcomes
- Patient safety and quality clinical outcomes

THE PHYSICAL ENVIRONMENT

The object and color in the materials around us actually have a physical effect on us, on how we feel.
        —Florence Nightingale

Interventions and Practice Considerations

- Create and maintain an age-appropriate, safe sensory milieu that complies with neonatal best practices and best available evidence.
    - Best practice considerations for lighting include adjustable lighting with ambient lighting levels maintained between 10 lux and 600 lux

- Best practice recommendations for the auditory environment include continuous sound levels at less than or equal to 45 dB and maximum intermittent sound levels not to exceed 65 dB; promote parent–infant conversations and skin-to-skin experiences (optimal auditory input includes parental voice and parental biological sounds of the heartbeat, breathing sounds, etc.)
- Best practice considerations for tactile input promote skin-to-skin contact and other positive touch experiences; consistently and reliably manage all skin-piercing procedures for pain and pain-related stress
- Best practice considerations for gustatory and olfactory experiences include the exclusive use of mother's milk for mouth care; promote skin-to-skin care; manage noxious odors in and around the infant's microenvironment
- Best practice considerations for vestibular and proprioceptive experiences to include slow-contained movements, nesting supports, skin-to-skin care experiences
- Best practice considerations for visual experiences to include protecting the eyes from direct light, support parent–infant en face experiences
- Create and maintain a physical layout that protects privacy, provides for family presence, supports parenting activities, and promotes interpersonal experiences with the health care team
  - Best practice considerations for a space that accommodates clinical safety, continuous parent presence, auditory and visual privacy
- Ensure and maintain an aesthetic environment that reflects a respect for human dignity encompassing the patient, the family, and the staff
  - Best practice considerations include stress-reducing strategies as well as facilities for respite and socialization

The Evidence

THE SENSORY MILIEU

Touch is the first sensory system to emerge and allows us to discriminate quality and location of a stimulus on the skin surface and to explore and manipulate objects haptically, but also experience pleasure through positive hedonic experiences and gain an integrated sense of self (Morrison et al., 2010). A fetus of 8.5 weeks gestation will respond to a gentle stroking to the face (Arabin et al., 1996). Intrauterine tactile experiences via oscillations of lanugo hairs during fetal movement activate mechanoreceptors on fetal skin connected to specialized unmyelinated fibers that send impulses to paralimbic and limbic structures linked to oxytocin release and the stimulation of fetal growth hormones (Bystrova, 2009).

Nurturing touch is crucial for healthy neonatal development, first reported by Spitz (1945, 1946) who noted that infants cared for in an orphanage had high mortality rates in the first year of life despite having their "basic" needs met (basic needs defined as being clean, well fed, and warm). A paucity of nurturing touch has been linked to compromised somatic growth and biobehavioral development despite adequate nutrition (Kuhn & Schanberg, 1998). In identifying nurturing touch as a neonatal growth requirement, Kuhn and Schanberg (1998) tested supplemental tactile stimulation in a cohort of very premature infants using infant massage. The treated infants demonstrated marked weight gain, improved behavioral development, and a significant maturation of sympatho-adrenal function.

Care strategies that promote nurturing touch improve the hospitalized infant's short-term experience of care in the NICU, but also favorably impact their developmental trajectory. The first European Conference on Kangaroo Mother Care presented the increasing evidence on the benefits of kangaroo mother care for infants and families across all intensive care settings (Nyqvist et al., 2010). Conde-Agudelo and Díaz-Rossello (2014) authored the latest Cochrane Review synthesizing the evidence that kangaroo mother care reduces morbidity and mortality in low-birth-weight infants. Lowson et al. (2015) completed an economic analysis on the effectiveness of an intervention aimed at increasing breastfeeding and kangaroo mother care. Economic benefits included a decrease in hospital stay, a reduction in infections, as well as a reduction in the number of infants requiring emergency transports.

Feldman et al. (2014) evaluated the effect of a kangaroo mother care intervention on a cohort of 73 premature mother–infant dyads with 73 case-matched controls who received standard incubator care. The subjects were followed over the first 10 years of life to assess multiple physiologic, cognitive, parental mental health, and mother–child relational measures. The findings demonstrated the long-term effects of touch-based interventions in the NICU on the children's physiologic organization and behavioral control.

The chemical senses of taste and smell develop early in intrauterine life. Taste buds are evident in human embryos by the seventh week of gestation (Salihagic-Kadic & Predojevic, 2012). Sweet tastes stimulate swallowing in the human fetus, whereas a bitter or sour taste decreases fetal swallowing (Salihagic-Kadic & Predojevic, 2012). By 17 weeks gestation, taste cells are functionally mature and primary olfactory receptors are functional as early as 24 weeks gestation (Lipchock et al., 2011).

Amniotic fluid is freely ingested by the developing fetus and is comprised of various flavonoid and odorant molecules derived from the maternal diet that prime fetal learning for postnatal maternal chemo-recognition and food preferences—specifically breast milk (Ventura & Worobey, 2013). The "flavor" of amniotic fluid is experienced through the complete immersion of the retro-nasal and oral mucosa (inhalation and swallowing) by the amniotic fluid, which occurs after 6 months gestation, when the epithelial plugs lodged in the nasal passages dissolve (Lipchock et al., 2011).

Maternal odor and maternal flavors have shown to decrease infant crying as well as increased mouthing movements suggesting a role for maternal odor for soothing and feeding (Croes et al., 2012; Sullivan & Toubas, 1998). Yildiz et al. (2011) conducted a prospective experimental study to investigate the effect of breast milk odor on preterm infant's transition time from gavage feeding to total oral feeding. Their findings indicated that infants stimulated with breast milk odor during gavage feedings transitioned to oral feedings 3 days sooner than controls. In addition to the hedonic olfactory properties of breast milk, prenatal flavor experiences with the amniotic fluid prime the infant for his or her flavor experience with maternal milk (Mennella et al., 2001).

Mitchell et al. (2013) present the effects of daily kangaroo care on cardiorespiratory parameters in preterm infants and concluded that kangaroo care decreased the incidence of bradycardia and oxygen desaturations in preterm infants. A randomized controlled trial of kangaroo care by Ludington-Hoe et al. (2004) demonstrated an absence of apnea, bradycardia, and period breathing during kangaroo care. Both studies validate the preterm infant's responsiveness to maternally mediated sensory stimulation, including odor and taste corroborating the findings of Doucet et al. (2007) who described infant behavioral responses to odor masking and selective unmasking of maternal breast scent. Their study quantified the global maternal odor effects on neonatal behavior to include the modulation of arousal states, stimulation of rooting, sucking, and licking movements, as well as stimulating visual behaviors.

Providing maternal olfactory and gustatory experiences in the NICU has demonstrated clinical utility and beneficence. In addition to providing this pleasant sensory experience, protecting infants from noxious exposures is equally needed. Bartocci et al. (2001) reported changes in cerebral hemodynamics in response to unpleasant odors (adhesive remover and a detergent product) by a cohort of preterm infants. Although the authors state they are unsure of the biologic relevance of their findings, the exposure is at the very least stressful. Paccauda et al. (2012) analyzed incubator atmosphere following the application of ethanol-based hand sanitizers and report that the inner atmosphere was highly polluted by alcohol vapors and recommend that staff delay entry into the incubator space until the hand sanitizer vapors have completely evaporated.

The structures responsible for hearing and vestibular function develop in tandem within the inner ear. The auditory system and cochlea become functional around 25 weeks gestation with ongoing development extending over the first decade of life (Eldredge & Salamy, 1996; Graven & Browne, 2008; Lasky & Williams, 2005; Ruben, 1995). Intrauterine low-frequency sounds meet the requirements of the developing cochlea. These low-frequency sound waves (vascular sounds, borborygmi, and muted maternal vocalizations, for example) support the necessary fine tuning of the highly specialized inner hair cells of the cochlea, preparing the hearing apparatus for eventual exposure to higher frequency sound waves associated with human speech (McMahon, Wintermark, & Lahav, 2012).

Adverse outcomes related to noxious sound exposure in the NICU include hypoxemia, blood-pressure fluctuations, sleep disturbances, an increase in behavioral and physiologic stress responses, as well as language, attention, and cognitive deficits observed in the former preterm patient population (American Academy of Pediatrics [AAP], 1997; Lahav & Skoe, 2014; Lasky & Williams, 2005; Wachman & Lahav, 2011). The incidence of hearing loss or hearing impairment among NICU graduates is estimated to be 10-fold greater than that of their term counterparts (Clark-Gambelunghe & Clark, 2015). The acoustic gap between the womb and NICU environments is illustrated in Table 5.2 (Lahav & Skoe, 2014).

TABLE 5.2   An Acoustic Gap Between the NICU and the Womb Environments
(Creative Commons Attribution License)

	Womb	NICU
Primary mode of hearing	Bone conduction	Air conduction
Sound transmission medium	Fluid	Air
Sound attenuation	Attenuation provided by maternal tissue and fluids	Direct exposure to sound source
Frequency range of sound exposure	Primarily low frequency (< 500 Hz)	Broad spectrum
Ambient noise dosage	Restricted daily exposure to noise	Excessive daily exposure to noise (e.g., alarms, white noise, and multi-talker babble)
Most prevalent sounds in environment	Maternal vocalizations, biological sounds (e.g., heartbeat, digestive noises)	Electronic, unnatural, nonbiological sounds
Exposure to language	High-quality stimuli, primarily from mother	Poor-quality stimuli during nonvisiting hours, primarily from multi-talker babble
Complexity of prevalent sounds in environment	Rhythmic, periodic, organized, predictable (e.g., heartbeat)	Aperiodic (e.g., white noise), unorganized, unpredictable (e.g., alarms)

Source: Lahav and Skoe (2014).

The vestibular system shares the inner-ear sensory end organs and together with central neurons of the brainstem, cerebellum, thalamus, and cortex computes an estimate of head and body positions in space (Beraneck et al., 2014). As the fetus enjoys a relatively gravity-free environment in utero, this unrestricted movement stimulates the developing vestibular structures generating vestibular motor reflexes in response to the varied fetal positions and movement patterns. These reflexes continue to develop postnatally calibrating the gravity information during critical periods of development (Jamon, 2014). Vestibular evoked myogenic potentials (VEMP) are prolonged in preterm infants and may reflect neurodevelopmental impairment (Eshaghi et al., 2014). Vestibular dysfunction is implicated in the motor and mental developmental delays observed in late preterm infants (Ecevit et al., 2012).

It is imperative that the auditory environment of the NICU acknowledges and responds to the vulnerabilities of the patient population served. Architectural redesigns ranging from single-patient rooms to more modest modifications, such as continuous monitoring of sound levels, the installation of sound-absorbing ceiling tiles and soft vinyl flooring have yielded a decrease in NICU noise levels (Chen et al., 2009; Krueger et al., 2007; Shahheidari & Homer, 2012). Carvalhais et al. (2015) evaluated the effectiveness of a staff-training program on noise reduction with disappointing results and the authors recommend that a training intervention needs to be part of a larger quality improvement initiative. These findings are similar to the work of Liu (2010), who introduced a quality improvement aimed at noise reduction in two open-unit-design neonatal centers sponsored by Neonatal Intensive Care Quality Collaboration. The take away message is that, at least for sound reduction, a more comprehensive intervention is required in order to achieve the desired results.

Neurosensory systems develop in an ordered, sequential fashion beginning with the tactile system and ending with the visual system, which becomes fully functional over the first 2 to 3 years of postnatal life (Graven, 2011; Graven & Browne, 2008). Visual system development is complex and particularly susceptible to pre- and postnatal nutrition as well as postnatal visual stimulation (Brémond-Gignac et al., 2011). NICU care can negatively impact visual development by interfering with endogenous brain cell activity, sleep deprivation and sleep fragmentation, as well as exposing the vulnerable ocular structures to intense light (Graven, 2011). Protective care strategies that support sleep (such as cycled lighting, maintaining ambient light and sound levels within recommended ranges) can minimize the deleterious effect of the NICU environment on the developing visual system (Guyer et al., 2012; Shahheidari & Homer, 2012).

THE PHYSICAL LAYOUT

The eighth edition of the recommended standards for newborn ICU design has updated the minimum space, clearance, and privacy requirements for an infant's bed space in the NICU. The minimum space dimensions must equal 120 ft.^{2} (11.2 m^2) of clear floor space, which shall accommodate sufficient furnishings for parental presence in addition to the medical equipment and resources necessary to render safe intensive care (White et al., 2013).

Adequate space, which affords privacy to patients and their families (specifically described in the single-family room design), has been shown to increase parental involvement leading to a decrease in hospital stay and readmission rates as well as a reduction in hospital-acquired infections, enhanced infant medical progress, and better breastfeeding success (Domanico et al., 2011; Erdeve et al., 2008; Shahheidari & Homer, 2012). The physical layout can be a challenge for staff, especially when patient assignments are dispersed across a wider geographic footprint; however, research suggests that the benefits to the patient and family impact the staff in a favorable way when the process to transition to a single-room design is thoughtful and comprehensive (Domanico et al., 2010; Stevens et al., 2010).

Although the physical dimensions of the patient's bedspace are an important piece in creating a healing environment and supporting family presence at the bedside, single-patient room design is just the tip of the iceberg. Franck et al. (2015) report a link between overnight accommodations and hospital experience, where families who stayed at a Ronald McDonald House had more positive overall experience scores than families who stayed in other accommodations (to include sleeping at the bedside and sleeping at home). These findings highlight the more complex needs of the family in crisis with a critically ill, hospitalized infant. Promoting positive psychosocial outcomes of infant–parent dyads requires interventions aimed at minimizing isolation and separation and focuses on family-centered, developmentally, and age-appropriate care—*family* presence and participation are crucial (Obeidat et al., 2009).

THE AESTHETICS

Nightingale articulated the importance of aesthetics in the healing process by drawing attention to how sensory impressions of the environment impacted the patient's recovery, both physically and mentally (Nightingale, 1969). Ulrich (1984) was one of the first researchers to publish the influence of aesthetics on the recovery of a cohort of surgical patients. In his seminal work, patients whose recovery room window provided a view of a natural scene had a shorter postoperative hospital stay and utilized fewer analgesics than their matched controls who recovered in similar rooms; however, their windows faced a brick building. An aesthetic design for a healing environment integrates the sensory milieu with the physical layout creating a space that honors the holistic human dimensions of those that inhabit the space (Schweitzer et al., 2004; Wikstrom, Westerlund, & Erkkila, 2012).

The importance of aesthetics in the NICU relate to how the environment influences the adults that occupy the space and how the space conveys a commitment to wholeness, healing, and dignity for the patient, the family, and the staff (Figure 5.1).

Ulrich's theory of supportive design (1997) suggests that a hospital environment that provides the occupants with a sense of control, access to social supports, and positive distractions will positively impact health and recovery by reducing the stress and distress experienced by patients, families, and staff. Aesthetic sensory impressions of art, nature, and natural lighting have been identified as powerful sources of well-being, relief, and hope for patients and their families as well

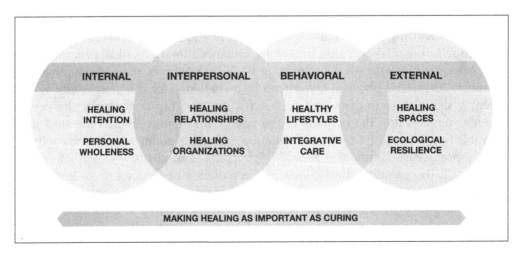

FIGURE 5.1   Optimal Healing Environments (OHE) Framework from Samueli Institute.

Reprinted with permission from the Samueli Institute: www.samueliInstitute.org
Source: Sakallaris, MacAllister, Voss, Smith, and Jonas (2015).

as enhancing staff motivation and engagement (Timmerman & Uhrenfeldt, 2014; Timmermann, Uhrenfeldt, & Birkelund, 2015; Wilkstrom et al., 2012).

Cost Analysis

Integrating the sensory, spacial, and aesthetic components of the physical environment points to a NICU design model that will have economic, clinical, and psychosocial benefits for patients, families, and staff. Shepley et al. (2014) present the cost implications of a single-family design NICU compared with quantifiable benefits. The authors conclude that the investment in new NICU construction to have a majority of single-family rooms is recouped after the first year with substantial savings in subsequent years. Building well-designed NICUs improve outcomes for the most fragile of patient populations and favorably impacts parent and staff satisfaction, all resulting in significant dollar savings (Shepley et al., 2014). Hospital-based environmental exposures to include the physical layout, the light and sound levels, the availability of social interactions with parents and clinicians, as well as chemical exposures from various medical equipment employed in the NICU poses a threat to neurodevelopmental outcomes of the individuals served in this environment (Santos et al., 2015). Managing and mitigating these noxious exposures is crucial in reducing the societal costs associated with prematurity and improving long-term developmental outcomes (Institute of Medicine [IOM], 2007; Pickler, McGrath, Reyna, Tubbs-Cooley et al., 2013).

Recommendations for the Physical Environment (Table 5.3)

TABLE 5.3   Major Practice Recommendations and Implementation Strategies—Sensory Milieu, Space, and Aesthetics

Sensory Milieu	
Recommendations	**Implementation Strategy**
1. Maintain sound levels within the recommended range and develop and implement noise reduction protocols (Pickler, McGrath, Reyna, Tubbs-Cooley et al., 2013; Ramesh et al., 2013; Swathi et al., 2014)	a. Collect baseline sound levels (either purchase a sound meter OR download a decibel reader app to your smartphone) b. Collect decibel readings at various locations within your unit and record location and baseline sound levels c. Share results with the team using multiple modes of communication (e-mail, posted graphs in staff lounge and staff restrooms/locker rooms) d. Outline an improvement strategy (e.g., we will reduce our ambient sound levels by 10% within 3 months). Consider employing a PDSA model for improvement (see Figure 5.2) e. On a weekly basis recollect sound level data (in the same locations as baseline), record and post to staff. SHARE TRENDING RESULTS—good or bad!

(continued)

TABLE 5.3   Major Practice Recommendations and Implementation Strategies—Sensory Milieu,
Space, and Aesthetics   *(continued)*

Sensory Milieu	
Recommendations	**Implementation Strategy**
	f. Consider sharing snippets from evidence-based resources regarding the impact of noise on patients and staff—do not be afraid to be creative; creativity will engage your colleagues and engagement is the first step in changing behaviors and practice.
2. Maintain light levels within the recommended range and provide cycled or day/night lighting in the NICU (Borniger et al., 2014; Guyer et al., 2012; Morag & Ohlsson, 2013; Pickler, McGrath, Reyna, Tubbs-Cooley et al., 2013; Vásquez-Ruiz et al., 2014)	a. Collect baseline light levels in various locations in your unit (don't forget to get eye level with the patient; this will give you good insight into the infant's lived lighting experience) b. Identify areas for improvement (do all the lights have dimmers? Are they working? Is the ambient lighting indirect or direct?) Talk with environmental services or biomed for innovative fiscally responsible solutions c. Initiate a practice improvement plan to introduce a cycled lighting practice standard to your unit d. Review your current practice in protecting infant's eyes from direct light—identify areas for improvement e. Consider replicating practice improvements already described in the literature (i.e., Guyer et al., 2012) f. Improvement strategies that are integrated into existing workflow processes OR creating reminders and redundancies in the workflow will help with practice adoption
3. Sensory input is age-appropriate; dose and duration of sensory input is guided by infant's behavioral and physiologic responses (Conde-Agudelo & Díaz-Rossello, 2014; Jefferies & CPS, 2012; Krueger, 2010; Medoff-Cooper et al., 2015)	a. Consider annual competency-based staff education on verbal and nonverbal communication styles used by neonates and infants to include autonomic, motoric and state expressions of engagement and disengagement b. Outline a process and action plan for managing disengagement cues during care interactions (see Table 5.4). c. Based on an individualized assessment of a patient's sensory stimulus preferences, integrate positive sensory experiences into the infant's daily care plan (e.g., kangaroo care, oral care with colostrum/breast milk, the use of familial scented devices clothes) d. Create a "practice pause" after applying hand sanitizer to allow the ethanol to evaporate before entering the infant's incubator
Space	
Recommendations	**Implementation Strategy**
1. Establish a dedicated space for family at the bedside that facilitates partnership, protects privacy, and	a. Critique your current bedspace dimensions, arrangement, and organization; identify existing challenges to accommodating parent presence and ensuring privacy safely

(continued)

TABLE 5.3   Major Practice Recommendations and Implementation Strategies—Sensory Milieu, Space, and Aesthetics   *(continued)*

Space	
Recommendations	**Implementation Strategy**
promotes parenting (Cleveland, 2008; Shahheidari & Homer, 2012; Vazquez & Cong, 2014)	b. Draft a redesign of the space that you think may work better (within the limitations of your existing footprint) c. Use the PDSA method to evaluate your design; share your results with peers and leaders (see Figure 5.2) d. Identify resources that will enhance the space, based on your evaluation e. Outline a cost–benefit analysis with the help of peers and leaders f. Collaborate with leadership to outline and address space opportunities and limitations g. Consider publishing/presenting your improvement project
Aesthetics	
Recommendations	**Implementation Strategy**

1. Create an aesthetic environ that honors the holistic and human dimensions of those that inhabit the space; integrates stress-reducing strategies (e.g., art, music); and facilitates social interactions for patients, families, and professionals (Huisman et al., 2012)[a]	a. Draft a survey/questionnaire for parents, visitors, and staff about the existing space aesthetics focusing on the following dimensions:
	  i. Lighting—e.g., The brightness, is lighting adjustable? Is there indirect lighting, natural lighting? On a scale from 1–10, how does the current lighting environment feel (1 = very cold and sterile to 10 = very warm and soothing)
	  ii. Color—e.g., Is everything white or a variation on pale palettes of blue or green? What colors would you like to see? How would you use color in the existing space? On a scale from 1–10, how does the current color scheme feel (1 = very cold and sterile to 10 = very warm and soothing)
	  iii. Texture—e.g., Are all the surfaces smooth and flat? How would texture enhance the space? On a scale from 1–10, how does the current textural dimensions feel (1 = very cold and sterile to 10 = very warm and soothing)
	  iv. Sound—e.g., Is the space very noisy? What are the sources of excess noise? Is there an opportunity to introduce sound-absorbing curtains/tiles to reduce noise and enhance the color and textural components of the space? On a scale from 1–10, how does the current sound environment feel (1 = very noisy and stressful to 10 = very quiet and calming)

(continued)

TABLE 5.3 Major Practice Recommendations and Implementation Strategies—Sensory Milieu, Space, and Aesthetics *(continued)*

Aesthetics	
Recommendations	Implementation Strategy
	v. Positive distractions—e.g., Are there any positive distractions in the space (art/music), not just in the hallways or the lobby, but in the actual care area? What are your thoughts about some positive distractions that might work in your space? Is there a music school nearby that might be interested in some community service in the unit? On a scale from 1–10, how does the current space use positive distraction (1 = bland space with no positive distractions to 10 = very rich space with positive distraction) vi. Furnishings—e.g., Is there enough furniture? What kind of furnishings are available? What would you like to see in the space? Are there furnishings that could serve a dual purpose? On a scale from 1–10, how accommodating are the existing furnishings (1 = very few and not accommodating to 10 = plentiful and accommodating) b. Analyze the responses—Are there themes? What are the budgetary limitations? Are there other resources available? (see Figure 5.2) c. Use the PDSA model to test out various change options d. After implementing your cost-conscious changes, resurvey e. Publish results

^aThese are just examples and samples of questions to be asked; many low-budget options with dual purposes are available to enhance the aesthetics of your care space—creativity and thinking outside of the box are key!
NICU, neonatal intensive care unit; PDSA, Plan-Do-Study-Act.

■ THE HUMAN ENVIRONMENT

A health care team is like a sports team, except ... instead of points we are dealing with people's lives. Like any great team, it is essential to know the roles and responsibilities of each of the players and to have trust in one another. It is vital to have that team learn together, and practice together so that when the game truly matters they can each play their best with trust and understanding leading to more positive outcomes.
> —Dr. Kyu Rhee, Health and Human Resources,
> Chief Public Health Officer (Nandiwada & Dang-Vu, 2010)

Interventions and Practice Considerations

- Create and maintain transdisciplinary collaboration
  - Best practice considerations include moving away from silos to synergies within interprofessional teams proficient in evidence-based practice and

quality improvement methodologies. This is exemplified in collaborative, interprofessional rounds, practice councils, and other initiatives aimed at improving patient care and service delivery through interprofessional collaboration.

- Create and maintain a culture of caring that transcends all facets of the NICU experience to ensure the consistently reliable provision of safe quality age-appropriate care
- Best practice considerations include implementing caring practice standards for patients and families (e.g., compliance with hand hygiene, adherence to pain- and stress-prevention practices, responsive attention to patients' distress [regardless if they are your patient or not]) as well as caring practices for each other (e.g., supporting individual and peer accountability to meet unit best practice standards; assisting colleagues in daily work; supporting peer reflection, practice improvement and development).
- Create and maintain respectful verbal and nonverbal communications with patients, families, and colleagues.
  - Best practice considerations include integrating teamwork training into new hire-orientation and annual competency-based education for staff; outlining communications and behavior that undermines a culture of safety; ensuring accountability for expected communication/behaviors.

The Evidence

Collaboration, caring, and communication in a NICU are the building blocks for a culture of safety. A culture of safety in a NICU consists of shared values, attitudes, perceptions, and patterns of behavior that convey the level of organizational and individual commitment, attention, and action in reducing patient harm (Profit et al., 2012a). The consistently reliable provision of trauma-informed, age-appropriate care is quality and patient safety as the priority, and requires individual and organizational commitment to that end—*first do no harm* (Coughlin, 2014). Interprofessional collaboration improves patient outcomes in an efficient and effective way using innovative models of care and when combined with a systematic, across-the-board approach to education and training, not only improves collaboration, but enables the team to sustain the gains (Martin et al., 2010; Murphy et al., 2015).

Potentially better practices in collaboration include clear, shared purpose, goals, and values; effective communication among and between teams and team members; walking the talk and role modeling the expected behaviors and practices; nurturing trust and respect; and a commitment to conflict management (Ohlinger et al., 2003). There is no easy road to creating and sustaining collaboration. Using the Plan-Do-Study-Act (PDSA) model for improvement, Brown et al. (2003) discovered that the initial hurdle for a team beginning the journey toward collaboration is getting past individuals' resistance to change and embracing patience and persistence—the journey to a new reality is made up of many tiny steps.

Evidence-based programs, models, and principles aimed at improving patient safety include the Team Strategies and Tools to Enhance Performance and Patient Safety (TeamSTEPPS) program, the "Just Culture Model," and principles of the High Reliability Organization (HRO; Bondurant et al., 2015; Samra et al., 2011). These resources facilitate a paradigm shift from an individual to a team orientation as well as build skills and staff competencies in using improvement methodologies to achieve consistency and reliability in the provision of safe, quality, and age-appropriate care (Bondurant et al., 2015; Samra et al., 2011).

Effective communication encourages collaboration and teamwork and prevents errors. According to The Joint Commission, compromised communication is a critical factor in 65% of sentinel events (The Joint Commission on Accreditation of Healthcare Organizations, 2007). Barriers to effective communication include personality differences, hierarchical structures, disruptive behavior, generational differences, inter- and intraprofessional rivalries, concerns regarding clinical responsibility, and complexity of care, to name a few (O'Daniel & Rosenstein, 2008). Inadequate information sharing regarding an infant's response to various pain- and stress-management strategies or parental presence and planned parental participation in care will have unintended consequences to the patient and family, compromise quality and safety, and increase the possibility of a prolonged hospital stay.

Creating environments that ensure open communication requires a commitment from leadership, the development of communication protocols or checklists that will transcend hierarchical boundaries, and the development of team-based training that encourage assertiveness, interprofessional communication, and teamwork (Profit et al., 2012a; Reader et al., 2007; Samra et al., 2011). Benchmarking your current culture, or "the way we do things here," using the Safety Attitudes Questionnaire (Figure 5.3) provides a vehicle to quantify and benchmark opportunities for improvement in collaboration, communication, and teamwork (Profit et al., 2012b).

Establishing collaborative relationships in the NICU begins with caring and trust. This work is not easy and takes authentic commitment to a patient-driven model of care. Nursing is positioned at the center of the patient experience of care and has a profound opportunity to cultivate collaborative, interprofessional relationships that will improve patient and family outcomes as well as energize health care professionals and remind us all why we chose the path to care (Duffy, 2009). Interprofessional-, collaborative-, relationship-centered leadership cultivates a culture of inclusion, facilitates effective and complete communication, and upholds professional standards to preserve patient and professional safety and quality of care (Duffy, 2009).

Cost Analysis

The economic benefits of a healthy human environment are related to the improved outcomes associated with effective collaboration, communication, and caring. These improved outcomes include a decrease in medical errors, improved care coordination, which can influence length of stay, and of course the benefits of an engaged and empowered health care team (Samra et al., 2011).

Recommendations for the Human Environment (Table 5.4)

TABLE 5.4   Major Practice Recommendations and Implementation Strategies—Collaboration, Caring, and Communication

Collaboration	
Recommendations	**Implementation Strategy**

1. Establish at minimum weekly interprofessional/multidisciplinary patient care rounds with shared responsibility in problem solving and decision making to formulate holistic plans for patient care; team members assume complementary roles that facilitate cooperation and synergy (Ivers et al., 2012; Sneve et al., 2008; Terra, 2015)	a. Examine your current rounding practice, identify the various opportunities to integrate an interprofessional approach
	  i. Are team members present, but not participating?
	  ii. How are the patient care discussions captured?
	  iii. Who is responsible for follow-through?
	  iv. Does your current format give you the desired results?
	b. Outline a test of change using the PDSA model (see Figure 5.4)
	c. Implement test of change and evaluate, revise as indicated
	d. Audit and provide feedback
	e. Annually review and refine
	f. Measure impact and publish results

Caring	
Recommendations	**Implementation Strategy**
1. Introduce clinician mindfulness training—improves patient safety and relationship-based care; audit practice and provide feedback (Halifax, 2014; Sibinga & Wu, 2010)	a. Seek out a quality mindfulness training program b. Consider benchmarking select indicators before the training session and then evaluating the impact of the program intervention c. Utilize Halifax's acronym G.R.A.C.E. as a first step to introduce staff to the concept of mindfulness (see Table 5.6) d. Consider putting the acronym on business cards as a quick reference for staff e. Be sure to evaluate the effectiveness/impact of your intervention on staff, patients, families, etc. f. Publish/present your results
2. Empower and promote peer recognition in supporting each other as a team to "always doing the right thing" for the patient, family, and staff (LaSala & Bjarnason, 2010)	a. Review your facilities mission, vision, and values statement; how is team support represented; does it reflect your team's reality? b. Consider developing a unit-based vision statement that articulates the reality you want to create c. Develop a launch plan and celebration of your "new" identity—T-shirts, posters, acknowledgments to colleagues who are "walking the talk," etc. (e.g., DAISY awards; https://www.daisyfoundation.org/daisy-award) d. Consider comparing staff engagement survey results before and after this intervention (or identify other ways of measuring an intervention effect) e. Refresh/remind staff

(continued)

TABLE 5.4   Major Practice Recommendations and Implementation Strategies—Collaboration,
Caring, and Communication   *(continued)*

Communication	
Recommendations	**Implementation Strategy**

1. Establish communication standards that ensure quality, safety, and respect; audit practice and provide feedback (Gephart & Cholette, 2012; Ivers et al., 2012; Raymond & Harrison, 2014)	a. Review existing communication strategies and perform a failure modes and effects analysis (see FMEA resource link in Resource section)
	   i. Failure modes: what could go wrong?
	   ii. Failure causes: why would the failure happen?
	   iii. Failure effects: what is the consequence of each failure?
	b. Consider existing communication tools (P.U.R.E. [see Figure 5.5] method of communication incorporated with SBAR
	c. Draft a test of change related to a specific communication challenge
	d. Test the new idea, evaluate, revise as indicated, implement
	e. Audit and provide feedback as indicated
	f. Publish results

2. Ensure parent/family communication (verbal, written, and behavioral) is unbiased, culturally and literacy sensitive, respectful and complete (Jones et al., 2007; Obeidat et al., 2009; Wigert et al., 2014)	a. Review current parent/family communication processes and resources b. Critically appraise the quality of these materials and identify opportunities for improvement c. Draft tests of change aimed at improving and standardizing parent/family communication d. Test the new idea, evaluate, revise as indicated, implement e. Audit and provide feedback as indicated f. Publish results
3. There is a zero tolerance policy for communication that compromises safety and/or undermines respectful relationships (Longo, 2010; O'Daniel & Rosenstein, 2008)	a. Review current practices aimed at addressing compromised communications (both at the staff and family level) b. Complete an FMEA c. Identify improvement opportunities d. Draft test of change e. Test the new idea (or obtain consensus), evaluate, revise as indicated, implement f. Audit and provide feedback as indicated g. Publish results

FMEA, Failure Modes and Effects Analysis; SBAR, situation, background, assessment, recommendation.

▨ THE ORGANIZATIONAL ENVIRONMENT

*Let whoever is in charge keep this simple question in [mind] (not, how
can I always do this right thing myself, but) how can I provide for this
right thing to be always done?*
　　　—Florence Nightingale

Interventions and Practice Considerations

- Create, maintain, and sustain a culture of care that reflects the standards for
  trauma-informed, age-appropriate care.
  - Best practice considerations include adoption and implementation of the
    2011 National Association of Neonatal Nurses (NANN) guidelines for
    age-appropriate care (Coughlin, 2011).
- Define, invest, and sustain the necessary human, material, and digital
  resources necessary to maintain the standards for trauma-informed, age-
  appropriate care.
  - Best practice considerations include integration of value-based financial
    models for nursing care and electronic medical record capabilities that
    adopt health predictive analytics.
- Create, empower and sustain a just culture of individual accountability
  across all individuals who interface with the NICU.
  - Best practice considerations include a shift from errors and outcomes to
    system design and managing behavioral choices.

The Evidence

The definition of the term "standard of care" is a diagnostic and treatment process
that a clinician should follow for a certain type of patient, illness, or clinical cir-
cumstance; in legal terms, the concept has evolved to what a minimally competent
clinician (or prudent clinician) in the same field would do in the same situation with
the same resources (Golec, 2009; Moffett & Moore, 2011). Standards of care strive
to maintain a level of consistency in practice across various clinical specialties by
setting an expectation for performance that is guided by evidence (Golec, 2009).
When care delivery deviates from the recommended standard of care or is inconsis-
tently applied (based on individual preferences or "beliefs"), other team members
may experience an overwhelming sense of powerlessness juxtaposed to their professional responsibility to "do no harm" (Golec, 2009).

Golec (2009) points out the importance of clarity and structure in defining standards across disciplines in an effort to achieve consistency. Coughlin et al. (2009)
define evidence-based core measure sets for developmental care in the NICU as a
vehicle to provide clear metrics for clinician actions and standardize disease-independent caring strategies that positively impact the infant–family dyad. In 2011,
NANN published the clinical practice guidelines for Age-Appropriate Care of the

Premature and Critically Ill Hospitalized Infants to outline and define the standard of development care in the NICU. Montirosso et al. (2012) concluded that very preterm infants who received quality developmental care during their hospital stay exhibited higher attention and regulation behaviors, less excitability and hypotonicity, and demonstrated lower stress/abstinence behaviors assessed with the NICU Network Neurobehavioral Scale (NNNS). Quality developmental care was defined by the core measures for age-appropriate care as well as features associated with the Neonatal Individualized Developmental Care Assessment Program (NIDCAP) model.

Despite these findings, NICUs struggle to adopt and integrate standards of care for developmentally supportive, age-appropriate practices (Goudarzi et al., 2015; Hendricks-Muñoz et al., 2010; Mosqueda et al., 2013; Valizadeh et al., 2013). Barriers to adoption and standardization include a lack of physician and leadership (transdisciplinary) buy-in, environmental limitations, poor staff engagement, resistance to change, a paucity of stakeholder conviction and commitment, minimal parental involvement, and restricted economic resources (Byrd et al., 2009; Hendricks-Muñoz & Prendergast, 2007; Mosqueda et al., 2013). The *Pursuing Perfection Initiative* of the Robert Wood Johnson Foundation and the Institute for Healthcare Improvement was able to demonstrate that when the performance bar is raised (meaning that practice expectations exceed levels that were previously thought to be unattainable), reaching perfection is not only possible but achievable when the practice aims are ambitious and evidence-based, and leadership is committed to getting the job done (Kabcenell et al., 2010).

Providing holistic, humanistic care in the NICU cannot be optional—as we take stock in the expanding body of evidence affirming the developmental and epigenetic vulnerabilities and susceptibilities of infants enduring early life adversity (Montirosso & Provenzi, 2015). Integrating and adhering to developmental, age-appropriate standards of care require a change of heart and mind to embrace and acknowledge our shared humanity with the tiny individuals we serve every day in NICUs across the globe (Coughlin, 2014; Goldstein, 2012).

Accountability is an obligation or willingness to accept responsibility or to account for one's actions (Figure 5.7). Accountability in health care ensures quality and safety in patient care delivery and continuous learning and improvement through the utilization of evidence-based practices and performance measurement tools; an increase in accountability results in a decrease in variability of practice (O'Hagan & Persaud, 2009).

Unfortunately, just because clinicians are aware of evidence-based practices does not mean that these practices will be adopted and implemented (Rangachari et al., 2013). The absence of clear, evidence-based standards will certainly make accountability difficult, but this difficulty is compounded when there are implementation barriers. Implementation research strives to understand phenomena in complex systems or "real-world" situations that impede or thwart implementation (Peters et al., 2013). Quality improvement methodologies, such as the PDSA cycle, are effective in facilitating implementation and promote accountability when there is stakeholder buy-in at the leadership and organizational levels.

Cost Analysis

Organizational culture plays a key role in quality improvement implementation and adoption, which impacts clinical and economic outcomes (Mahl et al., 2015; Samra et al., 2011). Improving quality and patient safety through the adoption of evidence-based practices in age-appropriate care will reduce length of stay, decrease morbidity, increase breastfeeding rates while enriching and engaging bedside clinicians (Coughlin, 2014).

Recommendations for the Organizational Environment (Table 5.5)

TABLE 5.5   Major Practice Recommendations and Implementation Strategies—Standards, Resources, and Accountability

Standards	
Recommendations	**Implementation Strategy**
1. Integrate the core measures for age-appropriate care into the culture of care in your NICU; begin with small tests of change and then expand and integrate the core principles of age-appropriate care across all care interactions and encounters in your NICU (Coughlin, 2014; Ploeg et al., 2014)	a. Create a multidisciplinary task force to review existing practice standards and guidelines b. Identify gaps between existing practice guidelines/standards and the core measures c. Draft a priority plan, include reasonable timelines, and identify responsible individuals d. Consider external expert consultation e. Initiate the PDSA model for testing change f. Measure, evaluate, revise, implement g. Monitor progress; engage leaders; establish performance metrics h. Measure and publish results

2. Integrate practice expectations for age-appropriate care into the annual performance evaluation for all disciplines/departments who interface with the neonatal/infant population (Ivers et al., 2012; Rangachari et al., 2013)	a. Review current performance metrics and identify how they connect to the work of age-appropriate care
	b. Create a task force to include leaders and staff and delineate specific behaviors that demonstrate adherence with the core measures for age-appropriate care
	c. Consider a phased approach based on your progress in transforming the culture; make sure to share performance expectations and behaviors with staff before the "go live" date for the revised performance evaluation tool
	d. Identify how staff will demonstrate the performance expectations/behaviors
	  i. Can a report be created from the EMR, for example, indicating the use of nonpharmacologic pain/stress interventions and can individuals pull a report on themselves?
	  ii. Could staff write up an exemplar each quarter describing how they have implemented the principles and practices of age-appropriate care?

(continued)

TABLE 5.5 Major Practice Recommendations and Implementation Strategies—Standards,
Resources, and Accountability *(continued)*

Standards	
Recommendations	**Implementation Strategy**

	e. Audit practices and provide feedback
	   i. Do the behaviors link to positive patient/family impact?
	   ii. Is there improved documentation that links to positive staff impact?
	f. Draft a test of change for the implementation
	g. Measure and publish/present results

Resources	
Recommendations	**Implementation Strategy**

1. Maintain and sustain human, material, and digital resources necessary to implement the age-appropriate care core measure standards (Doerhoff & Garrison, 2015; Rangachari et al., 2013)	a. Identify the resources needed to provide age-appropriate care consistently, reliably, and seamlessly in your environment across the following domains:
	   i. Human factors
	   ii. Material resources
	   iii. Digital capabilities
	b. Prioritize needs
	c. Develop a test of change for a select need
	   i. Make sure to include a reasonable timeframe and identify the responsible individual (cannot be the team, must be an individual)
	d. Revise and refine strategy
	e. Implement, audit, measure, and provide results to staff
	f. Publish/present results

Accountability	
Recommendations	**Implementation Strategy**

1. Adopt/adapt a "just culture" framework to ensure balanced accountability for the delivery of age-appropriate care at the individual and organizational level (Boysen, 2013; Frankel et al., 2006; Wyatt, 2013)	a. Review your existing culture:
	   i. Does it provide clarity around individual (see Figure 5.7) and organizational responsibilities for accountability (see Figure 5.6)
	   ii. Is the language easy to comprehend?
	   iii. Has the organization done a good job connecting the individual clinician with this organizational principle?
	b. Brainstorm on how to make accountability a lived reality in your NICU (remembering accountability is not about pointing the finger to others, but is about raising the bar on self performance)
	c. Discuss the merits and challenges of adopting or adapting a "just culture" framework
	d. Outline the steps necessary to realize individual accountability in your unit
	e. Develop a test of change to evaluate the effectiveness of your ideas
	f. Ensure cross disciplinary leadership support
	g. Consider expert consultation
	h. Audit and provide feedback to staff

EMR, electronic medical record; P-D-S-A, Plan-Do-Study-Act.

Tools and Resources for the Healing Environment

Failure Modes and Effects Analysis (FMEA) Tool: www.ihi.org/resources/
pages/tools/failuremodesandeffectsanalysistool.aspx
G.R.A.C.E. Script from Halifax 201 Creative Commons License:
creativecommons.org/licenses/by/3.0/legalcode (see Table 5.6)
Model for Improvement video clips:
(a) Clip 1: www.youtube.com/watch?v=SCYghxtioIY
(b) Clip 2: www.youtube.com/watch?v=6MIUqdulNwQ
(c) PDSA: www.youtube.com/watch?v=xzAp6ZV5ml4

TABLE 5.6   Setting the Stage for Compassion in the Clinical Encounter—G.R.A.C.E.

G = gather your attention	• Pause, breathe in, give yourself time to get grounded by gathering your attention • Invite yourself to be present and embodied, by sensing into a place of stability in your body • You can focus your attention on the breath, for example, or on a neutral part of the body, like the soles of your feet or your hands as they rest on each other • You can use this moment of grounding to interrupt your assumptions and expectations
R = recall your attention	• Remember what your service to the patient is really about: to relieve the individual's suffering and to act with integrity and preserve the integrity of the other • Recall the felt sense of why you have chosen to relieve the suffering of others and to serve in this way. This "touch in" can happen in a moment • Your motivation keeps you on track, morally grounded, and connected to the patient into your highest values
A = attune by checking in with yourself, then the patient	• First notice what is going on in your own mind and body. Then sense into the experience of your patient. This is an active process of bearing witness and inquiry, first involving yourself, then the patient • Give attention to your own somatic state, what the body is experiencing at this moment. Shift your attention to your affect extreme, and what emotions are present for you. Then shift to your cognitive stream, and notice what thoughts are present. Your sense of and insight into your internal experience can help you regulate biases that might be present in your perception of an attitude toward your patient • Now, sense into what the patient might be experiencing. Sense without judgment. Sense into not only what the patient is experiencing, but also how the patient might be seeing the situation, and experiencing you. • Open a space in which the encounter can unfold, in which you are present for whatever may arise, in yourself and in your patient. How you notice the patient, how you acknowledge your patient, how your patient notices you and acknowledges you, all constitute a kind of mutual exchange. The richer you make this mutual exchange, the more there is the capacity for unfolding.

(continued)

TABLE 5.6   Setting the Stage for Compassion in the Clinical Encounter—G.R.A.C.E.   *(continued)*

C = consider what will really serve your patient by being truly present with your patient and letting insights arise	• As the encounter with the patient unfolds, notice what the patient might be offering in this moment. What are you sensing, seeing, learning? Ask yourself: what will really serve here? • Draw on your expertise, knowledge, and experience, and at the same time, be open to seeing things in a fresh way • This is a diagnostic step, and the insights you have may fall outside of the medical category. Do not jump to conclusions too quickly
E = engage, enact ethically, and then end the interaction	*Part 1— Engage and Enact* • Compassionate action emerges from the sense of openness, connectedness, and discernment you have created. This action might be a recommendation, an open question about values, or even a proposal for how to spend the remaining time with this patient • You cocreate with the patient a dynamic, morally grounded situation, characterized by mutuality and trust, and consistent with your values and ethics; you draw on your professional expertise, intuition, and insight, and you look for common ground consistent with your values and supportive of mutual integrity • What emerges is principled compassion: mutual, respectful of all persons involved, and as well practical and actionable. These aspirations may not always be realized; there may be deeply rooted conflicts in goals and values that must be addressed from this place of stability and discernment *Part 2—End* • Mark the end of the interaction with your patient; release, let go, breathe out • Explicitly recognize internally when the encounter is over, so you can move cleanly to the next patient or task; this recognition can be marked by attention to your out-breath • Although the next step might be more than you expected would be possible or disappointingly small, notice that, acknowledge your work. Without acknowledging your own work, it will be difficult to let go of this encounter and move on

- **What is your aim:** (what are you trying to achieve)?

- **How will you know your change is an improvement** (what are the outcomes you are looking for, how will you measure success)?

- **What changes will you make that will result in the improvement?**

Every aim/goal will require multiple smaller tests of change

Describe your test of change (describe your new idea, based on evidence / best practice):	Person responsible	When to be done	Where to be done

Plan: *In order to actualize success, there has to be very clear expectations for accountability!*

List the tasks needed to set up this test of change	Person responsible	When to be done	Where to be done
Step 1			
Step 2			
Step 3			
Etc.			

Do: **Test your change with a small group of like-minded individuals**

Study: **Examine how your change worked: Did you expect the results you got? Are there things you need to revise?**

Act: **Revise your change based on your small test and evaluate again. Once you have worked out all the kinks, implement your change in a larger setting. CONTINUOUSLY RE-EVALUATE YOUR PRACTICE**

FIGURE 5.2   Sample PDSA (Plan-Do-Study-Act) worksheet.

Reprinted by permission from Caring Essentials.

Safety Attitudes: Frontline Perspectives from this Patient Care Area

I work in the (clinical area or patient care area where you typically spend your time):	This is in the
Department of:	Please complete this survey with respect to your experiences in this clinical area.

- Use number 2 pencil only.
- Erase cleanly any mark you wish to change.

Correct Mark ● Incorrect Marks

Not Applicable
Agree Strongly
Agree Slightly
Neutral
Disagree Slightly
Disagree Strongly

Please answer the following items with respect to your specific unit or clinical area. Choose your responses using the scale below:

A	B	C	D	E	X
Disagree Strongly	Disagree Slightly	Neutral	Agree Slightly	Agree Strongly	Not Applicable

1. Nurse input is well received in this clinical area.
2. In this clinical area, it is difficult to speak up if I perceive a problem with patient care.
3. Disagreements in this clinical area are resolved appropriately (i.e., not *who* is right, but *what* is best for the patient).
4. I have the support I need from other personnel to care for patients.
5. It is easy for personnel here to ask questions when there is something that they do not understand.
6. The physicians and nurses here work together as a well-coordinated team.
7. I would feel safe being treated here as a patient.
8. Medical errors are handled appropriately in this clinical area.
9. I know the proper channels to direct questions regarding patient safety in this clinical area.
10. I receive appropriate feedback about my performance.
11. In this clinical area, it is difficult to discuss errors.
12. I am encouraged by my colleagues to report any patient safety concerns I may have.
13. The culture in this clinical area makes it easy to learn from the errors of others.
14. My suggestions about safety would be acted upon if I expressed them to management.
15. I like my job.
16. Working here is like being part of a large family.
17. This is a good place to work.
18. I am proud to work in this clinical area.
19. Morale in this clinical area is high.
20. When my workload becomes excessive, my performance is impaired.
21. I am less effective at work when fatigued.
22. I am more likely to make errors in tense or hostile situations.
23. Fatigue impairs my performance during emergency situations (e.g. emergency resuscitation, seizure).
24. Management supports my daily efforts: Unit Mgt ⒶⒷⒸⒹⒺⓍ Hosp Mgt
25. Management doesn't knowingly compromise pt safety: Unit Mgt ⒶⒷⒸⒹⒺⓍ Hosp Mgt
26. Management is doing a good job: Unit Mgt ⒶⒷⒸⒹⒺⓍ Hosp Mgt
27. Problem personnel are dealt with constructively by our: Unit Mgt ⒶⒷⒸⒹⒺⓍ Hosp Mgt
28. I get adequate, timely info about events that might affect my work, from: Unit Mgt ⒶⒷⒸⒹⒺⓍ Hosp Mgt
29. The levels of staffing in this clinical area are sufficient to handle the number of patients.
30. This hospital does a good job of training new personnel.
31. All the necessary information for diagnostic and therapeutic decisions is routinely available to me.
32. Trainees in my discipline are adequately supervised.
33. I experience good collaboration with nurses in this clinical area.
34. I experience good collaboration with staff physicians in this clinical area.
35. I experience good collaboration with pharmacists in this clinical area.
36. Communication breakdowns that lead to delays in delivery of care are common.

BACKGROUND INFORMATION

Have you completed this survey before? ○ Yes ○ No ○ Don't Know

Today's Date (month/year): _____

Position: (mark only one)
- ○ Attending/Staff Physician
- ○ Fellow Physician
- ○ Resident Physician
- ○ Physician Assistant/Nurse Practitioner
- ○ Nurse Manager/Charge Nurse
- ○ Registered Nurse
- ○ Pharmacist
- ○ Therapist (RT, PT, OT, Speech)
- ○ Clinical Social Worker
- ○ Dietician/Nutritionist
- ○ Clinical Support (CMA, EMT, Nurses Aide, etc.)
- ○ Technologist/Technician (e.g., Surg., Lab, Rad.)
- ○ Admin Support (Clerk/Secretary/Receptionist)
- ○ Environmental Support (Housekeeper)
- ○ Other Manager (e.g., Clinic Manager)
- ○ Other: _____

Mark your gender: ○ Male ○ Female **Primarily** ○ Adult ○ Peds ○ Both
Years in specialty: ○ Less than 6 months ○ 6 to 11 mo. ○ 1 to 2 yrs ○ 3 to 4 yrs ○ 5 to 10 yrs ○ 11 to 20 yrs ○ 21 or more

Thank you for completing the survey - your time and participation are greatly appreciated.

PLEASE DO NOT WRITE IN THIS AREA

FIGURE 5.3 Safety attitudes and safety climate questionnaire.

Safety Attitudes and Safety Climate Questionnaire, The University of Texas at Austin. Reprinted with permission from Eric Thomas.

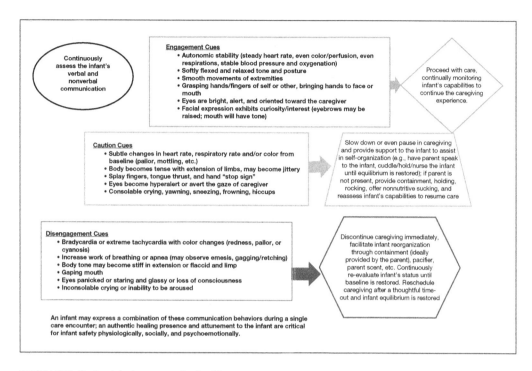

FIGURE 5.4   Infant cues sample algorithm.

P.U.R.E.	NICU Perinatal Care Coordination
P: Purposeful	• Perinatal nurse calls neonatal nurse to alert to possibility of high risk delivery. • High risk nursery notification slip is organized in SBAR format. • Obstetric and neonatal teams are aware of the reason for neonatal resuscitation team at delivary.
U: Unambiguous	• Perinatal team uses SBAR to alert NICU to delivery and faxes a written form, followed by phone call. • Team members needed at delivery is clear because of standard organizational procedure outlining who is to attend high-risk delivery. • Specific requests are clear.
R: Respectful	• Zero-tolerance policy for bullying or unprofessional behavior. • Culture of care that stresses importance of reporting disrespectful communication, does not allow retaliation. • Foster relationship-building across units and disciplines (joint break rooms, social events, set-aside time for team-building).
E: Effective	• Team de-briefing (NICU and perinatal staff) when outcomes are less than optimal. • Was conflict resolution necessary? • Was the patient outcome good? • Ongoing evaluation of process of communication during high-risk events.

FIGURE 5.5   Example of a P.U.R.E approach to communication.

SBAR, situation, background, assessment, recommendation.
Source: Gephart and Cholette (2012). Reprinted with permission from Elsevier.

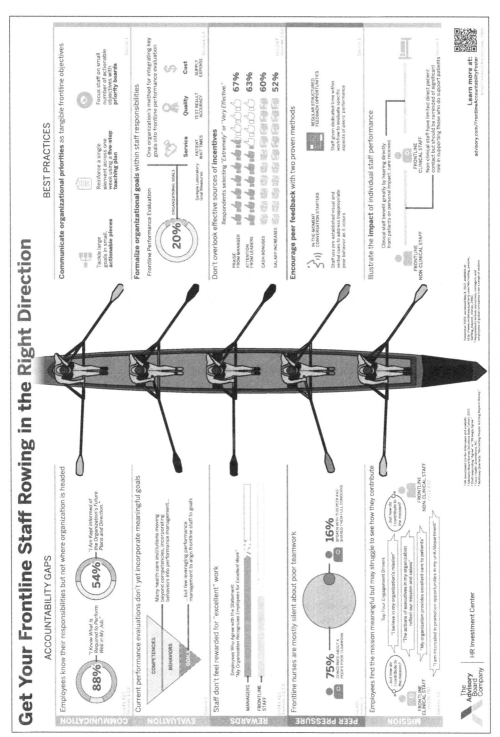

FIGURE 5.6 Frontline accountability, advisory board. Reprinted with Permission from the Advisory Board Company ©2012. All rights reserved.

How accountable are you? How are you doing in holding others accountable?

Read each of the following statements and indicate whether you agree or disagree. Then check your score at the end.

1. I clarify whether I am the owner or helper when accepting assignments from others.
   Always   Almost Always   Not Often Enough   Almost Never

2. I establish and communicate clear due-dates for assignments for which I am owner.
   Always   Almost Always   Not Often Enough   Almost Never

3. I return and report on status to others and rarely have people asking me where things stand.
   Always   Almost Always   Not Often Enough   Almost Never

4. When things I own are not meeting expectations, I acknowledge my responsibility for the lack of performance and make changes to get back on track.
   Always   Almost Always   Not Often Enough   Almost Never

5. I am conscious not to either over-do and over-own or under-do and under-own. I own my appropriate share of the load in our unit.
   Always   Almost Always   Not Often Enough   Almost Never

6. I clarify who the owner is when I make assignments to others.
   Always   Almost Always   Not Often Enough   Almost Never

7. I am clear on my expectations for "completion" of my assignments to others, including establishing agreed upon due-dates.
   Always   Almost Always   Not Often Enough   Almost Never

8. I establish mechanisms for those to whom I make assignments to return and report their status to me.
   Always   Almost Always   Not Often Enough   Almost Never

9. I address a lack of performance or results with others and work with them to establish a plan to get back on track.
   Always   Almost Always   Not Often Enough   Almost Never

10. I am careful to ensure that people on my team are not over-doing and over-owning or under-doing and under-owning and I make sure there is an appropriate load balancing in my group.
    Always   Almost Always   Not Often Enough   Almost Never

11. I make sure that a written recap is written in meetings I attend within the hospital.
    Always   Almost Always   Not Often Enough   Almost Never

Always	Almost Always	Not Often Enough	Almost Never	
x3	x2	x1	x0	Cumulative Score

Scoring
Give yourself 3 points for every question you answered "Always," 2 points for every question you answered "Almost Always," 1 point for those you answered "Not Often Enough," and 0 points for every question you answered "Almost Never."

Analysis

26–33 People know they can count on you to deliver or to ensure that your people do—nice work!

16–25 You are doing pretty well, but can still strengthen your accountability and/or that of your team.

0–15 Identify at least one item from this assessment that you can commit to doing and begin to increase the confidence others have in their ability to rely on you and/or your team to deliver!

FIGURE 5.7 Accountability self-assessment.

■ REFERENCES

American Academy of Pediatrics (AAP). (1997). Noise: A hazard for the fetus and newborn. *Pediatrics, 100*(4), 724–727.

Arabin, B., Bos, R., Rijlaarsdam, R., Mohnhaupt, A., & van Eyck, J. (1996). The onset of inter-human contacts: Longitudinal ultrasound observations in early twin pregnancies. *Ultrasound in Obstetrics & Gynecology: The Official Journal of the International Society of Ultrasound in Obstetrics and Gynecology, 8*(3), 166–173.

Bartocci, M., Winberg, J., Papendieck, G., Mustica, T., Serra, G., & Lagercrantz, H. (2001). Cerebral hemodynamic response to unpleasant odors in the preterm newborn measured by near-infrared spectroscopy. *Pediatric Research, 50*(3), 324–330.

Beraneck, M., Lambert, F. M., & Sadeghi, S. G. (2014). Functional development of the vestibular system: Sensorimotor pathways for stabilization of gaze and posture. In R. Romand & I. Varela-Nieto (Eds.), *Development of auditory and vestibular systems* (449–488). Waltham, MA: Academic Press.

Bondurant, P. G., Nielsen-Farrell, J., & Armstrong, L. (2015). The journey to high reliability in the NICU. *The Journal of Perinatal & Neonatal Nursing, 29*(2), 170–178.

Borniger, J. C., McHenry, Z. D., Abi Salloum, B. A., & Nelson, R. J. (2014). Exposure to dim light at night during early development increases adult anxiety-like responses. *Physiology & Behavior, 133*, 99–106.

Boysen, P. G. (2013). Just culture: A foundation for balanced accountability and patient safety. *The Ochsner Journal, 13*(3), 400–406.

Brémond-Gignac, D., Copin, H., Lapillonne, A., & Milazzo, S.; European Network of Study and Research in Eye Development. (2011). Visual development in infants: Physiological and pathological mechanisms. *Current Opinion in Ophthalmology, 22*(Suppl.), S1–S8.

Brown, M. S., Ohlinger, J., Rusk, C., Delmore, P., & Ittmann, P.; CARE Group. (2003). Implementing potentially better practices for multidisciplinary team building: Creating a neonatal intensive care unit culture of collaboration. *Pediatrics, 111*(4, Pt. 2), e482–e488.

Byrd, P. J., Gonzales, I., & Parsons, V. (2009). Exploring barriers to pain management in newborn intensive care units: A pilot survey of NICU nurses. *Advances in Neonatal Care: Official Journal of the National Association of Neonatal Nurses, 9*(6), 299–306.

Bystrova, K. (2009). Novel mechanism of human fetal growth regulation: A potential role of lanugo, vernix caseosa and a second tactile system of unmyelinated low-threshold C-afferents. *Medical Hypotheses, 72*(2), 143–146.

Carvalhais, C., Santos, J., da Silva, M. V., & Xavier, A. (2015). Is there sufficient training of health care staff on noise reduction in neonatal intensive care units? A pilot study from neonoise project. *Journal of Toxicology and Environmental Health. Part A, 78*(13–14), 897–903.

Chen, H. L., Chen, C. H., Wu, C. C., Huang, H. J., Wang, T. M., & Hsu, C. C. (2009). The influence of neonatal intensive care unit design on sound level. *Pediatrics and Neonatology, 50*(6), 270–274.

Clark-Gambelunghe, M. B., & Clark, D. A. (2015). Sensory development. *Pediatric Clinics of North America, 62*(2), 367–384.

Cleveland, L. M. (2008). Parenting in the neonatal intensive care unit. *Journal of Obstetric, Gynecologic, and Neonatal Nursing: JOGNN/NAACOG, 37*(6), 666–691.

Conde-Agudelo, A., & Díaz-Rossello, J. L. (2014). Kangaroo mother care to reduce morbidity and mortality in low birthweight infants. *Cochrane Database of Systematic Reviews, 2014*(4), CD002771.

Coughlin, M. (2011). *Age-appropriate care of the premature and critically ill hospitalized infant: Guideline for practice.* Glenview, IL: National Association of Neonatal Nurses.

Coughlin, M. (2014). *Transformative nursing in the NICU: Trauma-informed, age-appropriate care.* New York, NY: Springer Publishing.

Coughlin, M., Gibbins, S., & Hoath, S. (2009). Core measures for developmentally supportive care in neonatal intensive care units: Theory, precedence and practice. *Journal of Advanced Nursing, 65*(10), 2239–2248.

Croes, M., Chen, W., Feijs, L., & Oetomo, S. B. (2012). *Olfactory stimulation in premature neonates: The relevance of early experience, presented at GLOBAL HEALTH 2012: The First International Conference on Global Health Challenges.* Venice, Italy: IARIA.

Doerhoff, R., & Garrison, B. (2015). Human factors in the NICU: A bedside nurse perspective. *The Journal of Perinatal & Neonatal Nursing, 29*(2), 162–169.

Domanico, R., Davis, D. K., Coleman, F., & Davis, B. O. (2010). Documenting the NICU design dilemma: Parent and staff perceptions of open ward versus single family room units. *Journal of Perinatology: Official Journal of the California Perinatal Association, 30*(5), 343–351.

Domanico, R., Davis, D. K., Coleman, F., & Davis, B. O. (2011). Documenting the NICU design dilemma: Comparative patient progress in open-ward and single family room units. *Journal of Perinatology: Official Journal of the California Perinatal Association, 31*(4), 281–288.

Doucet, S., Soussignan, R., Sagot, P., & Schaal, B. (2007). The "smellscape" of mother's breast: Effects of odor masking and selective unmasking on neonatal arousal, oral, and visual responses. *Developmental Psychobiology, 49*(2), 129–138.

Duffy, J. R. (2009). Quality and nursing practice. In J. R. Duffy (Ed.), *Quality caring in nursing* (pp. 3–25). New York, NY: Springer Publishing.

Ecevit, A., Anuk-Ince, D., Erbek, S., Ozkiraz, S., Kurt, A., Erbek, S. S., & Tarcan, A. (2012). Comparison of cervical vestibular evoked myogenic potentials between late preterm and term infants. *The Turkish Journal of Pediatrics, 54*(5), 509–514.

Eldredge, L., & Salamy, A. (1996). Functional auditory development in preterm and full term infants. *Early Human Development, 45*(3), 215–228.

Erdeve, O., Arsan, S., Yigit, S., Armangil, D., Atasay, B., & Korkmaz, A. (2008). The impact of individual room on rehospitalization and health service utilization in preterms after discharge. *Acta Paediatrica (Oslo, Norway: 1992), 97*(10), 1351–1357.

Eshaghi, Z., Jafari, Z., Shaibanizadeh, A., Jalaie, S., & Ghaseminejad, A. (2014). The effect of preterm birth on vestibular evoked myogenic potentials in children. *Medical Journal of the Islamic Republic of Iran, 28*, 75.

Feldman, R., Rosenthal, Z., & Eidelman, A. I. (2014). Maternal-preterm skin-to-skin contact enhances child physiologic organization and cognitive control across the first 10 years of life. *Biological Psychiatry, 75*(1), 56–64.

Franck, L. S., Ferguson, D., Fryda, S., & Rubin, N. (2015). The child and family hospital experience: Is it influenced by family accommodation? *Medical Care Research and Review, 72*(4), 419–437.

Frankel, A. S., Leonard, M. W., & Denham, C. R. (2006). Fair and just culture, team behavior, and leadership engagement: The tools to achieve high reliability. *Health Services Research, 41*(4, Pt. 2), 1690–1709.

Gephart, S. M., & Cholette, M. (2012). P.U.R.E. communication: A strategy to improve care-coordination for high risk birth. *Newborn and Infant Nursing Reviews, 12*(2), 109–114.

Goldstein, R. F. (2012). Developmental care for premature infants: A state of mind. *Pediatrics, 129*(5), e1322–e1323.

Golec, L. (2009). The art of inconsistency: Evidence-based practice my way. *Journal of Perinatology: Official Journal of the California Perinatal Association, 29*(9), 600–602.

Goudarzi, Z., Rahimi, O., Khalessi, N., Soleimani, F., Mohammadi, N., & Shamshiri, A. (2015). The rate of developmental care delivery in neonatal intensive care unit. *Iran Journal of Critical Care Nursing, 8*(2), 117–124.

Graven, S. N. (2011). Early visual development: Implications for the neonatal intensive care unit and care. *Clinics in Perinatology, 38*(4), 671–683.

Graven, S. N., & Browne, J. V. (2008). Auditory development in the fetus and infant. *Newborn & Infant Nursing Reviews, 8*(4), 187–193.

Guyer, C., Huber, R., Fontijn, J., Bucher, H. U., Nicolai, H., Werner, H.,…Jenni, O. G. (2012). Cycled light exposure reduces fussing and crying in very preterm infants. *Pediatrics, 130*(1), e145–e151.

Halifax, J. (2014). G.R.A.C.E. for nurses: Cultivating compassion in nurse/patient interactions. *Journal of Nursing Education and Practice, 4*(1), 121–128.

Hendricks-Muñoz, K. D., Louie, M., Li, Y., Chhun, N., Prendergast, C. C., & Ankola, P. (2010). Factors that influence neonatal nursing perceptions of family-centered care and developmental care practices. *American Journal of Perinatology, 27*(3), 193–200.

Hendricks-Muñoz, K. D., & Prendergast, C. C. (2007). Barriers to provision of developmental care in the neonatal intensive care unit: Neonatal nursing perceptions. *American Journal of Perinatology, 24*(2), 71–77.

Huisman, E. R. C. M., Morales, E., van Hoof, J., & Kort, H. S. M. (2012). Healing environment: A review of the impact of physical environmental factors on users. *Building and Environment, 58*, 70–80.

Institute of Medicine (IOM). (2007). *Preterm birth: Causes, consequences, and prevention* (R. R Behrman & A. S. Butler, Eds.). Washington, DC: National Academies Press.

Ivers, N., Jamtvedt, G., Flottorp, S., Young, J. M., Odgaard-Jensen, J., French, S. D.,… Oxman, A. D. (2012). Audit and feedback: Effects on professional practice and healthcare outcomes. *Cochrane Database of Systematic Reviews, 2012*(6), CD000259.

Jamon, M. (2014). The development of vestibular system and related functions in mammals: Impact of gravity. *Frontiers in Integrative Neuroscience, 8*, 11.

Jefferies, A. L.; Canadian Paediatric Society, Fetus and Newborn Committee. (2012). Kangaroo care for the preterm infant and family. *Paediatrics & Child Health, 17*(3), 141–146.

The Joint Commission on Accreditation of Healthcare Organizations (TJC). (2007). *Communication as critical factor in sentinel events.* Retrieved from http://www.synergia .com/healthcare/communication.html

Jones, L., Woodhouse, D., & Rowe, J. (2007). Effective nurse parent communication: A study of parents' perceptions in the NICU environment. *Patient Education and Counseling, 69*(1–3), 206–212.

Kabcenell, A., Nolan, T. W., Martin, L. A., & Gill, Y. (2010). *The pursuing perfection initiative: Lessons on transforming healthcare.* IHI Innovation series white paper. Cambridge, MA: Institute for Healthcare Improvement.

Krueger, C. (2010). Exposure to maternal voice in preterm infants: A review. *Advances in Neonatal Care: Official Journal of the National Association of Neonatal Nurses, 10*(1), 13–18; quiz 19.

Krueger, C., Schue, S., & Parker, L. (2007). Neonatal intensive care unit sound levels before and after structural reconstruction. *MCN. The American Journal of Maternal Child Nursing, 32*(6), 358–362.

Kuhn, C. M., & Schanberg, S. M. (1998). Responses to maternal separation: Mechanisms and mediators. *International Journal of Developmental Neuroscience: The official Journal of the International Society for Developmental Neuroscience, 16*(3–4), 261–270.

LaSala, C. A., & Bjarnason, D. (2010). Creating workplace environments that support moral courage. *The Online Journal of Issues in Nursing, 15*(3), manuscript 4. doi:10.3912/OJIN .Vol15No03Man04

Lasky, R. E., & Williams, A. L. (2005). The development of the auditory system from conception to term. *NeoReviews, 6*(3), e141–e152.

Lahav, A., & Skoe, E. (2014). An acoustic gap between the NICU and womb: A potential risk for compromised neuroplasticity of the auditory system in preterm infants. *Frontiers in Neuroscience, 8,* 381.

Lipchock, S. V., Reed, D. R., & Mennella, J. A. (2011). The gustatory and olfactory systems during infancy: Implications for development of feeding behaviors in the high-risk neonate. *Clinics in Perinatology, 38*(4), 627–641.

Liu, W. F.; NIC/Q 2005 Physical Environment Exploratory Group. (2010). The impact of a noise reduction quality improvement project upon sound levels in the open-unit-design neonatal intensive care unit. *Journal of Perinatology: Official Journal of the California Perinatal Association, 30*(7), 489–496.

Longo, J. (2010). Combating disruptive behaviors: Strategies to promote a healthy work environment. *The Online Journal of Issues in Nursing, 15*(1), manuscript 5. doi:10.3912/ OJIN.Vol15No01Man05

Lowson, K., Offer, C., Watson, J., McGuire, B., & Renfrew, M. J. (2015). The economic benefits of increasing kangaroo skin-to-skin care and breastfeeding in neonatal units: Analysis of a pragmatic intervention in clinical practice. *International Breastfeeding Journal, 10,* 11.

Ludington-Hoe, S. M., Anderson, G. C., Swinth, J. Y., Thompson, C., & Hadeed, A. J. (2004). Randomized controlled trial of kangaroo care: Cardiorespiratory and thermal effects on healthy preterm infants. *Neonatal Network, 23*(3), 39–48.

Mahl, S., Lee, S. K., Baker, G. R., Cronin, C. M., Stevens, B., & Ye, X. Y.; Canadian Institutes of Health Research Team in Maternal-Infant Care. (2015). The association of organizational culture and quality improvement implementation with neonatal outcomes in the NICU. *Journal of Pediatric Health Care: Official Publication of National Association of Pediatric Nurse Associates & Practitioners, 29*(5), 435–441.

Martin, J. S., Ummenhofer, W., Manser, T., & Spirig, R. (2010). Interprofessional collaboration among nurses and physicians: Making a difference in patient outcome. *Swiss Medical Weekly, September 1,* 140: w13062. doi:10.4414/smw.2010.13062

McMahon, E., Wintermark, P., & Lahav, A. (2012). Auditory brain development in premature infants: The importance of early experience. *Annals of the New York Academy of Sciences, 1252,* 17–24.

Medoff-Cooper, B., Rankin, K., Li, Z., Liu, L., & White-Traut, R. (2015). Multisensory intervention for preterm infants improves sucking organization. *Advances in Neonatal Care: Official Journal of the National Association of Neonatal Nurses, 15*(2), 142–149.

Mennella, J. A., Jagnow, C. P., & Beauchamp, G. K. (2001). Prenatal and postnatal flavor learning by human infants. *Pediatrics, 107*(6), E88.

Mitchell, A. J., Yates, C., Williams, K., & Hall, R. W. (2013). Effects of daily kangaroo care on cardiorespiratory parameters in preterm infants. *Journal of Neonatal-Perinatal Medicine, 6*(3), 243–249.

Moffett, P., & Moore, G. (2011). The standard of care: Legal history and definitions: The bad and good news. *The Western Journal of Emergency Medicine, 12*(1), 109–112.

Montirosso, R., Del Prete, A., Bellù, R., Tronick, E., & Borgatti, R.; Neonatal Adequate Care for Quality of Life (NEO-ACQUA) Study Group. (2012). Level of NICU quality of developmental care and neurobehavioral performance in very preterm infants. *Pediatrics, 129*(5), e1129–e1137.

Montirosso, R., & Provenzi, L. (2015). Implications of epigenetics and stress regulation on research and developmental care of preterm infants. *Journal of Obstetric, Gynecologic, and Neonatal Nursing: JOGNN/NAACOG, 44*(2), 174–182.

Morag, I., & Ohlsson, A. (2013). Cycled light in the intensive care unit for preterm and low birth weight infants. *Cochrane Database of Systematic Reviews, 2013*(8), CD006982.

Morrison, I., Löken, L. S., & Olausson, H. (2010). The skin as a social organ. *Experimental Brain Research, 204*(3), 305–314.

Mosqueda, R., Castilla, Y., Perapoch, J., Lora, D., López-Maestro, M., & Pallás, C. (2013). Necessary resources and barriers perceived by professionals in the implementation of the NIDCAP. *Early Human Development, 89*(9), 649–653.

Murphy, T., Laptook, A., & Bender, J. (2015). Sustained improvements in neonatal intensive care unit safety attitudes after teamwork training. *Journal of Patient Safety.* Advance online publication. doi:10.1097/PTS.0000000000000191

Nandiwada, D. R., & Dang-Vu, C. (2010). Transdisciplinary health care education: Training team players. *Journal of Health Care for the Poor and Underserved, 21,* 26–34.

Nightingale, F. (1860/1969). *Notes on nursing: What it is and what it is not.* Mineola, NY: Dover Publications.

Nyqvist, K. H., Anderson, G. C., Bergman, N., Cattaneo, A., Charpak, N., Davanzo, R., ... Widström, A. M.; Expert Group of the International Network on Kangaroo Mother Care. (2010). State of the art and recommendations. Kangaroo mother care: Application in a high-tech environment. *Acta Paediatrica (Oslo, Norway: 1992), 99*(6), 812–819.

Obeidat, H. M., Bond, E. A., & Callister, L. C. (2009). The parental experience of having an infant in the newborn intensive care unit. *The Journal of Perinatal Education, 18*(3), 23–29.

O'Daniel, M., & Rosenstein, A. H. (2008). Professional communication and team collaboration. In R. G. Hughes (Ed.), *Patient safety and quality: An evidence-based handbook for nurses* (pp. 271–284). Rockville, MD: Agency for Healthcare Research and Quality.

O'Hagan, J., & Persaud, D. (2009). Creating a culture of accountability in health care. *The Health Care Manager, 28*(2), 124–133.

Ohlinger, J., Brown, M. S., Laudert, S., Swanson, S., & Fofah, O.; CARE Group. (2003). Development of potentially better practices for the neonatal intensive care unit as a culture of collaboration: Communication, accountability, respect, and empowerment. *Pediatrics, 111*(4 Pt. 2), e471–e481.

Paccauda, C., Vernez, D., Berodec, M., Charrière, N., Moessinger, A., & Laubscher, B. (2012). Hand-disinfectant alcoholic vapors in incubators. *Journal of Neonatal-Perinatal Medicine, 4*(1), 15–19.

Peters, D. H., Adam, T., Alonge, O., Agyepong, I. A., & Tran, N. (2013). Implementation research: What it is and how to do it. *British Medical Journal (Clinical Research Ed.), 347*, f6753.

Pickler, R. H., McGrath, J. M., Reyna, B. A., Tubbs-Cooley, H. L., Best, A. M., Lewis, M.,… Wetzel, P. A. (2013). Effects of the neonatal intensive care unit environment on preterm infant oral feeding. *Research and Reports in Neonatology, 2013*(3), 15–20.

Ploeg, J., Markle-Reid, M., Davies, B., Higuchi, K., Gifford, W., Bajnok, I.,… Bookey-Bassett, S. (2014). Spreading and sustaining best practices for home care of older adults: A grounded theory of study. *Implementation Science, 9*, 162. Retrieved from http://www.implementationscience.com/content/9/1/162

Profit, J., Etchegaray, J., Petersen, L. A., Sexton, J. B., Hysong, S. J., Mei, M., & Thomas, E. J. (2012a). Neonatal intensive care unit safety culture varies widely. *Archives of Disease in Childhood. Fetal and Neonatal Edition, 97*(2), F120–F126.

Profit, J., Etchegaray, J., Petersen, L. A., Sexton, J. B., Hysong, S. J., Mei, M., & Thomas, E. J. (2012b). The Safety Attitudes Questionnaire as a tool for benchmarking safety culture in the NICU. *Archives of Disease in Childhood. Fetal and Neonatal Edition, 97*(2), F127–F132.

Ramesh, A., Denzil, S. B., Linda, R., Josephine, P. K., Nagapoornima, M., Suman Rao, P. N., & Swarna Rekha, A. (2013). Maintaining reduced noise levels in a resource-constrained neonatal intensive care unit by operant conditioning. *Indian Pediatrics, 50*(3), 279–282.

Rangachari, P., Rissing, P., & Rethemeyer, K. (2013). Awareness of evidence-based practices alone does not translate to implementation: Insights from implementation research. *Quality Management in Health Care, 22*(2), 117–125.

Raymond, M., & Harrison, M. C. (2014). The structured communication tool SBAR (Situation, Background, Assessment and Recommendation) improves communication in neonatology. *South African Medical Journal = Suid-Afrikaanse tydskrif vir geneeskunde, 104*(12), 850–852.

Reader, T. W., Flin, R., Mearns, K., & Cuthbertson, B. H. (2007). Interdisciplinary communication in the intensive care unit. *British Journal of Anaesthesia, 98*(3), 347–352.

Ruben, R. J. (1995). The ontogeny of human hearing. *International Journal of Pediatric Otorhinolaryngology, 32*(Suppl.), S199–S204.

Sakallaris, B. R., MacAllister, L., Voss, M., Smith, K., & Jonas, W. B. (2015). Optimal healing environments. *Global Advances in Health and Medicine, 4*(3), 40–45.

Salihagic-Kadic, A., & Predojevic, M. (2012). What we have learned from fetal neurophysiology? *Donald School Journal of Ultrasound in Obstetrics and Gynecology, 6*(2), 179–188.

Samra, H. A., McGrath, J. M., & Rollins, W. (2011). Patient safety in the NICU: A comprehensive review. *The Journal of Perinatal & Neonatal Nursing, 25*(2), 123–132.

Santos, J., Pearce, S. E., & Stroustrup, A. (2015). Impact of hospital-based environmental exposures on neurodevelopmental outcomes of preterm infants. *Current Opinions in Pediatrics, 27*(2), 254–260.

Schweitzer, M., Gilpin, L., & Frampton, S. (2004). Healing spaces: Elements of environmental design that make an impact on health. *Journal of Alternative and Complementary Medicine, 10*(Suppl. 1), S71–S83.

Shahheidari, M., & Homer, C. (2012). Impact of the design of neonatal intensive care units on neonates, staff, and families: A systematic literature review. *The Journal of Perinatal & Neonatal Nursing, 26*(3), 260–6; quiz 267.

Shepley, M. M., Smith, J. A., Sadler, B. L., & White, R. D. (2014). The business case for building better neonatal intensive care units. *Journal of Perinatology: Official Journal of the California Perinatal Association, 34*(11), 811–815.

Sibinga, E. M., & Wu, A. W. (2010). Clinician mindfulness and patient safety. *Journal American Medical Association, 304*(22), 2532–2533.

Sneve, J., Kattelmann, K., Ren, C., & Stevens, D. C. (2008). Implementation of a multidisciplinary team that includes a registered dietitian in a neonatal intensive care unit improved nutrition outcomes. *Nutrition in Clinical Practice: Official Publication of the American Society for Parenteral and Enteral Nutrition, 23*(6), 630–634.

Spitz, R. A. (1945). Hospitalism. In R. S. Eissler (Ed.), *The psychoanalytic study of the child volume I* (pp. 53–74). New York, NY: International Universities Press.

Spitz, R. A. (1946). Hospitalism: A follow-up report. In R. S. Eissler (Ed.), *The psychoanalytic study of the child volume II* (pp. 113–117). New York, NY: International Universities Press.

Stevens, D. C., Helseth, C. C., Khan, M. A., Munson, D. P., & Smith, T. J. (2010). Neonatal intensive care nursery staff perceive enhanced workplace quality with the single-family room design. *Journal of Perinatology: Official Journal of the California Perinatal Association, 30*(5), 352–358.

Sullivan, R. M., & Toubas, P. (1998). Clinical usefulness of maternal odor in newborns: Soothing and feeding preparatory responses. *Biology of the Neonate, 74*(6), 402–408.

Swanson, K. M., & Wojnar, D. M. (2004). Optimal healing environments in nursing. *Journal of Alternative and Complementary Medicine, 10*(Suppl. 1), S43–S48.

Swathi, S., Ramesh, A., Nagapoornima, M., Fernandes, L. M., Jisina, C., Rao, P. N., & Swarnarekha, A. (2014). Sustaining a "culture of silence" in the neonatal intensive care unit during nonemergency situations: A grounded theory on ensuring adherence to behavioral modification to reduce noise levels. *International Journal of Qualitative Studies on Health and Well-Being, 9*, 22523.

Terra, S. M. (2015). Interdisciplinary rounds: The key to communication, collaboration, and agreement on plan of care. *Professional Case Management, 20*(6), 299–307; quiz 308.

Timmerman, C. & Uhrenfeldt, L. (2014). Patients' experiences of well-being in the physical hospital environment: A systematic review of qualitative evidence protocol. *The JBI Database of Systematic Reviews and Implementation Reports, 2*(12), 67–78. Retrieved from http://joannabriggslibrary.org/index.php/jbisrir/article/view/1537/2304

Timmermann, C., Uhrenfeldt, L., & Birkelund, R. (2015). Room for caring: Patients' experiences of well-being, relief and hope during serious illness. *Scandinavian Journal of Caring Sciences, 29*(3), 426–434.

Ulrich, R. S. (1984). View through a window may influence recovery from surgery. *Science, 224*(4647), 420–421.

Ulrich, R. S. (1997). A theory of supportive design for healthcare facilities. *Journal of Healthcare Design: Proceedings from the. Symposium on Healthcare Design. Symposium on Healthcare Design, 9*, 3–7; discussion 21.

Valizadeh, L., Asadollahi, M., Mostafa Gharebaghi, M., & Gholami, F. (2013). The congruence of nurses' performance with developmental care standards in neonatal intensive care units. *Journal of Caring Sciences, 2*(1), 61–71.

Vásquez-Ruiz, S., Maya-Barrios, J. A., Torres-Narváez, P., Vega-Martínez, B. R., Rojas-Granados, A., Escobar, C., & Angeles-Castellanos, M. (2014). A light/dark cycle in the NICU accelerates body weight gain and shortens time to discharge in preterm infants. *Early Human Development, 90*(9), 535–540.

Ventura, A. K., & Worobey, J. (2013). Early influences on the development of food preferences. *Current Biology, 23*(9), R401–R408.

Wachman, E. M., & Lahav, A. (2011). The effects of noise on preterm infants in the NICU. *Archives of Disease in Childhood. Fetal and Neonatal Edition, 96*(4), F305–F309.

White, R. D., Smith, J. A., & Shepley, M. M.; Committee to Establish Recommended Standards for Newborn ICU Design. (2013). Recommended standards for newborn ICU design, eighth edition. *Journal of Perinatology: Official Journal of the California Perinatal Association, 33*(Suppl. 1), S2–16.

Wigert, H., Dellenmark Blom, M., & Bry, K. (2014). Parents experiences of communication with neonatal intensive care unit staff: an interview study. *BMC Pediatrics, 14*, 304. Retrieved from http://bmcpediatr.biomedcentral.com/articles/10.1186/s12887-014-0304-5

Wikstrom, B-M., Westerlund, E., & Erkkila, J. (2012). The healthcare environment—the importance of aesthetic surroundings: Health professionals' experiences from a surgical ward in Finland. *Open Journal of Nursing, 2*, 188–195. Retrieved from http://dx.doi.org/10.4236/ojn.2012.23029

Wyatt, R. M. (2013). *Blameless or blameworthy errors-does your organization make a distinction?* Retrieved from http://www.jointcommission.org/jc_physician_blog/blameless_or_blameworthy_errors

Yildiz, A., Arikan, D., Gözüm, S., Tastekin, A., & Budancamanak, I. (2011). The effect of the odor of breast milk on the time needed for transition from gavage to total oral feeding in preterm infants. *Journal of Nursing Scholarship: An Official Publication of Sigma Theta Tau International Honor Society of Nursing/Sigma Theta Tau, 43*(3), 265–273.

CHAPTER 6

Guidelines for Pain and Stress Prevention, Assessment, Management, and the Family

Pain is an inseparable part of everyday life. It is universal, protective, and crucial for survival. Pain can have profound deleterious and disruptive effects on the quality of life.
    —K. J. S. Anand

This guideline presents the latest evidence-based research, along with clinical practice recommendations and implementation strategies related to the prevention, assessment, and management of pain and stress in the neonatal intensive care unit (NICU) as well as the role of the family within this context (as detailed in Table 6.1).

■ GUIDELINE OBJECTIVES

- To define the criteria and recommendations for best practice in the prevention, assessment, and management of pain and stress in the NICU
- To present the evidence that supports these criteria and best practice recommendations
- To present clinical practice strategies that facilitate adoption and integration of evidence-based best practices in pain and stress prevention, assessment, and management in the neonatal intensive care.

■ MAJOR OUTCOMES CONSIDERED

The impact of the consistently reliable application of the pain and stress core measure attributes and criteria on the NICU patient, family, and staff includes:

- Physiologic, psychosocial, and psychoemotional outcomes
- Patient safety and quality clinical outcomes

TABLE 6.1 Attributes and Criteria of the Pain and Stress Core Measure

Attributes	Criteria
Prevention of pain and stress is an expressed goal in the daily management of the hospitalized infant	1. Painful and/or stressful daily activities are critically reviewed, revised, and modified based on the infant's current health status 2. Each infant will have an individualized pain and stress prevention care plan that will be reviewed daily with the interprofessional team (to include the family) 3. A unit-specific pain and stress prevention policy will address strategies to manage disease-specific pain (abdominal, pulmonary, neurologic etc.) as well as pain and or distress associated with hunger, gas, pruritus, and other discomforts associated with hospitalization and critical illness
Pain and/or stress is assessed, managed, and reassessed before, during, and after all procedures until the infant returns to his or her baseline level of comfort; interventions and infant responses to stress-relieving and pain-management interventions are documented	1. A valid, age-appropriate, contextually accurate pain assessment tool is used for all patient care encounters throughout the hospital stay 2. Pain and stress assessments guide all caregiving activities; caregiving activities are adapted and modified based on infant biobehavioral cues 3. Nonpharmacologic and/or pharmacologic pain and/or stress-relieving strategies are consistently and reliably provided for ALL painful and/or stressful procedures; the procedure, pain/stress management intervention(s), and infant response(s) are documented
Family is involved, informed, and participates in the pain and stress management of their hospitalized infant(s); all participation and observations are documented	1. Parent education regarding infant pain and stress cues is provided within the first week of NICU admission; learning is validated 2. Parents are partners in pain and stress assessment of their infant(s). Parent observations are recorded and integrated into the individualized pain and stress prevention plan 3. Parents are encouraged, empowered, and supported to advocate for and provide comfort to their hospitalized infant(s)

■ PAIN AND STRESS PREVENTION

You must unlearn what you have learned...about pain...
     —G. Waddell (1987)

Interventions and Practice Considerations

1. Create a pain and stress prevention policy and practice guideline that is age-appropriate and contextually responsive to the variety of pain and stress experiences that occur in the NICU.
   - Best practice considerations must address accountability in adhering to the established policy, guidelines, and practice expectations for pain and stress prevention.
2. Develop procedural pain-prevention bundles for frequently occurring procedures (e.g., feeding tube insertion, needle sticks, dressing changes)

- Best practice considerations must include expectations related to comprehensive documentation of the painful procedure, the pain and pain-related stress prevention interventions, and the infant's response(s) and return to preprocedural biobehavioral baseline.
3. Collaborate with family on scheduling medically necessary procedures to ensure parent presence and participation in the pain and pain-related stress prevention care plan.
   - Best practice considerations focus on facilitating parental presence to support and comfort the infant during these procedures consistently and reliably.

The Evidence

The deleterious effects of unmanaged or undermanaged pain in the neonatal patient population impact the physiologic, behavioral, and cognitive integrity of the developing human (Hall & Anand, 2014). Allodynia, visceral hyperalgesia, an increased risk for fibromyalgia in adulthood, alterations in neuroendocrine functionality and stress responsivity, impaired visual-motor integration, reduced cortical thickness at school age, poor postnatal growth, and long-term abnormalities in white matter microstructure as well as lower IQ have been demonstrated with a failure to treat pain effectively in the neonatal patient population (Grunau, 2013; Hall & Anand, 2014; Low & Schweinhardt, 2012; Provenzi et al., 2015; Ranger et al., 2013; Vinall et al., 2012, 2014). Procedural pain-related stress is emerging as a significant factor in long-term outcomes of very preterm infants as it has been also associated with alterations in brain microstructure and stress hormone levels as well as poorer cognitive, motor, and behavioral neurodevelopmental outcomes (Vinall & Grunau, 2014).

With approximately 500,000 neonates in the United States alone requiring neonatal intensive care, the ramifications of unmanaged or undermanaged pain and pain-related stress pose a significant threat to the quality of life for individuals, families, and society at large. Understanding not only neurobiological vulnerabilities but also the human susceptibilities of these fragile individuals is a moral imperative in order to effectively and consistently respond to the physiologic and psychoemotional suffering too often endured by this unique patient population. Simons et al. (2003) estimate that only one third of infants undergoing NICU procedures receive appropriate analgesic therapy. Pain prevention and management are important components of quality health care (Anand, 2001). Employing a systematic approach to pain prevention with clear, standardized performance expectations and documentation criteria are paramount in improving pain prevention practices and mitigating short-term and long-term morbidity (Furdon, Eastman, Benjamin, & Horgan, 1998; Hall & Anand, 2014; Sharek, Powers, Koehn, & Anand, 2006; Simons et al., 2003; Walker, 2014).

The most effective way to prevent pain is to reduce the number of procedures routinely performed in the NICU (American Academy of Pediatrics [AAP] & the

Canadian Pediatric Society, 2006). Suggested strategies include the use of noninvasive technologies to collect biologically relevant data (e.g., using transcutaneous methods for blood gas analysis as well as employing transcutaneous bilirubinometry), critically reviewing the clinical necessity for routine laboratory and radiographic work, and minimizing the number of repeat procedures performed after failed attempts (e.g., defer IV insertion to a more experienced colleague after two failed attempts versus three failed attempts; AAP & the Canadian Pediatric Society, 2006; Meek, 2012). When a blood specimen is clinically necessary, employing venipuncture versus heel lance technique should be the standard as venipuncture has been shown to decrease cry characteristics as well as significantly reduce overall pain scores (Larsson, Tannfeldt, Lagercrantz, & Olsson, 1998; Shah & Ohlsson, 2012). Hall and Anand (2014) recommend placing a peripheral arterial or central venous catheter in patients who require more than three to four heel sticks per day and include the caveat that adequate analgesia is employed during line placement.

Pain and stress prevention care plans, protocols, and clinical practice guidelines provide a unique way of maintaining awareness of the detrimental effects of undermanaged and unmanaged pain and stress in the NICU. The AAP and the Canadian Pediatric Society recommend that every health care facility caring for neonates implement an effective pain prevention program that includes routinely assessing pain, minimizing the number of painful procedures performed, effectively using pharmacological and nonpharmacological therapies for the prevention of pain associated with routine minor procedures, and eliminating pain associated with surgery and other major procedures (AAP & the Canadian Pediatric Society, 2006; Anand, 2001; Barrington, Batton, Finley, Wallman, & The Canadian Pediatric Society Fetus and Newborn Committee, 2007; Harrison, Bueno, & Reszel, 2015). Yin et al. (2015) describe an effective "atraumatic heel-stick procedure" using a pain prevention bundle approach, which included a combination of non-nutritive sucking (NNS) with sucrose and facilitated tucking (FT). The heel-stick procedure can be atraumatic when conducted while the infant is stable and quiet, appropriately positioned, and offered FT, oral sucrose, and NNS before gently beginning this common NICU procedure (Yin et al., 2015).

Cost Analysis

Untreated or undertreated pain and pain-related stress result in longer hospital stays, increasing the patients' risk for additional hospital-acquired complications as well as undermining their developmental trajectory and long-term potential as productive, healthy human beings (Furdon et al., 1998). The consistently reliable prevention of neonatal pain and pain-related stress not only results in financial gains but ensures the delivery of high quality, patient-centered care that will positively impact clinical, socio-emotional, motor, behavioral, and cognitive outcomes (Institute of Medicine [IOM], 2007).

Recommendations for Pain and Stress Prevention (Table 6.2)

TABLE 6.2   Major Practice Recommendations and Implementation Strategies for Pain and Stress Prevention

Prevention	
Recommendation	**Implementation Strategy**
1. Create individualized pain-prevention care plans to be reviewed daily with the family and health care team; care plan will include a patient-centered strategy to determine the clinical necessity of laboratory, radiographic, and invasive procedures (to include medical device replacement procedures, dressing changes, etc.)	a. Review current practice around "routine" procedures—identify how the current practice can be individualized b. Review current documentation of procedures, pain/stress prevention interventions associated with these procedures, and how the patient's response to procedures is reflected in the medical record c. Review current practice around parental involvement with "routine" procedures (parent presence, parent knowledge, parent participation) d. Begin by selecting one frequently occurring procedure and draft a test of change to improve the individualization of that procedure for each patient e. Draft a pain prevention care plan (Figure 6.1) f. Implement and evaluate this test of change, refine and then apply this new practice approach to other routine procedures g. Measure the interval change (using big data, staff/parent interview, questionnaires etc.), report results to the team, publish and/or present your outcomes h. Continually evaluate and reevaluate your pain prevention strategies
2. Create pain prevention bundles for common painful procedures (e.g., feeding tube insertion, immunization, heel stick, venipuncture, endotracheal suctioning); each bundle to include a resource card with evidence-based best practices, specific procedural steps, and requisite equipment to implement the pain prevention bundle	a. Identify common painful procedures in your NICU b. Identify evidence-based best practices for management of procedural pain and pain-related stress (Table 6.3), also refer to National Association of Neonatal Nurses (NANN) Newborn Pain Assessment and Management Guideline for Practice (Walden & Gibbins, 2012) c. Begin by selecting one common painful procedure and identify effective evidence-based strategies for pain prevention; create a test of change for the use of a pain prevention bundle for your selected procedure d. Physically and/or visually create a bundle for your selected procedure that you will test (include the procedure related resources as well as pain prevention strategies (e.g., pacifier and sweet solution) (Figure 6.2) e. Consider placing bundle elements in a baggie with a brief questionnaire to users as part of the evaluation (Figure 6.3) f. Implement and evaluate this test of change, refine, revise, and apply this new practice approach to other common painful procedures g. Develop a documentation strategy that is comprehensive and streamlined (you may need to test various versions using the same "test of change" methodology) h. Measure the interval change (using big data, staff/parent interview, questionnaires etc.), report results to the team, publish and/or present your outcomes i. Continually evaluate and reevaluate your pain prevention strategies

(continued)

TABLE 6.2 Major Practice Recommendations and Implementation Strategies for Pain and Stress Prevention *(continued)*

Prevention	
Recommendation	**Implementation Strategy**
3. Establish a unit-specific pain prevention policy to address procedural pain and pain-related stress, disease specific pain, as well as the pain and distress associated with hunger, gas, pruritus, and other discomforts of hospitalization and critical illness	a. Review your existing pain and pain-related stress policy b. Identify gaps in your existing policy related to procedural pain, disease pain, and other types of pain associated with and experienced by hospitalized neonates/infants c. Review the existing literature for best practices in addressing the various dimensions of pain experienced by the NICU patient population d. In the absence of existing literature and/or practice guidelines and protocols, develop guidelines and practice strategies to address specific pain/distress experiences e. There is a paucity of evidence based strategies addressing the various dimensions of the pain experience in the NICU, specifically around hunger, gas pain, constipation, etc. f. Evaluate the effectiveness of your strategies using quantifiable methods, report results to the team, publish and/or present your outcomes. g. Continually evaluate and re-evaluate your pain prevention strategies and publish the results.
4. Develop a process to audit pain prevention practices and instill individual and peer accountability for the consistent, reliable provision of pain prevention measures	a. If it is not documented, it is not done. Review existing documentation practices around pain prevention b. Audit existing documentation indices for pain prevention c. Are these indices telling the full story of your patient's experience and the care you have provided? d. Meet with your informatics nurse to explore creative but complete ways to capture your pain prevention practices e. Using the PDSA methodology, test your revised documentation strategy, evaluate, revise, and retest f. Consider bi-weekly to monthly audit of documentation. g. Measure the interval change(s), report results to the team, publish and/or present your outcomes h. Address discrepancies in documentation/practice expectations i. Continually evaluate and re-evaluate your pain prevention documentation strategy

NICU, neonatal intensive care unit; PDSA, Plan-Do-Study-Act.

Tools and Parent Resources

TABLE 6.3 Common NICU Procedures and Evidence-Based Prevention and Management Strategies

Procedure	Prevention/Management Strategy
Heel-stick	• Nonnutritive sucking (with sweet solution and facilitated tucking) (Anand, 2001; Liaw et al., 2013; Yin et al., 2015) • Nonnutritive sucking and facilitated tucking (Anand, 2001; Liaw et al., 2012; Pillai Riddell et al., 2011) • Facilitated tucking (Anand, 2001; Hartley, Miller, & Gephart, 2015; Obeidat, Kahalaf, Callister, & Froelicher, 2009) • Skin-to-skin holding (Anand, 2001; Pillai Riddell et al., 2011; Johnson et al., 2014) • Breastfeeding or breast milk (Shah, Herbozo, Aliwalas, & Shah, 2012) • Sucrose/glucose 20% to 30% (Anand, 2001; Bueno et al., 2013; Cignacco et al., 2012; Stevens, Yamada, Lee, & Ohlsson, 2013) • Vibration (Baba, McGrath, & Liu, 2010) • Rocking/holding (Pillai Riddell et al., 2011)
Feeding-tube insertion	• Sucrose/glucose 20% to 30% (Bueno et al., 2013; McCullough, Halton, Mowbray, & Macfarlane, 2008; Pandey, Datta, & Rehan, 2013; Stevens et al., 2013) • Nonnutritive sucking with sucrose (Kristoffersen, Skogvoll, & Hafström, 2011) • Slow gentle technique with lubrication (Anand, 2001; Haxhija, Rosegger, & Prechtl, 1995)
Endotracheal suctioning	• Facilitated tucking, swaddling, containment (Anand, 2001; Hartley et al., 2015; Obeidat et al., 2009; Peyrovi, Alinejad-Naeini, Mohagheghi, & Mehran, 2014; Ward-Larson, Horn, & Gosnell, 2004) • Four-handed care (Cone, Pickler, Grap, McGrath, & Wiley, 2013) • Music therapy (Chou, Wang, Chen, & Pai, 2003)
Vaccination	• Facilitated tucking (Kucukoglu, Kurt, & Aytekin, 2015; Obeidat et al., 2009;) • Sucrose/glucose 20% to 30% (Bueno et al., 2013; Stevens et al., 2013) • Vibration (Taddio et al., 2015) • Educating staff (Pillai Riddell et al., 2015) • Parent presence (Pillai Riddell et al., 2015) • Consider acetaminophen (Walden & Gibbins, 2012)
Venipuncture	• Facilitated tucking (Hartley et al., 2015; Lopez et al., 2015; Obeidat et al., 2009; Pillai Riddell et al., 2011) • Sucrose/glucose 20% to 30% (Bueno et al., 2013; Stevens et al., 2013) • Skin-to-skin (Johnston et al., 2014; Pillai Riddell et al., 2011) • Breastfeeding or breast milk (Shah et al., 2012) • Rocking/holding (Pillai Riddell et al., 2011)
Arterial puncture	• Sweet solution (Bueno et al., 2013) • Nonnutritive sucking (with and without sucrose) (Bueno et al., 2013; Pillai Riddell et al., 2011; Walden & Gibbins, 2012) • Facilitated tucking (Pillai Riddell et al., 2011) • Rocking/holding (Pillai Riddell et al., 2011)

(continued)

TABLE 6.3   Common NICU Procedures and Evidence-Based Prevention and Management Strategies
(continued)

Procedure	Prevention/Management Strategy
Needle puncture	• Nonnutritive sucking with sucrose/sweet solution (Anand, 2001; Bueno et al., 2013; Johnston et al., 2014; Pillai Riddell et al., 2011; Stevens et al., 2013)
Eye examination for retinopathy of prematurity (ROP)	• Local anesthetic eye drops (Dempsey & McCreery, 2011) • Sucrose (Stevens et al., 2013)
Lumbar puncture	• Sucrose or breast milk with nonnutritive sucking (Lago et al., 2009) • EMLA cream (Taddio, Ohlsson, Einarson, Stevens, & Koren, 1998) • Subcutaneous infiltration of lidocaine (Anand, 2001; Gorchynski, Everett, & Prebil, 2008; Pinheiro, Furdon, & Ochoa, 1993)
Tape removal	• Nonnutritive sucking (with and without sucrose) (Walden & Gibbins, 2012)
Diaper change	• Nonnutritive sucking (with and without sucrose) (Walden & Gibbins, 2012) • Skin-to-skin (Walden & Gibbins, 2012) • Postural support (Comaru & Miura, 2009; Walden & Gibbins, 2012)
Umbilical catheterization	• Nonnutritive sucking (with and without sucrose/breast milk) (Walden & Gibbins, 2012) • Positioning and containment (Walden & Gibbins, 2012) • Gentle technique (Walden & Gibbins, 2012)
Percutaneous venous/ arterial line placement	• Nonnutritive sucking (with and without sucrose/breast milk) (Walden & Gibbins, 2012) • Positioning and containment (Walden & Gibbins, 2012) • Gentle technique (Walden & Gibbins, 2012) • Topical anesthetic (Anand, 2001; Menon, Anand, & McIntosh, 1998; Walden & Gibbins, 2012) • Consider subcutaneous infiltration of lidocaine (Anand, 2001) • Consider opioids (Anand, 2001; Walden & Gibbins, 2012)
Central venous line placement	• Nonnutritive sucking (with and without sucrose/breast milk) (Walden & Gibbins, 2012) • Positioning and containment (Walden & Gibbins, 2012) • Gentle technique (Walden & Gibbins, 2012) • Topical anesthetic (Anand, 2001; Menon et al., 1998; Walden & Gibbins, 2012) • Consider subcutaneous infiltration of lidocaine (Anand, 2001) • Consider opioids (Anand, 2001; Walden & Gibbins, 2012) • Consider general anesthesia (Anand, 2001)
Endotracheal tube placement	• Employ rapid sequence induction for ALL nonemergent endotracheal intubations (specifically excluding resuscitation in the delivery room where intravenous access may not be available) (Allen, 2012; Lago et al., 2009; Kumar, Denson, & Mancuso, 2010)

(continued)

TABLE 6.3   Common NICU Procedures and Evidence-Based Prevention and Management Strategies
(*continued*)

Procedure	Prevention/Management Strategy
Chest tube insertion	• Nonnutritive sucking (with and without sucrose/breast milk) (Anand, 2001; Walden & Gibbins, 2012) • Consider subcutaneous infiltration of lidocaine (Anand, 2001) • Consider opioids (Anand, 2001; Lago et al., 2009; Walden & Gibbins, 2012) • Consider the use of short-acting anesthetic agents (Anand, 2001; Lago et al., 2009)

Patient Identification	
Procedure	Personalized Pain and Pain-Related Stress Prevention Tactics
Feeding tube insertion	Baby X is able to tolerate this procedure when provided with a pacifier with sweet solution while being held by a parent
Heel stick	Baby X tolerates this procedure best when in skin-to-skin contact with parent

FIGURE 6.1   Sample pain prevention care plan.

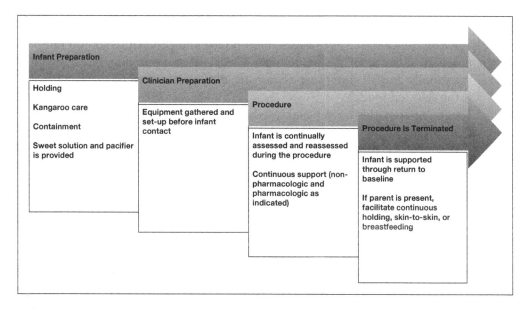

FIGURE 6.2   Sample pain prevention process steps.

Pain Prevention Bundle Feedback

- Did you use the pain prevention resources in the bundle?   Y   N
- Was it helpful to have these resources packaged together at the bedside?   Y   N
- Would you like to see this type of resource available for other procedures?   Y   N
- Which procedures? _____

FIGURE 6.3   Sample for pain prevention bundle feedback.

◼ PAIN AND STRESS ASSESSMENT, MANAGEMENT, AND REASSESSMENT

The experience of pain is not limited to physical sensations.
   —Anonymous

Interventions and Practice Considerations

1. Ensure that the pain/stress assessment tools employed have demonstrated reliability and validity and are contextually accurate for the patient population served in your NICU.
   - Best practice considerations must ensure that pain and stress assessment scores that indicate pain and/or stress are promptly and effectively treated using the appropriate pharmacologic and/or nonpharmacologic intervention(s).
   - An evidence-based pain assessment policy and procedure should be available to all NICU stakeholders (clinicians and parents), be reviewed annually and all staff must demonstrate competence in the correct use of the selected tool(s).
2. Caregiving activities must be adapted and modified based on infant biobehavioral cues of pain and/or stress.
   - Best practice considerations include competency in recognizing an infant's biobehavioral cues of pain and stress; in situations in which an infant is unable to verbally and/or nonverbally communicate his or her experience of pain/distress and/or stress due to his or her severity of illness, gestational immaturity, or level of consciousness/sedation, a protocol must outline pain and stress assessment strategies for this vulnerable group of individuals.
   - Responding sensitively and consistently to an infant's biobehavioral cues of stress and pain is a crucial best practice strategy to prevent lifelong morbidity associated with unmanaged or undermanaged pain and stress.
   - Best practice for humane, quality caring includes empathizing with the infant's experience of care to avoid unnecessary suffering.

3. Nonpharmacologic and/or pharmacologic pain and/or stress relieving strategies are consistently and reliably provided for ALL painful and/or stressful procedures, used to mange disease-specific pain as well as other painful or distressing circumstances (e.g., hunger pain, gas pain, constipation, pruritus).
   - Best practice considerations include establishing clearly defined procedural pain management strategies, protocols for addressing disease-specific conditions such as necrotizing enterocolitis, pneumothoraxes, surgical pain, and so on, as well as evidence-based guidelines to address other types of pain and distress for the hospitalized individual.
   - Best practices also address documentation requirements that describe the patient's pain/stress/distress experience to include the procedure, disease-specific context or physical discomfort, the pain and stress management intervention(s), the patient's response(s), and the patient's return to his or her baseline level of comfort (quantified by physical description, vital sign parameters/big data and pain assessment score[s]).
4. Clinician accountability to the pain and stress prevention/management guidelines and practice expectations must be clearly articulated and include a method for auditing practice, acknowledging excellence, and addressing compliance concerns.
   - Best practices in staff accountability include creating a culture of shared responsibility for patient outcomes, developing staff skills in providing real-time feedback with peers, and linking staff performance with organizational goals and achievements.

The Evidence

Consistently assessing and managing pain, pain-related stress and distress in the hospitalized infant remains a challenge in the NICU despite a plethora of assessment tools and an ever-expanding body of evidence related to effective pharmacologic and nonpharmacologic interventions. Infants receiving neonatal intensive care experience a median of 75 painful procedures during their hospital stay and on average 10 painful procedures per NICU day (Carbajal et al., 2008). Repeated and prolonged pain experiences during early-life alter pain-processing capabilities, compromise long-term development, and have been linked to a heightened vulnerability for chronic pain in NICU survivors (Grunau, 2013; Grunau, Holsti, & Peters, 2006; Hatfield, 2014; Low & Schweinhardt 2012).

The cerebral cortex is functionally mature with thalamocortical connections established by 22 weeks gestation; by 24 to 26 weeks the peripheral nervous system and ascending pain pathways are mature, however, the descending modulatory pain pathways remain immature until about 6 to 8 months of postnatal life (Hatfield, 2014; Walker, 2014). The clinical implications of this developmental reality is a hypersensitivity to pain and even nonpainful touch, a global motor response that become more discriminatory as the gestational age matures, and a prolonged experience of pain due to immature descending pathways designed to modulate the pain experience (Grunau et al., 2006; Hatfield, 2014; Johnston, Fernandes, & Campbell-Yeo, 2011). The long-term implications of undermanaged neonatal pain are a public health issue with ethical as well as economic implications related to neuronal and genomic alterations that affect the infant's developmental trajectory (Hatfield, Meyers, & Messing, 2013; Ranger & Grunau, 2014; Vinall & Grunau, 2014).

NICU clinicians grapple with competing priorities, time constraints, and the challenge of accurately and safely perceiving and interpreting the pain and stress experience of this vulnerable patient population. Although the stage has been set by a substantive body of evidence regarding a functional, responsive, and sensitive pain system in neonates, there continues to be remnants of skepticism and extreme caution that hinders consistent and effective infant pain management in the NICU (Rodkey & Pillai Riddell, 2013). Clinician concerns include the safety and long-term implications associated with various pharmacologic pain management interventions, as well as the accuracy of their pain assessments in preverbal individuals (Cong, Delaney, & Vazquez, 2013; Gibbins et al., 2015). Understanding clinician concerns enables organizations to identify knowledge and practice gaps to resolve the pervasive inconsistencies of infant pain, stress, and distress management in the NICU (Cong et al., 2013; Gibbins et al., 2015). Prevention must be the priority for pain management (AAP & the Canadian Pediatric Society, 2006; Hall & Anand, 2014; Walter-Nicolet, Annequin, Biran, Mitanchez, & Tourniaire, 2010). Surveillance procedures or "routine" lab work should be avoided and when a procedure is deemed necessary, a consistent focus on modifying the procedure to ensure pain prevention is required (Hall & Anand, 2014; Walter-Nicolet et al., 2010). Interprofessional awareness of pain is critical for excellence in managing infant pain and stress and is supported through integrated computerized pain evaluation modules and other reminders and redundancies in the environment of care (Mazars et al., 2012).

Tissue damage during critical and sensitive periods of development not only alters long-term pain sensitivity but increases risk for behavioral problems associated with methylation of the serotonin transporter gene—findings that have far-reaching implications, including safety and quality-of-life issues (Chau et al., 2014; Li & Baccei, 2011; Walker, Beggs, & Baccei, 2015). Accurate pain, stress, and distress assessment in preverbal individuals demands mindfulness, presence, and attunement framed by a systematic process that ensures consistency and reliability in the provision of effective, evidence-based pain, stress, and distress management strategies. Using the Plan-Do-Study-Act (PDSA) model for improvement, safety and quality-minded professionals will ensure the use of a contextually appropriate pain assessment tool; outline clear documentation criteria related to the pain event (to include the effectiveness of the pain management strategy, the patients' response to the pain management intervention and their return to baseline); adopt evidence-based best practices in pain, stress, and distress management; and establish accountability metrics for success and sustainability (Reavey et al., 2014; Walden & Gibbins, 2012).

Physical pain and stress are an ever-present reality in the NICU; however, it is not the only source of distress for this vulnerable population. Emotional pain and stress are often underrecognized in infants. Infants are completely dependent on adult caregivers to recognize and respond to their needs. When their needs are not met, infants experience prolonged periods of intense emotional arousal, which translates into traumatic or damaging stress in the absence of comfort from an adult caregiver, preferentially maternal care (Montirosso & Provenzi, 2015; Wotherspoon, Hawkins, & Gough, 2009). Emotional neglect is more damaging than other forms of maltreatment, and, yes, being separated from mother, having a life-threatening illness, and requiring frequent painful procedures can be viewed as "maltreatment" when one considers what the neonatal brain is wired to experience and expect during the first year of life (Coughlin, 2014; Karr-Morse & Wiley, 2012; Montirosso & Provenzi, 2015; Shonkoff & Garner, 2012; Wotherspoon & Gough, 2008). Crying is an infant's principal mode of communicating negative emotions, including pain, fear, and anger (Chóliz, Fernández-Abascal, & Martínez-Sánchez, 2012). When a hospitalized infant needs assistance, unlike an adult counterpart who can press the call light for a nurse, the infant relies on crying (if able) to communicate his or her needs. This "cry for help" can often go unheeded in a busy NICU with competing priorities and can even result in the infant being labeled as "fussy" or "spoiled." Needless to say, not responding to an infant's cry for help consistently and reliably is a quality and safety concern that is overshadowed by preconceived notions about the meaning of infant crying. The idea of "crying it out" has been a principle in child rearing and caregiving that is only now being questioned (Narvaez, 2011). Excessive crying not only wastes precious calories and consumes limited oxygen resources in the critically ill/convalescing infant, but when adults are unresponsive to the distressed infant, this alters their emotional regulatory development and alters their relational capabilities (Calkins & Hill, 2009; Narvaez, 2011; Schore, 2001; Soltis, 2004). Infant crying aims to reduce the risk of isolation or the withdrawal of parental care (Soltis, 2004). Esposito et al. (2013) demonstrated the positive effect of maternal infant carrying on beat-to-beat heart rate variability, sleep state, and cry. Caregiver interactions play a critical role in an infant's developing emotion regulation, which is intimately linked to mental health and well-being across the life span (Calkins & Hill, 2009).

Cost Analysis

Routine practices rarely reflect best practice in patient-centered care; they are convenient practices focused on clinician rituals based on a default setting giving the illusion of efficiency. NICU "routines" are often painful, stressful, or distressing to the patient and must be *routinely* reexamined, within the context of each patient, as to clinical relevance and patient impact (both short term and long term). True, authentic patient-centered care must be the primacy of the service we provide in the NICU in order to ensure humane, ethical care that reduces needless suffering (both physical and emotional) for the sake of clinician convenience. Patient-centered care underpins pain and stress prevention and management. Patient-centered care is not about the disease, it is not about the technology, and it is not about the physician, the nurse, or the hospital—it is care that is respectful and responsive to individual patient preferences, needs, and values—and this is where the challenge lies in caring for pre-verbal individuals (Epstein, Fiscella, Lesser, & Stange, 2010; Epstein & Street, 2011).

In the United States alone, the incremental costs of health care due to pain approaches $300 billion (IOM, 2011). When examining life-cycle factors associated with chronic pain, prematurity has been an identified risk factor (IOM, 2011). Littlejohn, Pang, Power, Macfarlane, and Jones (2012) examined the relationship between prematurity and chronic widespread pain in adults and although the results were not statistically significant, they did identify an increased risk for chronic widespread pain in very low birth weight survivors linking early-life adversity with adult chronic pain. Additional economic implications of unmanaged or undermanaged neonatal pain and stress are related to the effect of pain and stress on the developing neuronal architecture impacting the individual's developmental trajectory and, consequently, developmental potential (Doesburg et al., 2013; Low & Schweinhardt, 2012; Valeri, Holsti, & Linhares, 2015; Vinall & Grunau, 2014).

■ Recommendations for Pain and Stress Assessment, Management and Reassessment (Table 6.4)

TABLE 6.4   Major Practice Recommendations and Implementation Strategies—Assessment, Management, and Reassessment

Assessment	
Recommendation	**Implementation Strategy**
1. Use a validated, age-appropriate, and contextually accurate pain assessment tool(s)	a. Examine the demographic features of the patient population served in your NICU (e.g., medical vs. surgical, ELGA vs. LPT vs. Term) b. Review validated pain assessment tools that align with your patient population (you may need more than one tool if you serve a diverse patient population) c. Provide competency-based education on the selected pain assessment tool(s) to ALL NICU clinicians (MDs, RNs, Rehab professionals, etc.) (see Figure 6.4) d. Develop a modified education session on infant pain and stress behaviors for parents e. Audit accuracy of pain assessments (at a minimum quarterly); graph, trend, and share audit results
2. Link pain assessment outcomes with pain management interventions (both pharmacologic and nonpharmacologic)	a. Obtain consensus with the interprofessional team with specific pain management strategies across the spectrum of pain assessment scores (acknowledging a commitment to pain prevention for known painful procedures) b. Consider using an algorithmic approach c. Outline a documentation strategy that captures the patient's experience d. Audit practice compliance; graph, trend, and share audit results e. Consider publishing your results (positive or negative) in order to expand the available knowledge of both effective and ineffective strategies

(continued)

TABLE 6.4   Major Practice Recommendations and Implementation Strategies—Assessment, Management, and Reassessment   *(continued)*

Assessment	
Recommendation	**Implementation Strategy**
3. When physical pain has been ruled out, assess and respond to the emotional distress	a. Outline a care algorithm for the distressed infant (see Figure 6.5) b. Communicate algorithm with care team (to include the parents) c. Measure the impact of the care algorithm on key indicators (i.e., alarm data, big data, growth, parent–infant attachment/empowerment) d. Audit practice compliance e. Consider publishing your results (positive or negative) in order to expand the available knowledge of both effective and ineffective strategies
4. Provide annual competency-based education for ALL clinicians who provide hands-on care in the NICU	a. Include multimodal, competency-based education on pain prevention, assessment, and management for ALL new hires to the NICU (see Figure 6.6) b. Audit practice; graph, trend, and share audit results quarterly c. Integrate performance expectations around pain prevention, assessment, and management into the annual staff evaluation

Management	
Recommendation	**Implementation Strategy**
1. Determine the clinical necessity of the planned procedure; how will the information gained influence care?	a. Review patient status and need for various painful procedures with each shift change b. Obtain consensus with interprofessional team (to include consulting colleagues) about criteria to define medical necessity c. Test the review process with criteria using PDSA methodology; revise, refine, implement d. Publish results
2. Ensure the environment is suitable for the procedure (quiet, calm, appropriate lighting, etc.)	a. Develop a procedure checklist that incorporates the environmental dimensions as well as preparatory components for a successful procedure (see Figure 6.4)
3. Implement the appropriate sedation, analgesia, anesthesia and nonpharmacologic intervention making sure to allow sufficient time for the selected pain management strategy to be effective	a. Integrate a pain management reference guide (i.e., Table 6.3) into the EMR/MAR/CPOE system b. Integrate a computerized pain evaluation module into the CPOE c. Consider a procedure "time-out" until pain management intervention has been deemed effective d. Ensure ALL staff have demonstrated competence and knowledge about the various pain management strategies; review at a minimum annually e. Audit medical records and resolve knowledge and practice gaps promptly to avoid unnecessary suffering

(continued)

TABLE 6.4   Major Practice Recommendations and Implementation Strategies—Assessment, Management, and Reassessment   *(continued)*

Management	
Recommendation	**Implementation Strategy**
4. Make an action plan should the procedure fail or if the pain management strategy is ineffective.	a. Expert proficiency in various technical skills develops over time, however, this development cannot be at the expense of the patient. Identify who the technical experts are on the unit for the various anticipated shift procedures b. Inform these individuals at the beginning of the shift of their role as back-up support for their peers to avoid unnecessary pain and stress to the patients c. Before initiating a technically challenging procedure, verbally outline a back-up plan with parents and peers d. Provide the infant with a "time-out" between procedure attempts e. Limiting the number of attempts per clinician, deferring to the technical expert following two failed attempts f. Ensure that the pain management intervention has achieved the desired results BEFORE beginning the procedure g. Guarantee that the appropriate combination of pain management strategies are at the bedside and readily available to redose/retreat the infant during the procedure to eliminate unnecessary pain and stress for the infant

Reassessment	
Recommendation	**Implementation Strategy**
1. Reassess pain continuously throughout any given procedure and continue to assess for pain/stress until the infant's biobehavioral status returns to his or her baseline level of comfort.	a. Ensure that the EMR supports dynamic documentation of pain assessment and intervention, if not, devise a model to test on paper b. Evaluate, refine, and revise your documentation strategy c. Contact your informatics professional to integrate into your system d. Audit practice compliance, consider comparing documentation with big data e. Publish your results (both positive and negative)

CPOE, computerized physician order entry; EMR, electronic medical record; ELGA, extremely low gestational age; LPT, late preterm; MAR, medication administration record; PDSA, Plan-Do-Study-Act.

Tools and Parent Resources

PARENT RESOURCES
1. Hand to Hold: handtohold.org/support/nicu-support
2. March of Dime: www.marchofdimes.org/complications/the-nicu.aspx
3. National Association of Neonatal Nurses (NANN): babystepstohome.com

CLINICIAN TOOLS

The following resources may help you begin to transform your pain and stress assessment and management practices (Figures 6.4, 6.5, and 6.6):

VERIFICATION
1. Patient identification has been verified with two indicators .... ☐
2. Clinical necessity of the procedure has been discussed with the health care team and family and is confirmed .... ☐
3. Parent(s) present at the bedside .... ☐
   a. If not, parent is aware of the procedure .... ☐

Clinician Signature: _____   Date and Time: _____

COMMUNICATION
1. Action plan has been outlined if procedure is unsuccessful .... ☐
2. Pain and stress prevention interventions have been reviewed .... ☐
3. If parents are at the bedside, the pain and stress prevention strategy has been reviewed with them and they have acknowledged their role in the procedure for pain and stress prevention.... ☐

PREPARATION
1. Timing of the procedure coincides with awake/alert state of the infant .... ☐
2. Procedure equipment is gathered at the bedside BEFORE the patient is disturbed .... ☐
3. Pain and stress prevention supplies are gathered at the bedside BEFORE the patient is disturbed .... ☐
4. The environment (lighting and sound) have been adjusted to optimize procedural success and infant comfort .... ☐

TIME-OUT
1. Person performing the procedure initiated the time-out verbally .... ☐
2. All other activity ceased .... ☐
3. Second person (either health care provider or parent) verbally verified the procedure with the person performing the procedure.. ☐

Clinician Signature: _____   Date and Time: _____

PROCEDURE
1. Initiate pain prevention intervention, ensuring sufficient time for the selected pain management strategy to be effective prior to beginning the procedure .... ☐
2. Once pain prevention is confirmed effective, begin the procedure .... ☐
3. Continually evaluate the infant for level of comfort... ☐
4. Repeat pain prevention intervention guided by infant's biobehavioral pain score .... ☐
5. Document procedure outcome (successful vs. not successful)................................ ☐
6. Document infant's pain and stress management experience (successful vs. not successful) ☐

Clinician Signature: _____   Date and Time: _____

FIGURE 6.4   Sample pre-procedure verification checklist for bedside procedures.

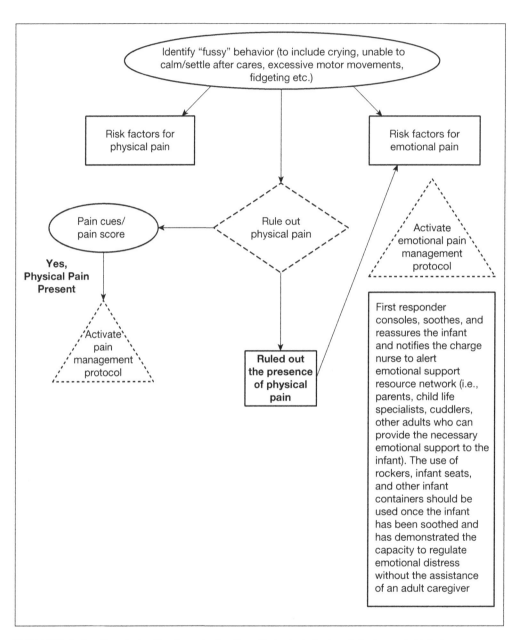

FIGURE 6.5   Sample algorithm for evaluating "fussy" behavior in the hospitalized preverbal infant.

Reproduced with permission from Caring Essentials Collaborative, LLC.

Step	Action	Demonstrated Mode of Competence	Complete ✓
1	Participate in pain prevention, assessment, management education	Attendance/ completion certificate	☐
2	Review the unit's procedural pain prevention, assessment, and management guidelines	Sign-off	☐
3	Perform pain assessment on select training videos using the designated, validated neonatal pain assessment tool (scores are validated by expert observer)	Observation/score validation with expert observer	Video 1: _____ ☐ Video 2: _____ ☐ Video 3: _____ ☐
4	Mock-up return demonstration of appropriate prevention, assessment, and management of procedural pain across three painful procedures (heel stick, NG tube insertion, other)	Observation checklist	Scenario 1: ☐ Scenario 2: ☐ Scenario 3: ☐
5	Undergo three observations of procedural pain prevention and management in three separate procedural pain situations	Observation	Date: _____ ☐ Date: _____ ☐ Date: _____ ☐
6	Document painful procedures (heel stick, needle stick, feeding tube insertion, etc.) along with the appropriate nonpharmacologic/ pharmacologic intervention in the EMR	Quarterly chart audit	Date: _____ ☐ Date: _____ ☐ Date: _____ ☐ Date: _____ ☐
7	Document pain reassessments in the medical record until the infant has returned to their baseline level of comfort	Quarterly chart audit	Date: _____ ☐ Date: _____ ☐ Date: _____ ☐ Date: _____ ☐
8	When parent(s) is/are present at the bedside, document parental participation in the management of the infant's procedural pain in the EMR	Chart audit	☐

Clinician: _____   _____   _____

Printed name   Signature   Date

Observer: _____   _____   _____

Printed name   Signature   Date

FIGURE 6.6   Sample pain prevention, assessment, and management in the NICU competency.

EMR, electronic medical record; NG, nasogastric.

■ THE FAMILY AND PAIN AND STRESS

It is easy to get a thousand prescriptions but hard to get one single remedy.
> —Chinese proverb

Interventions and Practice Considerations

1. Family education regarding infant pain and stress cues is provided, validated, and reinforced over the hospital stay.
   - Best practice considerations include: (a) acknowledging the important role of the parents in comforting their child; (b) ensuring parents receive accurate education/information about what pain and stress looks like in their infant; and finally (c) applying this knowledge so that the mother/father can parent their hospitalized infant and partner with the clinical staff to ensure consistent pain and stress prevention and management.
2. Parents are informed and involved in the pain and stress prevention and management plan of care for their hospitalized infant.
   - Best practice considerations focus on partnerships with parents to develop an effective and realistic pain and stress prevention plan of care in which parents play a crucial role; parent involvement and the infant's responses to parent-driven pain and stress management interventions are documented.
3. The family is encouraged, empowered, and supported in providing comfort to their infant throughout the hospital stay.
   - Best practice considerations include unrestricted parental access to the hospitalized infant, access to education regarding effective pain and stress prevention and management strategies, and parental implementation of various effective nonpharmacologic pain and stress interventions.

The Evidence

Parents have insufficient information and understanding of their hospitalized infant's pain experience and this paucity of knowledge as well as limited involvement in supporting their infant is a source of parental stress (Franck, Cox, Allen, & Winter, 2004). Cleveland (2008) identified the following needs of NICU parents: (a) a need for accurate information and inclusion in their infant's care; (b) a need to watch over and protect their infant; (c) a need for contact with their infant; (d) a need to be perceived positively by the nursery staff; (e) a need for individualized care for their infant; and (f) a need for a therapeutic relationship with the nursing staff. Nursing behaviors that will support parents in meeting these needs include the provision of emotional support, empowering the parents, creating a welcoming environment with supportive family-focused policies, and providing parent education with an opportunity to implement the new skills through guided partnership and mentoring (Cleveland, 2008). In a phenomenological study performed by Simons, Franck, and Roberson (2002) examining parent and nurse perceptions of parent involvement in their child's pain care, the findings indicated significant disparity; where nurses felt there was adequate parental involvement, parents described feelings of frustration with what was perceived as a passive parent role in caring for their child's pain. The nurse–parent relationship in the NICU is critical in facilitating parent attachment, empowerment, and overall satisfaction with their hospital experience of care (Axelin et al., 2015; Reis, Rempel, Scott, Brady-Fryer, & Van Aerde, 2010). In general, nurses acknowledge the important role of the parents in effective infant pain management; however, this acknowledgment does not consistently lead to parental involvement in practice. In a recent focus group of international NICU nurses exploring nurses' experiences and perceptions of parental participation in infant pain management, the majority of nurses preferred to control infant pain management or modestly share some control with parents (Axelin et al., 2015).

The evidence points to parental need to understand and recognize their infants pain and stress cues and to be involved during painful procedures to provide comfort and solace for their infant. Although education and participation may not necessarily reduce parental stress, taking an active role in supporting their infant during painful procedures increased parent role identity and satisfaction with staff in managing their infant's pain (Franck et al., 2011). Following up on the original cohort from Franck et al. (2011), the researchers uncovered parental desires for more information about neonatal pain and pain management and to receive this information sooner than later during the NICU stay (Franck, Oulton, & Bruce, 2012).

In addition to timely comprehensive information about infant pain care, it is also important to understand parental differences (mothers vs. fathers) in knowledge and pain perception. In a recent survey of 80 parents (57 mothers and 23 fathers), mothers indicated a higher degree of self-efficacy than fathers in helping their baby get into a quiet sleep despite their pain experience and also revealed a higher preference to hold their baby as soon as possible after a painful procedure than fathers (Vazquez, Cong, & DeJong, 2015). Educating, empowering, and involving parents in their infant's pain care during the NICU stay builds confidence and competence in parenting and validates parental role identity (Cleveland, 2008; Franck et al., 2004, 2011, 2012; Vazquez et al., 2015). Parent involvement with infant pain care will not respond to a one-size-fits-all approach. Mothers as well as fathers exhibit different levels of involvement with their infant's care. Axelin, Lehtonen, Pelander, and Salanterä (2010), in a descriptive exploratory study with post intervention interviews looking at how mothers use opportunities to participate in their infant's pain care using facilitated talk, discovered individual preferences and styles in parenting and supporting their infant during painful procedures.

The majority of NICUs provide some type of education for parents regarding infant pain assessment and management. The challenge is in the delivery and the translation of that information into something that can be applied in real time. Taddio et al. (2014) evaluated the efficacy of a parent-directed instructional pamphlet about needle pain and discovered that only 21% of the pamphlet recipients actually read the material. Farkas et al. (2015) completed a scoping review of publicly available educational videos regarding pediatric needle pain and were able to identify 25 relevant educational videos; the authors acknowledge that they need to further evaluate whether or not this form of education meets the target audience and how to facilitate access engagement and translation of the learned material.

The use of information prescriptions (IRx) was evaluated with a cohort of mothers of inpatient NICU patients; the mothers who were randomized to receive the information prescription reported a higher level of satisfaction regarding the information that they received suggesting that this may be a valuable vehicle to educate NICU parents (Oliver et al., 2011). Regardless of the specific educational modality employed to educate NICU parents about infant pain care, a systematic and standardized approach needs to be employed. Mobile technology combined with traditional modalities for education can be integrated into a competency-based package of learning specifically designed to meet the individual needs of NICU parents (Brett, Staniszewska, Newburn, Jones, & Taylor, 2011).

Cost Analysis

In 2007, the Institute of Medicine published *Preterm Birth: Causes, Consequences, and Prevention* revealing that the annual societal cost associated with preterm birth in the United States in 2005 was $26.2 billion. Eliminating unmanaged and undermanaged pain in the NICU will favorably impact short- and long-term outcomes of this vulnerable patient population and certainly reduce some of this economic burden. The creators of the Creating Opportunities for Parent Empowerment (COPE) program for NICU parents report a cost savings of at least $4,864 per infant in addition to improving parent and infant outcomes (Melnyk & Feinstein, 2009). Increasing parental presence, participation, and caregiving in the NICU enhances maternal caregiving, promotes breastfeeding, and validates parental role identity—all of which improve the post-NICU discharge success for the infant–family dyad (Hane et al., 2015; Melnyk et al., 2006; Welch et al., 2015).

◾ Recommendations for Family Involvement in the Pain and Stress Prevention and Management (Table 6.5)

TABLE 6.5   Major Practice Recommendations and Implementation Strategies—Education, Partnership, and Advocacy and Empowerment

Education	
Recommendation	**Implementation Strategy**
1. Multimodal parent education on infant pain and stress cues, effective pain and stress interventions, as well as common procedures that benefit from parental involvement are provided within the first week of NICU admission	a. Review existing parent education resources and critically appraise/evaluate their effectiveness (Figure 6.7) b. Revise or develop parent teaching resources as indicated by evaluation criteria (see Figures 6.8 and 6.9) c. Consider partnering with former NICU parents and evaluate in-house patient education resources to develop culturally and literacy sensitive parent education materials d. Evaluate efficacy of education resources; audit parental participation with education resources and address gaps e. Publish results (both positive and negative) f. Annually review to ensure most up-to-date information is being provided

2. Provide simulated and then real-time return demonstration of competence in assessing and intervening on pain and stress cues	a. Integrate in the education resources opportunities for return demonstration of learning:
	   i. Have parents score a series of infant facial expressions and discuss results
	   ii. Have parents return demonstrate a facilitated tuck, holding in arms, and skin-to-skin holding for selected procedures (e.g., heel stick, vaccination, feeding tube insertion) using a doll and mocked up various NICU equipment (see Figure 6.10)
	 b. Disseminate certificates of completion; celebrate skill achievement
	 c. Evaluate the effectiveness of the return demonstration with questionnaires, parent interviews, parent participation, and presence, etc.
	 d. Revise process as indicated
	 e. Publish results

Partnership	
Recommendation	**Implementation Strategy**

1. Review the daily and weekly plan of care with parents to facilitate parent presence and foster communication and partnerships between parents and the clinical team	a. Develop a parent communication system/process to ensure consistent communication—collaborate with information technology specialists in your facility to explore options
	   i. Notification system via mobile device
	   ii. Telephone communication schedule
	   iii. Bedside whiteboard
	 b. Get input and feedback from family regarding their preferred communication mode

(continued)

TABLE 6.5   Major Practice Recommendations and Implementation Strategies—Education, Partnership, and Advocacy and Empowerment   *(continued)*

Partnership	
Recommendation	**Implementation Strategy**
2. Ensure that the documentation solution used in your unit accommodates entries that reflect parent participation/involvement in infant pain and stress care	a. Draft a documentation strategy to capture parent participation in infant pain and stress care i. Drop-down menu (EMR) ii. Text-box entry (paper or EMR) iii. Time-stamp entry for accuracy (paper or EMR) b. Test the draft, revise as indicated, and implement in partnership with informatics professionals c. Audit documentation, trend and graph results, address gaps in documentation d. Publish results
3. Create a mechanism for parent feedback to ensure sensitive, individualized partnerships are being forged	a. Organize parent group discussions, use a "suggestion" box model, or schedule one-on-one meetings with parents b. Define a process for gathering feedback with each selected modality that is consistent and responsive to parents
Advocacy and Empowerment	
Recommendation	**Implementation Strategy**
1. Establish a practice culture dedicated to patient- and family-centered care	a. Consider various staff education and culture transformation programs to build staff engagement in patient-centered and family-centered care i. Quantum Caring program (www.caringessentials.org/qc) ii. COPE program (www.copeforhope.com/index.php) iii. Family Nurture Intervention (nurturescienceprogram.org/content/family-nurture-intervention) iv. NIDCAP Program (nidcap.org/en)
2. Establish a parent support group with former NICU parents	a. Reach out to local March of Dimes chapters and other community and national parent support organizations for guidance and assistance i. Hand to Hold (handtohold.org) ii. NICU Helping Hands (www.nicuhelpinghands.org/resources/national-organizations) iii. Preemie Parent Alliance (www.preemieparentalliance.wildapricot.org) iv. Grahams Foundation (grahamsfoundation.org).

(continued)

TABLE 6.5   Major Practice Recommendations and Implementation Strategies—Education, Partnership, and Advocacy and Empowerment   *(continued)*

Advocacy and Empowerment	
Recommendation	**Implementation Strategy**
3. Establish a unit-based family advocacy council	a. Collaborate with your hospital's patient advocacy group to develop a vision and mission statement for your unit-based council b. Recruit for a multidisciplinary team and include former NICU parents as council members (may be a subcommittee of your developmental care/quality or clinical practice council) c. Identify existing gaps in parent advocacy and empowerment in your unit. Here are some available tools: 　i. Hospital self-assessment of Patient and Family-Centered Care from the American Hospital Association: www.google.com/url?sa=t&rct=j&q=&esrc=s&source=web&cd=1&ved=0ahUKEwiEgla28brJAhUFqx4KHbUVDhIQFggiMAA&url=http%3A%2F%2Fwww.aha.org%2Fcontent%2F00–10%2Fassessment.pdf&usg=AFQjCNEEs1gUTS6hA2D8krAhgyOR-Jr9sA&sig2=JLgkjWXm-5f3NQTroSbCNwA 　ii. Family Voices Self-Assessment tool: www.familyvoices.org/admin/work_family_centered/files/fcca_FamilyTool.pdf 　iii. Institute for Patient- and Family-Centered Care: ipfcc.org/resources/other/index.html d. Schedule meetings, outline goals and objectives based on vision and mission statement as well as self-assessment e. Identify/define indicators that reflect parent empowerment to monitor progress and success f. Perform routine audits of your journey g. Publish your results

COPE, Creating Opportunities for Parent Empowerment; EMR, electronic medical record; NIDCAP, Newborn Individualized Developmental Care and Assessment Program.

Tools and Parent Resources

CLINICIAN RESOURCES

Parent Assessment of Infant Nociception (PAIN) Questionnaire: nursing.ucsf.edu/sites/nursing.ucsf.edu/files/Permission%20to%20use%20the%20PAIN%20Questionnaire%20and%20Guidelines.pdf

PARENT RESOURCES

Dr. Linda Franck, internationally renowned nurse researcher, has developed a multimedia resource for parents entitled "Comforting Your Baby in Intensive Care." This evidence-based resource is available for download free-of-charge from the following link: familynursing.ucsf.edu/resources-parents.

The following questions ask about your baby's stay in the neonatal unit

1. Approximately how often do you visit your baby in the neonatal unit? (CHOOSE ONE)
   - I stay all the time
   - Several times a day
   - Once daily
   - Every few weeks
   - Once a week

2. Please circle how seriously ill you think your baby is at the moment, with 0 = low risk of dying and 5 = high risk of dying. (CHOOSE ONE)

        0 1 2 3 4 5

The following questions ask about pain. Please feel free to add additional comments in the space provided.

3. My baby felt pain while in the neonatal unit. (CHOOSE ONE)
   - Yes
   - No
   - Don't know

4. Please circle how much pain you think your baby is feeling **at this moment**, with 0 = no pain and 10 = worst possible pain. (CHOOSE ONE)

        0 1 2 3 4 5 6 7 8 9 10

   No Pain   **Worst Pain**

5. Please circle the **worst** pain you think your baby has felt since admission to the neonatal unit. (CHOOSE ONE)

        0 1 2 3 4 5 6 7 8 9 10

   No Pain   **Worst Pain**

6. Please circle the **least** pain you think your baby has felt since admission to the neonatal unit. (CHOOSE ONE)

        0 1 2 3 4 5 6 7 8 9 10

   No Pain   **Worst Pain**

7. Please circle how much pain you **expected** your baby would have while in the neonatal unit. (CHOOSE ONE)

        0 1 2 3 4 5 6 7 8 9 10

   No Pain   **Worst Pain**

8. Please circle how much pain **relief** you expected your baby would have while in the neonatal unit. (CHOOSE ONE)

        0 1 2 3 4 5 6 7 8 9 10

   No Pain   **Worst Pain**

FIGURE 6.7   Sample of pain questionnaire.

Adapted and reprinted from Franck et al. (2004). Full questionnaire and permission are available at http://familynursing.ucsf.edu/sites/familynursing.ucsf.edu/files/Permission-use-PAIN-Questionnaire-Guidelines_6-21-16.pdf

It can be hard to tell the difference between pain and stress in babies. Remember all pain is stressful, but all stress is not pain—but both can change the way your baby's brain develops and works. Understanding what is happening to your baby will help you understand what your baby may be feeling.

Although babies are unable to tell us with words that they are in pain or are stressed, they are able to express their pain and stress in other ways. Changes in heart rate, breathing pattern, blood pressure, and oxygen saturation as well as facial expressions and body movements or the absence of body movements are all the ways babies tell us how they are feeling.

Illustration of the Pain Pathway

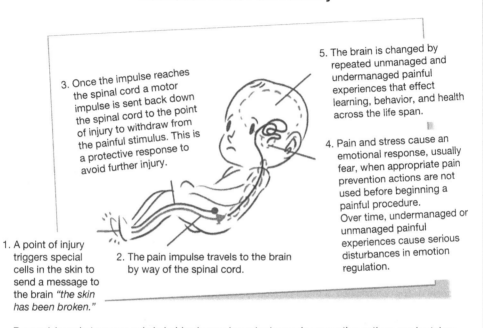

5. The brain is changed by repeated unmanaged and undermanaged painful experiences that effect learning, behavior, and health across the life span.

3. Once the impulse reaches the spinal cord a motor impulse is sent back down the spinal cord to the point of injury to withdraw from the painful stimulus. This is a protective response to avoid further injury.

4. Pain and stress cause an emotional response, usually fear, when appropriate pain prevention actions are not used before beginning a painful procedure.
Over time, undermanaged or unmanaged painful experiences cause serious disturbances in emotion regulation.

1. A point of injury triggers special cells in the skin to send a message to the brain *"the skin has been broken."*

2. The pain impulse travels to the brain by way of the spinal cord.

Recognizing what causes pain in babies is very important so pain prevention actions can be taken. Sometimes the most appropriate pain prevention action may need to be repeated while the procedure is still going on. "Reading" your baby's behaviors and changes in the usual vital signs will let you know if your baby is feeling pain and/or stress.

FIGURE 6.8   Sample parent pain and stress teaching sheet.

Source: © 2016 Caring Essentials Collaborative, LLC. All rights reserved.

Breastfeeding and breast milk feeding provide the perfect nutrition for your baby; however, your baby may not be able to take milk directly from the breast or bottle right away. Many babies begin feeding through a soft tube that is placed through the nose or mouth and advanced into your baby's stomach.

Your baby needs to be able to suck, swallow, and breath to breastfeed (or bottle feed). It will take time for your baby to build these skills but in the meantime your baby can have your breast milk (or formula) through the feeding tube. Even tiny amounts of breast milk started on the first or second day after birth helps your baby grow, can decrease your baby's risk of infection, and can shorten your baby's hospital stay!

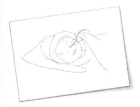

Feeding tubes are soft, flexible tubes that are placed into your baby's stomach through the nose or mouth. The tube is then secured to your baby's cheek with special tape so that it stays in place. This tube allows you and the health care team to provide milk to your baby until your baby is able to take milk by mouth (either by breastfeeding, bottle feeding, or a combination of both).

For longer-term tube feeding, some babies will have a gastrostomy tube (or G-tube) placed. A G-tube is a surgically placed tube that goes directly into your baby's stomach through an incision in the baby's belly. This is done in the operating room while your baby is under anesthesia. This type of feeding tube provides a safe way of feeding your baby when he or she needs more time to develop and mature. This is often a temporary measure and does not require surgery to be removed. This tube allows your baby to build his or her oral feeding skills without the stress of having to get in enough calories with each oral feeding.

Insertion and manipulations of these tube is uncomfortable and your baby will need comfort measures when the tube is inserted or manipulated. Providing some comfort measures prior to the procedure can reduce your baby's discomfort and distress. Research shows that skin-to-skin care, holding your baby, giving your baby a pacifier with a sweet solution (breastmilk, sucrose, or glucose) or any combination of these comfort measures are very effective in reducing your baby's pain during this procedure. Ask your baby's nurse about the pain and stress prevention plan for your baby and how you can be involved to support your baby during painful and stressful procedures.

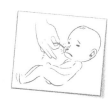

Build competence and confidence caring for your baby in the NICU; and discover your full parenting potential at www.caringessentials.org/family-use

FIGURE 6.9   Sample parent teaching sheet: Tube feeding insertion.

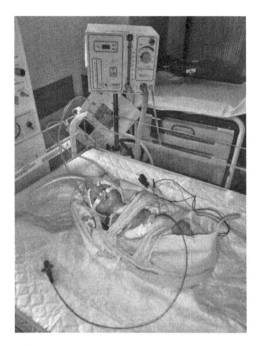

FIGURE 6.10   Mock-up doll for parent education.

At the end of the day, the most overwhelming key to a child's success is the positive involvement of parents.
          —Jane D. Hull

■ REFERENCES

Allen, K. A. (2012). Premedication for neonatal intubation: Which medications are recommended and why. *Advances in Neonatal Care, 12*(2), 107–111.

American Academy of Pediatrics and the Canadian Pediatric Society. (2006). Prevention and management of pain in the neonate: An update. *Pediatrics, 118*(5), 2231–2241.

Anand, K. J.; International Evidence-Based Group for Neonatal Pain. (2001). Consensus statement for the prevention and management of pain in the newborn. *Archives of Pediatrics & Adolescent Medicine, 155*(2), 173–180.

Axelin, A., Anderzén-Carlsson, A., Eriksson, M., Pölkki, T., Korhonen, A., & Franck, L. S. (2015). Neonatal intensive care nurses' perceptions of parental participation in infant pain management: A comparative focus group study. *The Journal of Perinatal & Neonatal Nursing, 29*(4), 363–374.

Axelin, A., Lehtonen, L., Pelander, T., & Salanterä, S. (2010). Mothers' different styles of involvement in preterm infant pain care. *Journal of Obstetric, Gynecologic, and Neonatal Nursing, 39*(4), 415–424.

Baba, L. R., McGrath, J. M., & Liu, J. (2010). The efficacy of mechanical vibration analgesia for relief of heel stick pain in neonates: A novel approach. *The Journal of Perinatal & Neonatal Nursing, 24*(3), 274–283.

Barrington, K. J., Batton, D. G., Finley, G. A., Wallman, C., & the Canadian Pediatric Society Fetus and Newborn Committee. (2007). Prevention and management of pain in the neonate: An update. *Pediatrics & Child Health, 12*(2), 137–138.

Brett, J., Staniszewska, S., Newburn, M., Jones, N., & Taylor, L. (2011). A systematic mapping review of effective interventions for communicating with, supporting and providing information to parents of preterm infants. *BMJ Open, 1*(1), e000023.

Bueno, M., Yamada, J., Harrison, D., Khan, S., Ohlsson, A., Adams-Webber, T., . . . Stevens, B. (2013). A systematic review and meta-analyses of nonsucrose sweet solutions for pain relief in neonates. *Pain Research & Management, 18*(3), 153–161.

Calkins, S. D., & Hill, A. (2009). Caregiver influences on emerging emotion regulation: Biological and environmental transactions in early development. In J. J. Gross (Ed.), *Handbook of emotion regulation* (pp. 229–248). New York, NY: Guilford.

Carbajal, R., Rousset, A., Danan, C., Coquery, S., Nolent, P., Ducrocq, S., . . . Bréart, G. (2008). Epidemiology and treatment of painful procedures in neonates in intensive care units. *Journal of the American Medical Association, 300*(1), 60–70.

Chau, C. M. Y., Ranger, M., Sulistyoningrum, D., Devlin, A. M., Oberlander, T. F., & Grunau, R. E. (2014). Neonatal pain and *COMT* Val158Met genotype in relation to serotonin transporter (*SLC6A4*) promoter methylation in very preterm children at school age. *Frontiers in Behavioral Neuroscience, 8*, 409. doi:http://dx.doi.org/10.3389%2Ffnbeh.2014.00409

Chóliz, M., Fernández-Abascal, E. G., & Martínez-Sánchez, F. (2012). Infant crying: Pattern of weeping, recognition of emotion and affective reactions in observers. *The Spanish Journal of Psychology, 15*(3), 978–988.

Chou, L. L., Wang, R. H., Chen, S. J., & Pai, L. (2003). Effects of music therapy on oxygen saturation in premature infants receiving endotracheal suctioning. *The Journal of Nursing Research, 11*(3), 209–216.

Cignacco, E. L., Sellam, G., Stoffel, L., Gerull, R., Nelle, M., Anand, K. J., & Engberg, S. (2012). Oral sucrose and "facilitated tucking" for repeated pain relief in preterms: A randomized controlled trial. *Pediatrics, 129*(2), 299–308.

Cleveland, L. M. (2008). Parenting in the neonatal intensive care unit. *Journal of Obstetric, Gynecologic, and Neonatal Nursing: JOGNN/NAACOG, 37*(6), 666–691.

Comaru, T., & Miura, E. (2009). Postural support improves distress and pain during diaper change in preterm infants. *Journal of Perinatology, 29*(7), 504–507.

Cone, S., Pickler, R. H., Grap, M. J., McGrath, J., & Wiley, P. M. (2013). Endotracheal suctioning in preterm infants using four-handed versus routine care. *Journal of Obstetric, Gynecologic, and Neonatal Nursing, 42*(1), 92–104.

Cong, X., Delaney, C., & Vazquez, V. (2013). Neonatal nurses' perceptions of pain assessment and management in NICUs: A national survey. *Advances in Neonatal Care, 13*(5), 353–360.

Coughlin, M. (2014). *Transformative nursing in the NICU: Trauma-informed, age-appropriate care*. New York, NY: Springer Publishing.

Dempsey, E., & McCreery, K. (2011). Local anaesthetic eye drops for prevention of pain in preterm infants undergoing screening for retinopathy of prematurity. *Cochrane Database of Systematic Reviews, 2011*(9), CD007645. doi:10.1002/14651858.CD007645.pub2

Doesburg, S. M., Chau, C. M., Cheung, T. P., Moiseev, A., Ribary, U., Herdman, A. T.,…Grunau, R. E. (2013). Neonatal pain-related stress, functional cortical activity and visual-perceptual abilities in school-age children born at extremely low gestational age. *Pain, 154*(10), 1946–1952.

Epstein, R. M., Fiscella, K., Lesser, C. S., & Stange, K. C. (2010). Why the nation needs a policy push on patient-centered health care. *Health Affairs (Project Hope), 29*(8), 1489–1495.

Epstein, R. M., & Street, R. L. (2011). The values and value of patient-centered care. *Annals of Family Medicine, 9*(2), 100–103.

Esposito, G., Yoshida, S., Ohnishi, R., Tsuneoka, Y., Rostagno, M. d. e. l. C., Yokota, S.,… Kuroda, K. O. (2013). Infant calming responses during maternal carrying in humans and mice. *Current Biology, 23*(9), 739–745.

Farkas, C., Solodiuk, L., Taddio, A., Franck, L., Berberich, F. R., LoChiatto, J., & Solodiuk, J. C. (2015). Publicly available online educational videos regarding pediatric needle pain: A scoping review. *The Clinical Journal of Pain, 31*(6), 591–598.

Franck, L. S., Cox, S., Allen, A., & Winter, I. (2004). Parental concern and distress about infant pain. *Archives of Disease in Childhood. Fetal and Neonatal Edition, 89*(1), F71–F75.

Franck, L. S., Oulton, K., & Bruce, E. (2012). Parental involvement in neonatal pain management: An empirical and conceptual update. *Journal of Nursing Scholarship, 44*(1), 45–54.

Franck, L. S., Oulton, K., Nderitu, S., Lim, M., Fang, S., & Kaiser, A. (2011). Parent involvement in pain management for NICU infants: A randomized controlled trial. *Pediatrics, 128*(3), 510–518.

Furdon, S. A., Eastman, M., Benjamin, K., & Horgan, M. J. (1998). Outcome measures after standardized pain management strategies in postoperative patients in the neonatal intensive care unit. *The Journal of Perinatal & Neonatal Nursing, 12*(1), 58–69.

Gibbins, S., Stevens, B., Dionne, K., Yamada, J., Pillai Riddell, R., McGrath, P.,…Johnston, C. (2015). Perceptions of health professionals on pain in extremely low gestational age infants. *Qualitative Health Research, 25*(6), 763–774.

Gorchynski, J., Everett, W., & Prebil, L. (2008). Underutilization of local anesthetics in infant lumbar punctures. *The Western Journal of Emergency Medicine, 9*(1), 9–12.

Grunau, R. E., Holsti, L., & Peters, J. W. (2006). Long-term consequences of pain in human neonates. *Seminars in Fetal & Neonatal Medicine, 11*(4), 268–275.

Grunau, R. E. (2013). Neonatal pain in very preterm infants: Long-term effects on brain, neurodevelopment and pain reactivity. *Rambam Maimonides Medical Journal, 4*(4), e0025.

Hall, R. W., & Anand, K. J. (2014). Pain management in newborns. *Clinics in Perinatology, 41*(4), 895–924.

Hane, A. A., Myers, M. M., Hofer, M. A., Ludwig, R. J., Halperin, M. S., Austin, J.,…Welch, M. G. (2015). Family nurture intervention improves the quality of maternal caregiving in the neonatal intensive care unit: Evidence from a randomized controlled trial. *Journal of Developmental and Behavioral Pediatrics, 36*(3), 188–196.

Harrison, D., Bueno, M., & Reszel, J. (2015). Prevention and management of pain and stress in the neonate. *Research and Reports in Neonatology, 5*, 9–16.

Hartley, K. A., Miller, C. S., & Gephart, S. M. (2015). Facilitated tucking to reduce pain in neonates: Evidence for best practice. *Advances in Neonatal Care, 15*(3), 201–208.

Hatfield, L. A. (2014). Neonatal pain: What's age got to do with it? *Surgical Neurology International, 5*(Suppl. 13), S479–S489.

Hatfield, L. A., Meyers, M. A., & Messing, T. M. (2013). A systematic review of the effects of repeated painful procedures in infants: Is there a potential to mitigate future pain responsivity? *Journal of Nursing Education and Practice, 3*(8), 99–112.

Haxhija, E. Q., Rosegger, H., & Prechtl, H. F. (1995). Vagal response to feeding tube insertion in preterm infants: Has the key been found? *Early Human Development, 41*(1), 15–25.

Institute of Medicine (IOM). (2007). *Preterm birth: Causes, consequences, and prevention.* Washington, DC: National Academies Press.

Institute of Medicine (IOM). (2011). *Relieving pain in America: A blueprint for transforming prevention, care, education, and research.* Washington, DC: National Academies Press.

Johnston, C., Campbell-Yeo, M., Fernandes, A., Inglis, D., Streiner, D., & Zee, R. (2014). Skin-to-skin care for procedural pain in neonates. *Cochrane Database of Systematic Reviews, 2014*(1), CD008435.

Johnston, C. C., Fernandes, A. M., & Campbell-Yeo, M. (2011). Pain in neonates is different. *Pain, 152*(3 Suppl.), S65–S73.

Karr-Morse, R., & Wiley, M. S. (2012). *Scared sick: The role of childhood trauma in adult disease.* New York, NY: Basic Books.

Kristoffersen, L., Skogvoll, E., & Hafström, M. (2011). Pain reduction on insertion of a feeding tube in preterm infants: A randomized controlled trial. *Pediatrics, 127*(6), e1449–e1454.

Kucukoglu, S., Kurt, S., & Aytekin, A. (2015). The effect of the facilitated tucking position in reducing vaccination-induced pain in newborns. *Italian Journal of Pediatrics, 41*, 61.

Kumar, P., Denson, S. E., & Mancuso, T. J.; Committee on Fetus and Newborn, Section on Anesthesiology and Pain Medicine. (2010). Premedication for nonemergency endotracheal intubation in the neonate. *Pediatrics, 125*(3), 608–615.

Lago, P., Garetti, E., Merazzi, D., Pieragostini, L., Ancora, G., Pirelli, A., & Bellieni, C. V.; Pain Study Group of the Italian Society of Neonatology. (2009). Guidelines for procedural pain in the newborn. *Acta Paediatrica, 98*(6), 932–939.

Larsson, B. A., Tannfeldt, G., Lagercrantz, H., & Olsson, G. L. (1998). Venipuncture is more effective and less painful than heel lancing for blood tests in neonates. *Pediatrics, 101*(5), 882–886.

Li, J., & Baccei, M. L. (2011). Neonatal tissue damage facilitates nociceptive synaptic input to the developing superficial dorsal horn via NGF-dependent mechanisms. *Pain, 152*(8), 1846–1855.

Liaw, J. J., Yang, L., Lee, C. M., Fan, H. C., Chang, Y. C., & Cheng, L. P. (2013). Effects of combined use of non-nutritive sucking, oral sucrose, and facilitated tucking on infant behavioural states across heel-stick procedures: A prospective, randomised controlled trial. *International Journal of Nursing Studies, 50*(7), 883–894.

Liaw, J. J., Yang, L., Katherine Wang, K. W., Chen, C. M., Chang, Y. C., & Yin, T. (2012). Non-nutritive sucking and facilitated tucking relieve preterm infant pain during heel-stick procedures: A prospective, randomised controlled crossover trial. *International Journal of Nursing Studies, 49*(3), 300–309.

Littlejohn, C., Pang, D., Power, C., Macfarlane, G. J., & Jones, G. T. (2012). Is there an association between preterm birth or low birthweight and chronic widespread pain? Results from the 1958 Birth Cohort Study. *European Journal of Pain, 16*(1), 134–139.

Lopez, O., Subramanian, P., Rahmat, N., Theam, L. C., Chinna, K., & Rosli, R. (2015). The effect of facilitated tucking on procedural pain control among premature babies. *Journal of Clinical Nursing, 24*(1–2), 183–191.

Low, L. A., & Schweinhardt, P. (2012). Early life adversity as a risk factor for fibromyalgia in later life. *Pain Research and Treatment, 2012,* 140832.

Mazars, N., Milési, C., Carbajal, R., Mesnage, R., Combes, C., Rideau Batista Novais, A., & Cambonie, G. (2012). Implementation of a neonatal pain management module in the computerized physician order entry system. *Annals of Intensive Care, 2*(1), 38.

McCullough, S., Halton, T., Mowbray, D., & Macfarlane, P. I. (2008). Lingual sucrose reduces the pain response to nasogastric tube insertion: A randomised clinical trial. *Archives of Disease in Childhood. Fetal and Neonatal Edition, 93*(2), F100–F103.

Meek, J. (2012). Options for procedural pain in newborn infants. *Archives of Disease in Childhood. Education and Practice Edition, 97*(1), 23–28.

Melnyk, B. M., & Feinstein, N. F. (2009). Reducing hospital expenditures with the COPE (Creating Opportunities for Parent Empowerment) program for parents and premature infants: An analysis of direct healthcare neonatal intensive care unit costs and savings. *Nursing Administration Quarterly, 33*(1), 32–37.

Melnyk, B. M., Feinstein, N. F., Alpert-Gillis, L., Fairbanks, E., Crean, H. F., Sinkin, R. A.,... Gross, S. J. (2006). Reducing premature infants' length of stay and improving parents' mental health outcomes with the Creating Opportunities for Parent Empowerment (COPE) neonatal intensive care unit program: A randomized, controlled trial. *Pediatrics, 118*(5), e1414–e1427.

Menon, G., Anand, K. J., & McIntosh, N. (1998). Practical approach to analgesia and sedation in the neonatal intensive care unit. *Seminars in Perinatology, 22*(5), 417–424.

Montirosso, R., & Provenzi, L. (2015). Implications of epigenetics and stress regulation on research and developmental care of preterm infants. *Journal of Obstetric, Gynecologic, and Neonatal Nursing, 44*(2), 174–182.

Narvaez, D. (2011, December). Dangers of "crying it out": Damaging children and their relationships for the long term. *Psychology Today.* Retrieved from https://www.psychologytoday.com/blog/moral-landscapes/201112/dangers-crying-it-out

Obeidat, H., Kahalaf, I., Callister, L. C., & Froelicher, E. S. (2009). Use of facilitated tucking for nonpharmacological pain management in preterm infants: A systematic review. *The Journal of Perinatal & Neonatal Nursing, 23*(4), 372–377.

Oliver, K. B., Lehmann, H. P., Wolff, A. C., Davidson, L. W., Donohue, P. K., Gilmore, M. M.,...Roderer, N. K. (2011). Evaluating information prescriptions in two clinical environments. *Journal of the Medical Library Association, 99*(3), 237–246.

Pandey, M., Datta, V., & Rehan, H. S. (2013). Role of sucrose in reducing painful response to orogastric tube insertion in preterm neonates. *Indian Journal of Pediatrics, 80*(6), 476–482.

Peyrovi, H., Alinejad-Naeini, M., Mohagheghi, P., & Mehran, A. (2014). The effect of facilitated tucking position during endotracheal suctioning on physiological responses and coping with stress in premature infants: A randomized controlled crossover study. *The Journal of Maternal-Fetal & Neonatal Medicine, 27*(15), 1555–1559.

Pillai Riddell, R. R., Racine, N. M., Turcotte, K., Uman, L. S., Horton, R.E., Din Osmun, L.,… Gerwitz-Stern, A. (2011). Non-pharmacological management of infant and young children procedural pain. *Cochrane Database of Systematic Reviews, 2011*(10), CD006275. doi:10.1002/14651858.CD006275.pub2

Pillai Riddell, R., Taddio, A., McMurtry, C. M., Shah, V., Noel, M., & Chambers, C. T.; HELPinKIDS&Adults Team. (2015). Process interventions for vaccine injections: Systematic review of randomized controlled trials and quasi-randomized controlled trials. *The Clinical Journal of Pain, 31*(10 Suppl.), S99–108.

Pinheiro, J. M., Furdon, S., & Ochoa, L. F. (1993). Role of local anesthesia during lumbar puncture in neonates. *Pediatrics, 91*(2), 379–382.

Provenzi, L., Fumagalli, M., Sirgiovanni, I., Giorda, R., Pozzoli, U., Morandi, F.,… Montirosso, R. (2015). Pain-related stress during the neonatal intensive care unit stay and SLC6A4 methylation in very preterm infants. *Frontiers in Behavioral Neuroscience, 9*, 99.

Ranger, M., Chau, C. M., Garg, A., Woodward, T. S., Beg, M. F., Bjornson, B.,…Grunau, R. E. (2013). Neonatal pain-related stress predicts cortical thickness at age 7 years in children born very preterm. *PloS One, 8*(10), e76702.

Ranger, M., & Grunau, R. E. (2014). Early repetitive pain in preterm infants in relation to the developing brain. *Pain Management, 4*(1), 57–67.

Reavey, D. A., Haney, B. M., Atchison, L., Anderson, B., Sandritter, T., & Pallotto, E. K. (2014). Improving pain assessment in the NICU: A quality improvement project. *Advances in Neonatal Care, 14*(3), 144–153.

Reis, M. D., Rempel, G. R., Scott, S. D., Brady-Fryer, B. A., & Van Aerde, J. (2010). Developing nurse/parent relationships in the NICU through negotiated partnership. *Journal of Obstetric, Gynecologic, and Neonatal Nursing, 39*(6), 675–683.

Rodkey, E. N., & Pillai Riddell, R. (2013). The infancy of infant pain research: The experimental origins of infant pain denial. *The Journal of Pain, 14*(4), 338–350.

Schore, A. N. (2001). The effects of early relational trauma on right brain development, affect regulation, and infant mental health. *Infant Mental Health Journal, 22*(1–2), 201–269.

Shah, P. S., Herbozo, C., Aliwalas, L. L., & Shah, V. S. (2012). Breastfeeding or breast milk for procedural pain in neonates. *Cochrane Database of Systematic Reviews, 2012*(12), CD004950.

Shah, V. S., & Ohlsson, A. (2011). Venepuncture versus heel lance for blood sampling in term neonates. *Cochrane Database of Systematic Reviews, 2011*(10), CD001452. doi:10.1002/14651858.CD001452.pub4

Sharek, P. J., Powers, R., Koehn, A., & Anand, K. J. (2006). Evaluation and development of potentially better practices to improve pain management of neonates. *Pediatrics, 118*(Suppl. 2), S78–S86.

Shonkoff, J. P., & Garner, A. S.; Committee on Psychosocial Aspects of Child and Family Health; Committee on Early Childhood, Adoption, and Dependent Care; Section on Developmental and Behavioral Pediatrics. (2012). The lifelong effects of early childhood adversity and toxic stress. *Pediatrics, 129*(1), e232–e246.

Simons, S. H., van Dijk, M., Anand, K. S., Roofthooft, D., van Lingen, R. A., & Tibboel, D. (2003). Do we still hurt newborn babies? A prospective study of procedural pain and analgesia in neonates. *Archives of Pediatrics & Adolescent Medicine, 157*(11), 1058–1064.

Simons, J., Franck, L., & Roberson, E. (2001). Parent involvement in children's pain care: Views of parents and nurses. *Journal of Advanced Nursing, 36*(4), 591–599.

Soltis, J. (2004). The signal functions of early infant crying. *The Behavioral and Brain Sciences, 27*(4), 443–458; discussion 459.

Stevens, B., Yamada, J., Lee, G. Y., & Ohlsson, A. (2013). Sucrose for analgesia in newborn infants undergoing painful procedures. *Cochrane Database of Systematic Reviews, 2013*(1), CD001069. doi:10.1002/14651858.CD001069.pub4

Taddio, A., MacDonald, N. E., Smart, S., Parikh, C., Allen, V., Halperin, B., & Shah, V. (2014). Impact of a parent-directed pamphlet about pain management during infant vaccinations on maternal knowledge and behavior. *Neonatal Network: NN, 33*(2), 74–82.

Taddio, A., Ohlsson, A., Einarson, T. R., Stevens, B., & Koren, G. (1998). A systematic review of lidocaine-prilocaine cream (EMLA) in the treatment of acute pain in neonates. *Pediatrics, 101*(2), E1.

Taddio, A., Shah, V., McMurtry, C. M., MacDonald, N. E., Ipp, M., Riddell, R. P., . . . Chambers, C. T.; HELPinKids&Adults Team. (2015). Procedural and physical interventions for vaccine injections: Systematic review of randomized controlled trials and quasi-randomized controlled trials. *The Clinical Journal of Pain, 31*(10 Suppl.), S20–S37.

Valeri, B. O., Holsti, L., & Linhares, M. B. (2015). Neonatal pain and developmental outcomes in children born preterm: A systematic review. *The Clinical Journal of Pain, 31*(4), 355–362.

Vazquez, V., Cong, X., & DeJong, A. (2015). Maternal and paternal knowledge and perceptions regarding infant pain in the NICU. *Neonatal Network, 34*(6), 337–344.

Vinall, J., & Grunau, R. E. (2014). Impact of repeated procedural pain-related stress in infants born very preterm. *Pediatric Research, 75*(5), 584–587.

Vinall, J., Miller, S. P., Bjornson, B. H., Fitzpatrick, K. P., Poskitt, K. J., Brant, R., . . . Grunau, R. E. (2014). Invasive procedures in preterm children: Brain and cognitive development at school age. *Pediatrics, 133*(3), 412–421.

Vinall, J., Miller, S. P., Chau, V., Brummelte, S., Synnes, A. R., & Grunau, R. E. (2012). Neonatal pain in relation to postnatal growth in infants born very preterm. *Pain, 153*(7), 1374–1381.

Waddell, G. (1987). 1987 Volvo award in clinical sciences. A new clinical model for the treatment of low-back pain. *Spine, 12*(7), 632–644.

Walden, M., & Gibbins, S. (2012). *Newborn pain assessment and management: Guideline for practice.* Glenview, IL: National Association of Neonatal Nurses.

Walker, S. M. (2014). Neonatal pain. *Paediatric Anaesthesia, 24*(1), 39–48.

Walker, S. M., Beggs, S., & Baccei, M. L. (2016). Persistent changes in peripheral and spinal nociceptive processing after early tissue injury. *Experimental Neurology, 275*(Pt. 2), 253–260.

Walter-Nicolet, E., Annequin, D., Biran, V., Mitanchez, D., & Tourniaire, B. (2010). Pain management in newborns: From prevention to treatment. *Paediatric Drugs, 12*(6), 353–365.

Ward-Larson, C., Horn, R. A., & Gosnell, F. (2004). The efficacy of facilitated tucking for relieving procedural pain of endotracheal suctioning in very low birthweight infants. *MCN. The American Journal of Maternal Child Nursing, 29*(3), 151–156; quiz 157.

Welch, M. G., Firestein, M. R., Austin, J., Hane, A. A., Stark, R. I., Hofer, M. A., . . . Myers, M. M. (2015). Family nurture intervention in the neonatal intensive care unit improves social-relatedness, attention, and neurodevelopment of preterm infants at 18 months in a randomized controlled trial. *Journal of Child Psychology and Psychiatry, and Allied Disciplines, 56*(11), 1202–1211.

Wotherspoon, E., Hawkins, E., & Gough, P. (2009). *Emotional trauma in infancy.* CECW Information Sheet #75E. Toronto, Canada: University of Toronto Factor-Inwentash Faculty of Social Work. Retrieved from www.cecw-cepb.ca/DocsEng/InfantTrauma75E.pdf

Wotherspoon, E., & Gough, P. (2008). *Assessing emotional neglect in infants.* CECW Information Sheet #59E. Toronto, Canada: University of Toronto, Faculty of Social Work.

Yin, T., Yang, L., Lee, T. Y., Li, C. C., Hua, Y. M., & Liaw, J. J. (2015). Development of atraumatic heel-stick procedures by combined treatment with non-nutritive sucking, oral sucrose, and facilitated tucking: A randomised, controlled trial. *International Journal of Nursing Studies, 52*(8), 1288–1299.

CHAPTER 7

Guidelines for Protected Sleep

The nicest thing for me is sleep, then at least I can dream.
        —Marilyn Monroe

This guideline presents the latest evidence-based research, along with clinical practice recommendations and implementation strategies related to protecting, supporting, and practicing safe sleep in the neonatal intensive care unit (Table 7.1).

TABLE 7.1   Attributes and Criteria of the Protected Sleep Core Measure

Attributes	Criteria
Practices that protect sleep integrity and support circadian/diurnal rhythmicity are integrated into the culture of care	1. Scheduled, nonemergent caregiving is contingent on the infant's sleep–wake state and adapted accordingly 2. Cycled lighting is provided to support circadian rhythms 3. Staff and family are competent in the assessment of infant sleep–wake states
Care strategies that support infant sleep are implemented in partnership with the family	1. Skin-to-skin care is an integral part of the daily care of eligible infants; length of sessions is documented in the medical record 2. An individualized sleep hygiene routine is an integral part of daily care 3. Supportive sleep routines are developed in partnership with family and documented to ensure consistency
Staff role -model compliance with recommended back to sleep safety practices for eligible infants	1. All staff are competent in the most current "back to sleep" recommendations from the AAP; competency is documented 2. There is a clear protocol and/or algorithm for the initiation of "back to sleep" practices 3. Parents demonstrate competency in "back to sleep" recommendations before infant discharge to home

AAP, American Academy of Pediatrics.

◼ GUIDELINE OBJECTIVES

- To define the criteria and recommendations for best practice in protecting, supporting, and practicing safe sleep in the neonatal intensive care unit (NICU)
- To present the evidence that supports the criteria and best practice recommendations for protected sleep in the NICU
- To present clinical practice strategies that facilitate adoption and integration of evidence-based best practices in protecting, supporting, and practicing safe sleep in the hospital

◼ MAJOR OUTCOMES CONSIDERED

The impact of the consistently reliable application of the protected sleep core measure attributes and criteria on the NICU patient, family, and staff includes:

- Physiologic, psychosocial, and psycho-emotional outcomes
- Patient safety and quality clinical outcomes

◼ PROTECTING SLEEP

Let her sleep for when she wakes, she will move mountains.
        —Napoléon Bonaparte

Interventions and Practice Considerations

1. Create and maintain an individualized approach to nonemergent caregiving guided by the infant's sleep–wake state
   - Best practice considerations include an individualized approach to care based on infant's readiness behaviors
2. Create and maintain cycled lighting in the patient care area
   - Best practice considerations include maintaining both day and night light levels within the recommended range, with nighttime levels in the lower range—avoid near darkness as well as continuous bright lighting in the patient care area
3. Create and maintain staff proficiency in assessing infant sleep–wake states
   - Best practice considerations include annual competency-based training (CBT) for all staff; include comprehensive sleep education and sleep–wake state assessment for all multidisciplinary new hires

The Evidence

Sleep is essential for homeostasis, neurosensory and motor system development, learning and memory, immune function, growth, as well as brain plasticity (Besedovsky, Lange, & Born, 2012; Born, Rasch, & Gais, 2006; Calciolari & Montirosso, 2011; Graven & Browne, 2008; Ibarro-Coronado et al., 2015; Miyamoto & Hensch, 2003; Peirano & Algarin, 2007; Watson & Buzsáki, 2015). Fetal sleep–wake cycles have been identified as early as 30 weeks gestation and the prevailing fetal sleep state is active sleep (Mirmiran, Maas, & Ariagno, 2003; Peirano, Algarín, & Uauy, 2003; Scher, Johnson, & Holditch-Davis, 2005). A term newborn infant requires 14 to 17 hours of sleep per day (Hirshkowitz et al., 2015) with 50% of the sleep time being spent in active sleep (rapid eye movement [REM]) and 50% quiet sleep (non-rapid eye movement [NREM]); however, in preterm infants up to 80% of their sleep cycle is spent in active sleep (REM) and their daily sleep requirement approaches 20 hours (Calciolari & Montirosso, 2011). The organization of sleep–wake states reflects brain maturation facilitating and enhancing our capability to process wakeful experiences and transform them into memories. These memories facilitate our *autonoetic awareness* or consciousness (which the human fetus is capable of, based on the presence of thalamocorticial and corticocortical spinal tracts by approximately 24 weeks gestation) (Fivush, 2011; Lagercrantz, 2014; Lagercrantz & Changeux, 2009, 2010). When we are awake or vigilant, we acquire a variety of inputs, some meaningful and others not so meaningful and these are processed at a neurobiological level while we sleep. Quiet sleep (NREM) is associated with the pre-consolidation phase, whereby meaningful events or inputs (skin-to-skin, sound of mother's voice) are separated from what has been referred to as "interference" inputs (such as light, noise, pain). Once this has taken place, the brain begins the consolidation phase, which occurs during active sleep (REM) and prepares the meaningful inputs for permanent storage into memory (Calciolari & Montirosso, 2011).

Infants make meaning out of the world through unconscious and involuntary processes related to how the environment and associated stimuli make them feel (Tronick & Beeghly, 2011). These "meaningful" events can be positive or negative, occur while the infant is awake (vigilant state) or in quiet sleep, and trigger learning (Graham, Fisher, & Pfeifer, 2013). These emotional memories are processed during active sleep (REM), the predominant sleep state of premature infants through term-corrected gestational age (Calciolari & Montirosso, 2011; Foreman, Thomas, & Blackburn, 2008; Groch, Zinke, Wilhelm, & Born, 2015), and lay the foundation for infants' behavioral and mental health trajectory. The valence of emotional events will influence the quality of sleep, impact sympathetic activity, and increase infant vulnerability to emotion dysregulation and subsequent mental health challenges (Delannoy, Mandai, Honoré, Kobayashi, & Sequeira, 2015; Graham, Pfeifer, Fisher, Carpenter, & Fair, 2015). Protecting sleep during neonatal intensive care is of paramount importance and encompasses caregiving modifications, environmental adaptations, as well as a focus on intersubjectivity and interpersonal experiences (Allen, 2012; Bertelle, Sevestre, Laou-Hap, Nagahapitiye, & Sizun, 2007;

Calciolari & Montirosso, 2011). In addition to sleep's role in processing exogenous events, sleep is critical for many intrinsic endogenous activities, specifically neurosensory development (Graven, 2006; Graven & Browne, 2008).

Assessing behavioral sleep–wake states guides an individualized approach to caregiving and thereby protects the sleeping infant and his or her developmental potential (Coughlin, 2011, 2014; Coughlin, Gibbins, & Hoath, 2009). Active sleep in both preterm and term infants presents with sporadic large body movements, irregular respirations, increased heart rate variability, and REMs; quiet sleep presents with eyes closed and no ocular movement observable, regular and rhythmic respirations that may include some abdominal movements, and limited motor activity (see Figure 7.1; Elder, Campbell, Larsen, & Galletly, 2011; Holditch-Davis & Edwards, 1998). Sleep–wake transitions and sleep organization are markers for neuromaturation and can predict short-term neurodevelopmental outcomes (Weisman et al., 2011). Sleep–wake cycling can be recorded and measured using continuous EEG monitoring in vulnerable infants in the NICU as demonstrated by Palmu, Kirjavainen, Stjerna, Salokivi, and Vanhatalo (2013) and Stevenson, Palmu, Wikström, Hellström-Westas, and Vanhatalo (2014). This potentially better practice in sleep–wake assessment provides NICU clinicians with real-time information to guide neuroprotective strategies, optimize care delivery, and improve infant outcomes (Scher, 2004).

Cycled lighting in the NICU has been shown to improve weight gain, decrease the length of hospital stay, reduce the amount of crying and fussing time, and has shown trends in a decreased incidence of retinopathy of prematurity when compared to infants nursed in environments of near darkness or continuous bright light (Guyer et al,. 2012; Morag & Ohlsson, 2013; Vasquez-Ruiz et al., 2014). Improved oxygen saturation as well as the emergence of a daily melatonin rhythm were additional outcomes associated with cycled lighting in the NICU (Vasquez-Ruiz et al., 2014).

Cost Analysis

The economic implications of protecting sleep in the NICU are related to the benefits described in the previous section, specifically better growth and a reduced hospital stay. The average daily cost of NICU care in the United States is in excess of $3,000, and this number does not begin to calculate the human costs associated with this traumatic life event; reducing the length of stay by adopting evidence-based practices that protect sleep are easily worth the effort.

Recommendations for Best Practices in Protecting Sleep in the NICU (Table 7.2)

TABLE 7.2   Major Practice Recommendations and Implementation Strategies—Protection of Sleep

Recommendations	Implementation Strategy
1. Develop an education module on sleep–wake states for parents and staff	a. Review your available education resources (instructor led, eLearning, mobile resources, pamphlets) b. Collect baseline knowledge levels from staff and parents (this will allow you to measure your success) c. Introduce education module and follow with a posttest to measure the impact of teaching d. Consider a practicum component to the teaching to allow application of the new knowledge e. Outline a plan for continuing education, integration to orientation across all disciplines

2. Define what constitutes nonemergent caregiving and develop an algorithm to guide clinicians in the clinical application of individualized care based on the infant's sleep–wake state	a. Establish a multidisciplinary task force to define nonemergent caregiving—task force attributes:
	  i. ≤10 persons
	  ii. Balance the power (equal number of staff to leader presence)
	  iii. Voluntary participation
	  iv. Bias for action—do not meet to meet, you meet to change!
	b. Test the definition using the PDSA method
	  i. Is it feasible?
	  ii. What kind of modifications were necessary to balance the infant's sleep needs with the clinician's needs?
	  iii. What outcomes or indicators tell you that your change is good, bad, or indifferent (big data, frequency of nuisance alarms, weight gain)?
	  iv. Decide and collect benchmark data
	c. Once you have refined your practice change idea, evaluate with a larger group of supportive staff
	  i. Reevaluate the findings
	  ii. Revise as indicated
	d. Draft clinical practice algorithm and practice guideline
	e. Implement new practice, monitor compliance, measure results
	f. Provide continual feedback to staff
	g. Publish and/or present results

3. Adopt a cycled lighting protocol (Guyer et al., 2012; Morag & Ohlsson, 2013; Vasquez-Ruiz et al., 2014)	a. Consider replicating the Guyer et al. (2012) study b. Collect baseline measurements of your current lighting levels (make sure to get readings from various locations in and adjacent to the patient care area) c. Draft a test of change using the PDSA method a. Clearly define your aim and your process/outcome measures d. Test your change idea, evaluate, revise, adopt e. Consider incorporating some reminders and redundancies to help staff sustain the practice over time (signage, fluctuating light levels before the change in light condition, a musical snippet, etc.) f. Report findings back to the team g. Publish and/or present results

PDSA, Plan-Do-Study-Act.

Sample Clinical Guide

The Neonatal Sleep-Wake Assessment tool (NeoSWAT) was developed as a teaching resource for neonatal clinicians (Figure 7.1).

	Neonatal Sleep-Wake Assessment Tool (Neo SWAT)			
Indicator	0	1	2	Total Score
Eyes	Lids closed with intermittent REM (rapid eye movement)	Lids closed; no REM observed	Lids open	
Respirations	Uneven respirations	Relatively regular and abdominal	Regular respirations, may be crying	
Facial expressions	Negative facial expressions (cry face or a frown)	Quiet facies, occasional sigh/startle	Interactive facies	
Motor activity	Sporadic motor movements, muscle tone low between movements	Tonic level of motor tone is maintained and motor activity is limited to startles or sighs	Motor activity varies but is usually high	
			Cumulative Score	

Score < 3: is in clear sleep state, do not disturb unless there is a medical emergency.

Score 3–6: if cares are indicated, infant should be aroused gently with soft vocalizations and firm but gentle tactile input to a non-vulnerable area (i.e., placing caregiver's hand on the infant's back); increase verbal and tactile input as the infant's arousal level rises.

Score > 6: infant is waking/awake and ready for cares.

FIGURE 7.1   Neonatal Sleep Wake Assessment Tool (neo SWAT).

■ SUPPORTING SLEEP

Without enough sleep, we all become tall 2-year-olds.
        —JoJo Jensen

Interventions and Practice Considerations

1. Create and maintain a systematic approach to the provision of skin-to-skin care in the NICU

- Best practice considerations include an evidence-based practice guideline with clearly articulated eligibility criteria; a documentation strategy that captures the dose-dependent effect of skin-to-skin care experiences; and, a systematic, competency-based process for establishing the standing transfer as the preferred infant transfer method for staff and parent
2. Create and maintain individualized sleep hygiene routines for all infants as they approach discharge, attain 4 months corrected gestational age, and/or demonstrate a decrease in their total sleep time
   - Best practice considerations include staff partnering with parents to create a sleep diary for their hospitalized infant and share sleep observations and sleep trends to inform bedtime routines
3. Engage and empower parents to outline bedtime and nap routines that will be sustained over time
   - Best practice considerations include modifying staff routines to meet the infant's needs and cultivating parent–infant rituals related to sleep to support this emotional and physiologic transition consistently

The Evidence

The body of evidence to support skin-to-skin care in the NICU is expansive. Benefits include a decreased risk for morbidity, mortality, hospital-acquired infection/sepsis, neurodevelopmental disabilities, and cardiovascular disease in adulthood, as well as improved growth, breastfeeding, and maternal attachment (Conde-Agudelo & Diaz-Rossello, 2014; Moore, Anderson, Bergman, & Dowswell, 2012). Additional studies demonstrate that skin-to-skin care accelerates brain maturation in premature infants, decreases cortisol levels in both mother and infant, and is an effective nonpharmacologic strategy to manage procedural pain (Kaffashi, Scher, Ludington-Hoe, & Loparo, 2013; Ludington-Hoe et al., 2006; Neu, Hazel, Robinson, Schmiege, & Laudenslager, 2014; Scher et al., 2009). The acceleration of brain maturation is quantified by a decrease in active sleep and an increase in quiet sleep; this very favorable outcome has been associated with quality sleep in preterm infants during skin-to-skin care (Ludington-Hoe et al., 2006). More organized sleep–wake cyclicity was observed in infants who received skin-to-skin care when compared to a control group receiving traditional care leading researchers to conclude that skin-to-skin care not only supported infant neurophysiologic development but also improved parental mood, behavior, and perceptions of self as an effective parent (Feldman, Eidelman, Sirota, & Weller, 2002; Jefferies et al., 2012). Prolonged sleep deprivation in mammals results in death. The implication for sleep deprivation in human neonates continues to unfold but sleep deprivation for this patient population has been linked with a lower pain threshold coupled with the fear and anxiety associated with maternal separation, and can interfere with the quantity and quality of sleep for this fragile population—adopting and integrating kangaroo mother care (aka skin to skin) is a profoundly effective, evidence-based intervention (Bonan, Pimentel Filho, Tristão, Jesus, & Campos Junior, 2015).

Mindell, Li, Sadeh, Kwon, and Goh (2015) recommend introducing sleep routines early in infancy to fully maximize the benefits of the bedtime routine. Harrison and Goodman (2015) conducted a retrospective study looking at trends in NICU admission and discovered that there is an increase in overall admission rates and that more than half of the newborns admitted were born at term gestation with a birthweight of at least 2,500 g. The average length of hospital stay for a very preterm infant ranges between 2 and 3 months (Numerato et al., 2015) and for late preterm and term infants the average length of stay can range between 7 and 45 days (based on the admitting diagnosis; Lusk et al., 2014; March of Dimes Perinatal Data Center, 2011). Once an infant has stabilized from their initial life-threatening condition, creating a bedtime routine with the family validates parental role identity and forms the foundation for the parent–infant lifelong relationship (Craig et al., 2015). After 4 months postnatal age, infant sleep time requirements decrease to approximately 12 to 15 hours per day (Hirshkowitz et al., 2015) and this transition in sleep requirements marks the beginning of sleep consolidation and napping. Implementing a bedtime routine for infants has been shown to improve latency to sleep onset, decrease the frequency and duration of night awakenings, improve sleep continuity, increase sleep time, in addition to improving maternal mood (Mindell, Telofski, Wiegand, & Kurtz, 2009; Staples, Bates, & Petersen, 2015). Mindell et al. (2015) observed a dose-dependent relationship between bedtime routines and improved sleep quality—demonstrating that consistency makes a big impact.

Daytime napping has demonstrated benefits across cognitive domains and language acquisition for infants up to 2 years of age; beyond 2 years, daytime napping had a negative effect on nighttime sleep quality and total sleep time (Gómez, Bootzin, & Nadel, 2006; Horvath, Liu, & Plunkett, 2015; Thorpe et al., 2015). Several NICUs have adopted "quiet time" initiatives, specifically aimed at reducing noise levels in the NICU but this quality improvement practice also serves as a vehicle to provide protected time for the infant to sleep or nap (Laubach, Wilhelm, & Carter, 2014; Ribeiro dos Santos et al., 2015). Creating an environment conducive to sleeping through the quiet time initiative not only decreases ambient noise levels but can also decrease nuisance alarms (Rolfes, Sealer, & Coughlin, 2014).

Developing supportive sleep routines in partnership with the NICU staff, parents cultivate a trusting parent–professional relationship while building parental confidence and competence in recognizing their infant's states, reading their infant's cues, and understanding their infant's unique capabilities (Bruns & McCollum, 2002; Tedder, 2008). A 2011 systematic review on the benefits of family-centered care for children with special health care needs indicates that it is the relationship between the family and the health care team that has the most significant impact for positive results (Kuhlthau et al., 2011). Parents want and need to care for their infant in the NICU and creating daily bedtime and napping routines solidifies parental role identity, decreases infant and parent stress, and prepares the infant–family dyad for transition to home (Cooper et al., 2007; Craig et al., 2015; Gooding et al., 2011).

Cost Analysis

As sleep is a critical part of brain maturation, the cost–benefit of protecting sleep in the NICU is well worth the investment. Linked to a decreased length of stay, morbidity, and mortality, efforts to support sleep are recouped with improved neurodevelopmental outcomes for this vulnerable population, smoother transitions to home, and a decrease in hospital readmissions (Bastani, Abadi, & Haghani, 2015).

Recommendations to Support Sleep in the NICU (Table 7.3)

TABLE 7.3   Major Practice Recommendations and Implementation Strategies—Supporting Sleep

Recommendations	Implementation Strategy
1. Standardize and formalize your skin-to-skin care practices (Coughlin, 2015)	a. Review your current skin-to-skin care practices and policy (Specifically, does your policy have clearly articulated eligibility criteria? Recommended infant transfer method? What are your documentation expectations? How are staff AND parents deemed competent in providing skin-to-skin care?) 　i. Consider performing a "failure modes and effects analysis" (Figure 7.2) 　ii. A key failure mode is an infant meeting eligibility criteria not receiving skin-to-skin care when the parents are present (the existing body of evidence is too powerful to defer a skin-to-skin time because of clinician time constraints; Davanzo et al., 2013) b. Revise your skin-to-skin care policy/guideline to reflect latest evidence and include eligibility criteria c. Educate parents and staff on the evidence-based benefits associated with kangaroo care d. Develop a competency-based training for parents and staff on the infant transfer (see Figures 7.3 and 7. 4)—remember, the best practice is the standing transfer (Ludington-Hoe 2008; Neu, Browne, & Vojir, 2000) e. Collect benchmark data regarding the frequency in which skin-to-skin care is currently documented; current transfer method (consider gauging staff confidence with the infant transfer; Coughlin, 2015) f. Initiate a test of change (PDSA); identify success indicators g. Report results to staff h. Audit practice compliance, documentation i. Publish and/or present results
2. Engage parents to keep a sleep diary of their infant to discover their infant's sleep routine and plan for nighttime rituals around sleep	a. Design a sleep diary that will reflect your unit's routines in partnership with a parent task force or modify the sample diary that accompanies this chapter b. Diary should include sleep time, feedings (maybe include type of feeding), tests, skin-to-skin times, and other activities c. Decide how the diary will be maintained (i.e., kept at the bedside, completed by the parents)

(continued)

TABLE 7.3   Major Practice Recommendations and Implementation Strategies—Supporting Sleep   *(continued)*

Recommendations	Implementation Strategy
	d. Once you have completed your draft diary, test it out with select parents e. Obtain feedback from parents and staff (how does the diary help the parent/the clinician/the baby?) i. Consider evaluating parent engagement as a result of this project using the NICU PREEMI (Samra et al., 2015) f. How does the diary information guide caregiving? How does it facilitate a bedtime routine for the infant–family dyad? g. Consider publishing and presenting your results

3. Partner with parents to develop a bedtime routine for their hospitalized infant(s)	a. Outline various activities that support sleep for the hospitalized infant (skin-to-skin care, swaddled bath, massage, holding, rocking, singing, reading a story, and so on)
	b. Share, discuss, mentor, and empower parents to adopt these various strategies into their parenting repertoire with their hospitalized infant
	c. Ask the parents if they would like to create a daytime and nighttime ritual to support their infant's sleep
	   i. Discuss how the staff can support these rituals
	   ii. Identify and resolve potential schedule conflicts
	   iii. Invite the parents to identify what times work best for them, what they can commit to based on their infant's sleep diary (consistency and routines support the infant's psychoemotional development and also validate parental role identity; Craig et al., 2015; Vasquez & Cong, 2014; Wigert, Hellström, & Berg, 2008)
	d. Implement the sleep time routines/rituals and evaluate the impact on the infant, parent, staff (consider survey/interview for the adults and for the infant, consider looking at big data, sleep time, growth, and so on)
	e. Refine plan as necessary
	f. Publish and/or present results

PREEMI, Parent Risk Evaluation & Engagement Model & Instrument.

Clinician and Parent Resources

Steps in the Process	Failure Mode	Failure Causes	Failure Effects	Likelihood of Occurrence (1–10)	Likelihood of Detection (1–10)	Severity (1–10)	Risk Priority Number (RPN)	Actions to Reduce Occurrence of Failure
1								
2								
3								
4								
5								
6								
7								
8								
9								
10								
11								
12								
13								
14								
15								
							Total RPN (sum of all RPNs)	

Failure Mode: What could go wrong?
Failure Causes: Why would the failure happen?
Failure Effects: What would be the consequences of failure?
Likelihood of Occurrence: 1–10, 10 = very likely to occur
Likelihood of Detection: 1–10, 10 = very unlikely to detect
Severity: 1–10, 10 = most severe effect
Risk Priority Number (RPN): Likelihood of Occurrence x Likelihood of Detection x Severity

FIGURE 7.2   Failure Modes and Effects Analysis template, retrieved from www.ihi.org/resources/pages/tools/failuremodesandeffectsanalysistool.aspx

Step	Action	Validation of Competence	Complete ☑
1	Completes parent education for kangaroo care in the NICU	Certificate of completion	☐
2	Reviews the unit protocol and understands the eligibility criteria for kangaroo care	Observation	☐
3	Mock-up return demonstration of the kangaroo care procedure for standing infant transfer and parent seated transfer with doll simulator	Observation	☐
4	Assess own infant's eligibility and readiness for kangaroo care.	Observation	☐
5	Prepare self for kangaroo care	Observation	☐
	a. Ensure proper attire for parent		
	b. Ensure parent personal needs are attended to prior to the session		
	c. Ensure comfortable, safe seating and privacy for the session		
6	Prepare infant for kangaroo care	Observation	☐
	a. Ensure proper attire for infant		
	b. Ensure infant's personal needs are attended to prior to the session		
	c. Ensure comfortable, safe seating and privacy for the session		
6	Perform transfer in accordance with parent preference and unit protocol	Observation	☐
7	Review safety plan once the parent is settled in kangaroo position (how will the parent access a clinician, when should the parent access the clinician)	Observation	☐
10	Perform return transfer in accordance with parent preference and unit protocol	Observation	☐
11	Support your infant's transition once in the incubator with gentle containment, soothing vocalizations, etc.	Observation & Documentation	☐

Parent: _____   _____   _____
    Printed name   *Signature*   *Date*

Observer: _____   _____   _____
    Printed name   *Signature*   *Date*

FIGURE 7.3   Sample kangaroo care parent competency checklist.

Step	Action	Demonstration Mode of Competence	Complete ☑
1	Complete learning module	Certificate of completion	☐
2	Mock-up return demonstration of kangaroo care (standing transfer and seated transfer)	Observation	☐
3	Assess infant's readiness for kangaroo care	Observation	☐
4	Assess parent's readiness for kangaroo care (parent must complete parent education module and comply with parent requirements in accordance with unit practice guideline)	Observation	☐
5	Prepare infant–parent dyad for kangaroo care	Observation	☐
	a. Ensure proper attire for parent and infant		
	b. Ensure parent personal needs are attended to prior to the session		
	c. Ensure comfortable, safe seating and privacy for the session		
6	Perform transfer in accordance with unit practice guideline	Observation	☐
7	Review safety plan with parent once infant–parent dyad is in kangaroo position (how will the parent access a clinician, when should the parent access the clinician)	Observation	☐
7	Document initiation time of kangaroo care session	Documentation	☐
8	Reassess dyad every 5 minutes x 3 then every 15 minutes x 2 then every 30 minutes (or as outlined in your unit practice guideline); record assessments	Documentation	☐
9	Document termination of kangaroo session and how the experience was tolerated by infant and parent	Documentation	☐
10	Prepare infant-parent dyad for infant transfer to incubator	Observation	☐
11	Perform return transfer in accordance with unit practice guideline	Observation	☐
12	Support infant's transition back to the incubator by monitoring/recording vital signs until they return to baseline	Observation and Documentation	☐

Clinician: _____ _____ _____
          Printed name   *Signature*   *Date*

Observer: _____ _____ _____
          Printed name   *Signature*   *Date*

FIGURE 7.4 Sample staff kangaroo care competency checklist.

▪ SAFE SLEEP

A mother's arms are made of tenderness and children sleep soundly in them.
> —Victor Hugo

Interventions and Practice Considerations

1. Create and maintain a systematic approach to staff competency-based education regarding the most recent safe sleep practice recommendations from the AAP
   - Best practice considerations include annual interdisciplinary training on the latest safe sleep practice recommendations with a pretest, posttest, and simulated return demonstration (this training should also be incorporated into new hire orientation)
2. Create and maintain a clear protocol and clinical algorithm outlining eligibility criteria for the initiation of safe sleep practices as well as the specific steps that define safe sleep practices in the NICU and home
   - Best practice considerations include a review of the literature regarding the latest recommendations to develop the protocol and algorithm, which will include documentation requirements and role-modeling expectations
3. Partner with parents and parent support resources to develop/adopt education materials for safe sleep practices in the hospital and home
   - Best practice considerations include using current, engaging teaching materials with parents and family members with a pre-/posttest to validate knowledge transfer and a real-time return demonstration of safe sleep practices for their baby

The Evidence

Although there are emerging new hypotheses challenging the pathogenesis of sudden infant death syndrome (SIDS) based on pathological findings and epidemiological risk factors (Goldwater, 2011), it is clear that the introduction of the "back to sleep" initiative in the 1990s has seen a decline in the mortality rate from SIDS by more than 50% (Kinney & Thach, 2009). In a recent breakdown of sudden unexpected infant death by cause, SIDS accounts for 45% of the infant deaths, with 24% of the deaths caused by accidental suffocation and strangulation in bed, and 31% of deaths from unknown causes (Centers for Disease Control and Prevention [CDC]/ National Center for Health Statistics [NCHS], National Vital Statistics System, Compressed Mortality File, 2013).

As seen in Figure 7.5 there was a dramatic decline in the SIDS rate in the wake of the Back-to-Sleep (BTS) campaign; however, these gains have leveled off and researchers are now reexamining the intrinsic and extrinsic risks associated with SIDS infants in the BTS era. Despite a statistically significant decrease in the

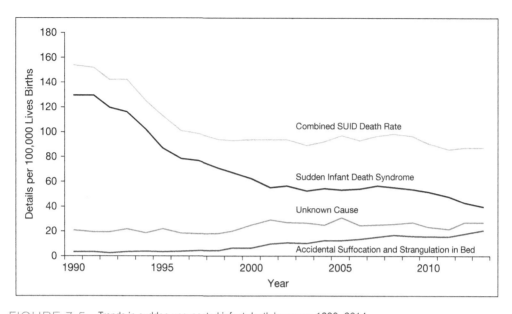

FIGURE 7.5   Trends in sudden unexpected infant death by cause, 1990–2014.

SUID, sudden unexpected infant death.

Source: Centers for Disease Control and Prevention/National Center for Health Statistics, National Vital Statistics System, Compressed Mortality File

percentage of SIDS infants positioned in prone for sleep (84%–48.5%), SIDS infants' bed sharing at the time of death increased from 19% to 40%, the percentage of SIDS infants found in an adult bed increased from 23% to 45% and SIDS victims born prematurely increased from 20% to 29% (Trachtenberg, Haas, Kinney, Stanley, & Krous, 2012).

Several researchers question the advances in neonatal care and the improved premature survival rates as contributing factors to the increase in premature SIDS victims and the overall plateaued SIDS rate (Garcia, Koschnitzky, & Ramirez, 2013). Although the mechanisms that place premature infants at higher risk are poorly understood, the risk for SIDS among premature infants remains significantly elevated (Malloy, 2013).

In a recent integrative review looking at whether or not nurses provide a safe sleep environment for infants in the hospital setting, Patton, Stiltner, Wright, and Kautz, (2015) conclude that some infants continue to be placed in positions that increase their risk for SIDS and that nurses are not following the 2011 AAP recommendations for a safe sleep environment. National and international surveys to NICU clinicians conclude that NICU discharge instructions regarding supine sleep positions at home are inconsistent, inappropriate, and in conflict with safe sleep recommendations (Aris et al., 2006; Dattani, Bhat, Rafferty, Hannam, & Greenough, 2011; Rao, May, Hannam, Rafferty, & Greenough, 2007). This global reality is a significant quality and safety concern. Organizations must take a systematic approach, adopting multimodal interventions to improve compliance with safe sleep practices in the neonatal intensive care unit and at home.

Gelfer, Cameron, Masters, and Kennedy (2013) report a statistically significant improvement in compliance with AAP safe sleep recommendations following a systematic approach integrating a NICU parent and staff education plan, developing a clinical algorithm (see Figure 7.6) for initiation of safe sleep practices, created bedside reminder cards, and implementing a post-discharge telephone reminder process for parents. In addition to the didactic NICU staff education, clinicians were also accountable to attend an annual skills evaluation on safe sleep role modeling; practice compliance was monitored with an audit tool that was completed randomly and unannounced by different members of the quality improvement (QI) project team facilitating feedback to staff as well as being a success metric (Gelfer et al., 2013). Voos, Terreros, Larimore, Leick-Rude, and Park (2015) report a 67% increase in safe sleep practice compliance following a revision and update of their NICU safe sleep policy combined with staff and parent education, adoption of a safe sleep checklist, and the use of infant sleep sacks.

Qureshi, Malkar, Splaingard, Khuhro, and Jadcherla (2015), using pH impedance methods and polysomnography analyzed the incidence of reflux in a cohort

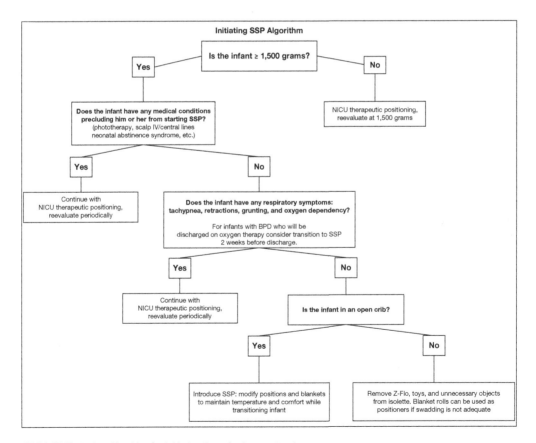

FIGURE 7.6   Algorithm for initiating the safe sleep protocol.

BPD, bronchopulmonary dysplasia; NICU, neonatal intensive care unit; SSP, safe sleep protocol.

Reprinted with permission from Dr. Polina Gelfer.

of preterm infants diagnosed with gastroesophageal reflux; positioned supine for sleep, the infants demonstrated a lower frequency of reflux events. In addition, there is no evidence to support the routine head-of-bed elevation in nonventilated, medically stable infants with suspected or even confirmed reflux and for infants with noncomplicated reflux, the general consensus is that no intervention is necessary (Corvaglia et al., 2013; Czinn & Blanchard, 2013; Pfister, 2012; Schurr & Findlater, 2012).

Following and role-modeling safe sleep practice recommendations consistently and reliably saves lives; however, hospital settings that serve the infant patient population continue to struggle to integrate these best practice strategies (AAP, 2011; Hitchcock, 2012; Lane, 2015). Leadership stakeholders must set the expectation and partner with clinicians and parents to achieve the desired goals for quality and patient safety (AAP, 2011; Hitchcock, 2012).

Cost Analysis

Although there may be costs associated with developing and managing the educational components of a safe sleep QI project, as well as sustaining the change through individual and organizational accountability, the benefit of decreased infant morbidity and mortality both inhospital and postdischarge is truly priceless.

Recommendations for Implementing Safe Sleep Practices in the NICU (Table 7.4)

TABLE 7.4   Major Practice Recommendations and Implementation Strategies—Safe Sleep

Recommendations	Implementation Strategy
1. Standardize safe sleep practice education across all disciplines and include a competency-based component for the role-modeling expectations (Gelfer et al., 2013)	a. Review the literature for the latest AAP recommendations for safe sleep b. Compare the evidence with your current policy/practice guideline and revise as indicated (be sure to include clearly defined eligibility criteria; Hwang et al., 2015) c. Develop an education plan that will present the evidence but also address misconceptions about "back to sleep" for the NICU patient (McMullen, Fioravanti, Brown, & Carey, 2016; Qureshi et al., 2015) d. Design a competency-based checklist that reflects clinicians' performance in role-modeling safe sleep; consider making this an annual competency until compliance is > 95% e. Record attendance and competency completions f. Audit practice compliance g. Outline a strategy to resolve compliance challenges h. Consider publishing/presenting your work

(continued)

TABLE 7.4   Major Practice Recommendations and Implementation Strategies—Safe Sleep   *(continued)*

Recommendations	Implementation Strategy

2. Define eligibility criteria for safe sleep practice initiation; include a clinical algorithm (Gelfer et al., 2013; Hwang et al., 2015)	a. Review the literature for the latest AAP recommendations for safe sleep
	b. Compare the evidence with your current policy/practice guideline and revise as indicated
	c. Consider a provider order to activate the safe sleep practice
	  i. Order should include safe sleep A, B, Cs: Alone, Back, Crib
	d. Test your change ideas, revise, and refine as indicated
	e. Review your documentation criteria related to safe sleep; revise to ensure that the practice can be audited
	f. Audit practice compliance
	g. Outline a strategy to resolve compliance challenges
	  i. Additional education (Lane, 2015)
	  ii. Disciplinary
	h. Consider publishing/presenting your work

3. Ensure that comprehensive, culturally congruent safe sleep education resources are available for all parents	a. Review your current available parent education resources/tools for safe sleep practices
	  i. Do they reflect the latest recommendations?
	  ii. Are they culturally sensitive for the families you serve?
	b. Consider expanding your resources to include multimodal teaching strategies
	c. Consider a competency-based checklist for parents performing safe sleep practices in the hospital and include this as a check off for discharge to home
	d. Integrate safe sleep practice into the parents nighttime/bedtime ritual with eligible infants; this could also serve as a checkoff

Tools and Patient Resources

PARENT RESOURCES

www.nichd.nih.gov/sts/about/Pages/default.aspx

www.firstcandle.org/new-moms-dads/bedtime-basics-for-babies

www.healthychildren.org/English/ages-stages/baby/sleep/Pages/A-Parents-Guide-to-Safe-Sleep.aspx

CLINICIAN RESOURCES

www.halosleep.com/in-hospital-sleepsack-program

AAP EXPANDED SAFE SLEEP RECOMMENDATIONS (2011)
1. Place infants to sleep on their backs (supine) from 32 weeks postconceptual age to 12 months of age
2. Use a firm sleep surface to decrease the risk of SIDS and suffocation

3. Caution parents not to share a bed with their infant while sleeping but encourage them to share the room (bed sharing is not recommended with siblings even in the case of twins)
4. Keep soft objects and loose items out of the crib; this includes bumper pads, wedges, ALL sleep positioners, blankets, and pillows
5. Give the infant a pacifier at naptime and bedtime (this has been shown to have a protective effect in reducing SIDS even for breastfeeding infants)
6. Avoid overheating the infant; dress the infant in one layer more than what a parent would be comfortable wearing
7. Teach women that breastfeeding helps reduce the risk of SIDS
8. Encourage tummy time while the infant is awake and alert and supervised by an adult
9. Encourage pregnant patients to get regular prenatal care to deep crease the risk of SIDS and SUID
10. Instruct women to avoid smoke exposure during pregnancy and following delivery
11. Caution women to avoid alcohol and illicit drug use during pregnancy and following delivery
12. Advise parents not to use cardiorespiratory monitors as these monitors have not been found to be effective in reducing SIDS risk
13. Urge parents to immunize the infant according to the AAP recommendations and to take him or her for regular well-child checks
14. Health care professionals, parents, and child care providers should follow SIDS risk reduction recommendations beginning at the infant's birth (caveat: full-term healthy infants)
15. Media and product manufacturers should follow safe sleep guidelines messaging and marketing their materials
16. The national campaign to reduce SIDS risk should focus on the infant's entire sleep environment not justly position
17. Ongoing SIDS research and surveillance are needed and this includes nursing research

■ REFERENCES

Allen, K. A. (2012). Promoting and protecting infant sleep. *Advances in Neonatal Care, 12*(50), 288–291.

American Academy of Pediatrics (2011). SIDS and other sleep-related infant deaths: Expansion of recommendations for a safe infant sleeping environment. *Pediatrics, 128*(5), 1031–1039.

Aris, C., Stevens, T. P., Lemura, C., Lipke, B., McMullen, S., Cote-Arsenault, D., & Consenstein, L. (2006). NICU nurses' knowledge and discharge teaching related to infant sleep position and risk of SIDS. *Advances in Neonatal Care, 6*(5), 281–294.

Bastani, F., Abadi, T. A., & Haghani, H. (2015). Effect of family-centered care on improving parental satisfaction and reducing re-admission among premature infants: A randomized controlled trial. *Journal of Clinical and Diagnostic Research, 9*(1), SC04–SC08.

Bertelle, V., Sevestre, A., Laou-Hap, K., Nagahapitiye, M. C., & Sizun, J. (2007). Sleep in the neonatal intensive care unit. *The Journal of Perinatal & Neonatal Nursing, 21*(2), 140–8; quiz 149.

Besedovsky, L., Lange, T., & Born, J. (2012). Sleep and immune function. *Pflü̈gers Archiv: European Journal of Physiology, 463*(1), 121–137.

Bonan, K. C., Pimentel Filho, J. d. a. C., Tristão, R. M., Jesus, J. A., & Campos Junior, D. (2015). Sleep deprivation, pain and prematurity: A review study. *Arquivos de Neuro-Psiquiatria, 73*(2), 147–154.

Born, J., Rasch, B., & Gais, S. (2006). Sleep to remember. *The Neuroscientist: A Review Journal Bringing Neurobiology, Neurology and Psychiatry, 12*(5), 410–424.

Bruns, D. A., & McCollum, J. A. (2002). Partnerships between mothers and professionals in the NICU: Caregiving, information exchange, and relationships. *Neonatal Network, 21*(7), 15–23.

Calciolari, G., & Montirosso, R. (2011). The sleep protection in the preterm infants. *The Journal of Maternal-Fetal & Neonatal Medicine: The Official Journal of the European Association of Perinatal Medicine, the Federation of Asia and Oceania Perinatal Societies, the International Society of Perinatal Obstetricians, 24*(Suppl. 1), 12–14.

Conde-Agudelo, A., & Díaz-Rossello, J. L. (2014). Kangaroo mother care to reduce morbidity and mortality in low birthweight infants. *Cochrane Database of Systematic Reviews, 2014*(4), CD002771.

Cooper, L. G., Gooding, J. S., Gallagher, J., Sternesky, L., Ledsky, R., & Berns, S. D. (2007). Impact of a family-centered care initiative on NICU care, staff and families. *Journal of Perinatology: Official Journal of the California Perinatal Association, 27*(Suppl. 2), S32–S37.

Corvaglia, L., Martini, S., Aceti, A., Arcuri, S., Rossini, R., & Faldella, G. (2013). Nonpharmacological management of gastroesophageal reflux in preterm infants. *Biomed Research International, 2013,* Article ID 141967. Retrieved from http://dx.doi .org/10.1155/2013/141967

Coughlin, M. (2015). The Sobreviver (survive) project. *Newborn & Infant Nursing Reviews, 15*(4), 169–173.

Coughlin, M. (2014). *Transformative nursing in the NICU: Trauma-informed, age-appropriate care.* New York, NY: Springer Publishing.

Coughlin, M. (2011). *Age-appropriate care of the premature and critically ill hospitalized infant: Guideline for practice.* Glenview, IL: National Association of Neonatal Nurses.

Coughlin, M., Gibbins, S., & Hoath, S. (2009). Core measures for developmentally supportive care in neonatal intensive care units: Theory, precedence and practice. *Journal of Advanced Nursing, 65*(10), 2239–2248.

Craig, J. W., Glick, C., Phillips, R., Hall, S. L., Smith, J., & Browne, J. (2015). Recommendations for involving the family in developmental care of the NICU baby. *Journal of Perinatology: Official Journal of the California Perinatal Association, 35*(Suppl. 1), S5–S8.

Czinn, S. J., & Blanchard, S. (2013). Gastroesophageal reflux disease in neonates and infants: When and how to treat. *Paediatric Drugs, 15*(1), 19–27.

Dattani, N., Bhat, R., Rafferty, G. F., Hannam, S., & Greenough, A. (2011). Survey of sleeping position recommendations for prematurely born infants. *European Journal of Pediatrics, 170*(2), 229–232.

Davanzo, R., Brovedani, P., Travan, L., Kennedy, J., Crocetta, A., Sanesi, C.,... De Cunto, A. (2013). Intermittent kangaroo mother care: A NICU protocol. *Journal of Human Lactation: Official Journal of International Lactation Consultant Association, 29*(3), 332–338.

Delannoy, J., Mandai, O., Honoré, J., Kobayashi, T., & Sequeira, H. (2015). Diurnal emotional states impact the sleep course. *PloS One, 10*(11), e0142721.

Elder, D. E., Campbell, A. J., Larsen, P. D., & Galletly, D. (2011). Respiratory variability in preterm and term infants: Effect of sleep state, position and age. *Respiratory Physiology & Neurobiology, 175*(2), 234–238.

Feldman, R., Eidelman, A. I., Sirota, L., & Weller, A. (2002). Comparison of skin-to-skin (kangaroo) and traditional care: Parenting outcomes and preterm infant development. *Pediatrics, 110*(1, Pt. 1), 16–26.

Fivush, R. (2011). The development of autobiographical memory. *Annual Review of Psychology, 62,* 559–582.

Foreman, S. W., Thomas, K. A., & Blackburn, S. T. (2008). Individual and gender differences matter in preterm infant state development. *Journal of Obstetric, Gynecologic, and Neonatal Nursing: JOGNN/NAACOG, 37*(6), 657–665.

Garcia, A. J., Koschnitzky, J. E., & Ramirez, J. M. (2013). The physiological determinants of sudden infant death syndrome. *Respiratory Physiology & Neurobiology, 189*(2), 288–300.

Gelfer, P., Cameron, R., Masters, K., & Kennedy, K. A. (2013). Integrating "back to sleep" recommendations into neonatal ICU practice. *Pediatrics, 131*(4), e1264–e1270.

Goldwater, P. N. (2011). A perspective on SIDS pathogenesis. The hypotheses: Plausibility and evidence. *BMC Medicine, 9*(64). Retrieved from http://bmcmedicine .biomedcentral.com/articles/10.1186/1741-7015-9-64

Gómez, R. L., Bootzin, R. R., & Nadel, L. (2006). Naps promote abstraction in language-learning infants. *Psychological Science, 17*(8), 670–674.

Gooding, J. S., Cooper, L. G., Blaine, A. I., Franck, L. S., Howse, J. L., & Berns, S. D. (2011). Family support and family-centered care in the neonatal intensive care unit: Origins, advances, impact. *Seminars in Perinatology, 35*(1), 20–28.

Graham, A. M., Fisher, P. A., & Pfeifer, J. H. (2013). What sleeping babies hear: A functional MRI study of interparental conflict and infants' emotion processing. *Psychological Science, 24*(5), 782–789.

Graham, A. M., Pfeifer, J. H., Fisher, P. A., Carpenter, S., & Fair, D. A. (2015). Early life stress is associated with default system integrity and emotionality during infancy. *Journal of Child Psychology and Psychiatry, and Allied Disciplines, 56*(11), 1212–1222.

Graven, S. (2006). Sleep and brain development. *Clinics in Perinatology, 33*(3), 693–706, vii.

Graven, S. N., & Browne, J. V. (2008). Sleep and brain development: The critical role of sleep in fetal and early neonatal brain development. *Newborn and Infant Nursing Reviews, 8*(4), 173–179.

Groch, S., Zinke, K., Wilhelm, I., & Born, J. (2015). Dissociating the contributions of slow-wave sleep and rapid eye movement sleep to emotional item and source memory. *Neurobiology of Learning and Memory, 122*, 122–130.

Guyer, C., Huber, R., Fontijn, J., Bucher, H. U., Nicolai, H., Werner, H., ... Jenni, O. G. (2012). Cycled light exposure reduces fussing and crying in very preterm infants. *Pediatrics, 130*(1), e145–e151.

Harrison, W., & Goodman, D. (2015). Epidemiologic trends in neonatal intensive care, 2007–2012. *Journal of the American Medical Association Pediatrics, 169*(9), 855–862.

Hirshkowitz, M., Whiton, K., Albert, S. M., Alessi, C., Bruni, O., DonCarlos, L., ... Adams Hillard, P. J. (2015). National Sleep Foundation's sleep time duration recommendations: Methodology and results summary. *Sleep Health, 1*, 40–43.

Hitchcock, S. (2012). Endorsing safe infant sleep: A call to action. *Nursing for Women's Health, 16*(5), 386–396.

Holditch-Davis, D., & Edwards, L. J. (1998). Modeling development of sleep-wake behaviors: Results of two cohorts of preterms. *Physiology and Behavior, 63*(3), 319–328.

Horvath, K., Liu, S., & Plunkett, K. (2015). A daytime nap facilitates generalization of word meanings in young toddlers. *Sleep*, July 24, pii: sp-00265–15. [Epub ahead of print].

Hwang, S. S., O'Sullivan, A., Fitzgerald, E., Melvin, P., Gorman, T., & Fiascone, J. M. (2015). Implementation of safe sleep practices in the neonatal intensive care unit. *Journal of Perinatology: Official Journal of the California Perinatal Association, 35*(10), 862–866.

Ibarro-Coronado, E. G., Pantaleon-Martinez, A. M., Velazquez-Moctezuma, J., Prospero-Garcia, O., Mendez-Diaz, M., Perez-Tapia, M., ... Morales-Montor, J. (2015). The bidirectional relationship between sleep and immunity against infections. *The Journal of Immunology Research, 2015*, Article ID 678164. Retrieved from http://dx.doi.org/10.1155/2015/678164

Jefferies, A. L.; Canadian Paediatric Society, Fetus and Newborn Committee. (2012). Kangaroo care for the preterm infant and family. *Paediatrics & Child Health, 17*(3), 141–146.

Kaffashi, F., Scher, M. S., Ludington-Hoe, S. M., & Loparo, K. A. (2013). An analysis of the kangaroo care intervention using neonatal EEG complexity: A preliminary study. *Clinical Neurophysiology: Official Journal of the International Federation of Clinical Neurophysiology, 124*(2), 238–246.

Kinney, H. C., & Thach, B. T. (2009). The sudden infant death syndrome. *The New England Journal of Medicine, 361*(8), 795–805.

Kuhlthau, K. A., Bloom, S., Van Cleave, J., Knapp, A. A., Romm, D., Klatka, K., ... Perrin, J. M. (2011). Evidence for family-centered care for children with special health care needs: A systematic review. *Academic Pediatrics, 11*(2), 136–143.

Lagercrantz, H. (2014). The emergence of consciousness: Science and ethics. *Seminars in Fetal and Neonatal Medicine, 19*(5) 300–305.

Lagercrantz, H., & Changeux, J. P. (2010). Basic consciousness of the newborn. *Seminars in Perinatology, 34*(3), 201–206.

Lagercrantz, H., & Changeux, J. P. (2009). The emergence of human consciousness: From fetal to neonatal life. *Pediatric Research, 65*(3), 255–260.

Lane, A. (2015). Good night, baby ... Sleep safely. *American Nurse Today, 10*(11), 8–10.

Laubach, V., Wilhelm, P., & Carter, K. (2014). Shhh...I'm growing: Noise in the NICU. *The Nursing Clinics of North America, 49*(3), 329–344.

Ludington-Hoe, S. M. (2008). A clinical guideline for implementation of kangaroo care with premature infants of 30 or more weeks' postmenstrual age. *Advances in Neonatal Care, 8*(3), s3–s23.

Ludington-Hoe, S. M., Johnson, M. W., Morgan, K., Lewis, T., Gutman, J., Wilson, P. D., & Scher, M. S. (2006). Neurophysiologic assessment of neonatal sleep organization: Preliminary results of a randomized, controlled trial of skin contact with preterm infants. *Pediatrics, 117*(5), e909–e923.

Lusk, L. A., Brown, E. G., Overcash, R. T., Grogan, T. R., Keller, R. L., Kim, J. H.,...DeUgarte, D. A.; University of California Fetal Consortium. (2014). Multi-institutional practice patterns and outcomes in uncomplicated gastroschisis: A report from the University of California Fetal Consortium (UCfC). *Journal of Pediatric Surgery, 49*(12), 1782–1786.

Malloy, M. H. (2013). Prematurity and sudden infant death syndrome: United States 2005–2007. *Journal of Perinatology: Official Journal of the California Perinatal Association, 33*(6), 470–475.

March of Dimes Perinatal Data Center (2011). Special care nursery admissions. *National Perinatal Information System/Quality Analytic Services.* Retrieved from https://www.marchofdimes.org/peristats/pdfdocs/nicu_summary_final.pdf

McMullen, S. L., Fioravanti, I. D., Brown, K., & Carey, M. G. (2016). Safe sleep for hospitalized infants. *MCN. The American Journal of Maternal Child Nursing, 41*(1), 43–50.

Mindell, J. A., Li, A. M., Sadeh, A., Kwon, R., & Goh, D. Y. (2015). Bedtime routines for young children: A dose-dependent association with sleep outcomes. *Sleep, 38*(5), 717–722.

Mindell, J. A., Telofski, L. S., Wiegand, B., & Kurtz, E. S. (2009). A nightly bedtime routine: Impact on sleep in young children and maternal mood. *Sleep, 32*(5), 599–606.

Mirmiran, M., Maas, Y. G., & Ariagno, R. L. (2003). Development of fetal and neonatal sleep and circadian rhythms. *Sleep Medicine Reviews, 7*(4), 321–334.

Miyamoto, H., & Hensch, T. K. (2003). Reciprocal interaction of sleep and synaptic plasticity. *Molecular Interventions, 3*(7), 404–417.

Moore, E. R., Anderson, G. C., Bergman, N., & Dowswell, T. (2012). Early skin-to-skin contact for mothers and their healthy newborn infants. *Cochrane Database of Systematic Reviews, 2012*(5), CD003519.

Morag, I., & Ohlsson, A. (2013). Cycled light in the intensive care unit for preterm and low birth weight infants. *Cochrane Database of Systematic Reviews, 2013*(8), CD006982.

Neu, M., Browne, J. V., & Vojir, C. (2000). The impact of two transfer techniques used during skin-to-skin care on the physiologic and behavioral responses of preterm infants. *Nursing Research, 49*(4), 215–223.

Neu, M., Hazel, N. A., Robinson, J., Schmiege, S. J., & Laudenslager, M. (2014). Effect of holding on co-regulation in preterm infants: A randomized controlled trial. *Early Human Development, 90*(3), 141–147.

Numerato, D., Fattore, G., Tediosi, F., Zanini, R., Peltola, M., Banks, H.,...Seppälä, T. T. (2015). Mortality and length of stay of very low birth weight and very preterm infants: A EuroHOPE study. *PloS One, 10*(6), e0131685.

Palmu, K., Kirjavainen, T., Stjerna, S., Salokivi, T., & Vanhatalo, S. (2013). Sleep wake cycling in early preterm infants: Comparison of polysomnographic recordings with a novel EEG-based index. *Clinical Neurophysiology: Official Journal of the International Federation of Clinical Neurophysiology, 124*(9), 1807–1814.

Patton, C., Stiltner, D., Wright, K. B., & Kautz, D. D. (2015). Do nurses provide a safe sleep environment for infants in the hospital setting? An integrative review. *Advances in Neonatal Care: Official Journal of the National Association of Neonatal Nurses, 15*(1), 8–22.

Peirano, P. D., & Algarín, C. R. (2007). Sleep in brain development. *Biological Research, 40*(4), 471–478.

Peirano, P., Algarín, C., & Uauy, R. (2003). Sleep-wake states and their regulatory mechanisms throughout early human development. *The Journal of Pediatrics, 143*(4 Suppl.), S70–S79.

Pfister, S. (2012, November). Evidence-based treatment of gastroesophageal reflux in neonates. *Nurse Currents*, 13–18. Retrieved from http://static.abbottnutrition.com/cms/ANHI2010/MEDIA/Nurse%20Currents-November2012-RefluxArticle.pdf

Qureshi, A., Malkar, M., Splaingard, M., Khuhro, A., & Jadcherla, S. (2015). The role of sleep in the modulation of gastroesophageal reflux and symptoms in NICU neonates. *Pediatric Neurology, 53*(3), 226–232.

Rao, H., May, C., Hannam, S., Rafferty, G. F., & Greenough, A. (2007). Survey of sleeping position recommendations for prematurely born infants on neonatal intensive care unit discharge. *European Journal of Pediatrics, 166*(8), 809–811.

Ribeiro dos Santos, B., Sbampato CaladoOrsi, K. C., Ferreira Gomes Balieiro, M. M., Hiromi Sato, M., Yoshiko Kakehashi, T., & Moreira Pinheiro, E. (2015). Effect of "quiet time" to reduce noise at the neonatal intensive care unit. *Escola Anna Nery Revista de Enfermagem, 19*(1), 102–106.

Rolfes, M., Sealer, H., & Coughlin, M. (2014, February). *Touch a life–impact a lifetime.* Poster session presented at the 27th Annual Gravens Conference on the Physical and Developmental Environment of the High Risk Infant, Clearwater Beach, FL.

Samra, H. A., McGrath, J. M., Fischer, S., Schumacher, B., Dutcher, J., & Hansen, J. (2015). The NICU Parent Risk Evaluation and Engagement Model and Instrument (PREEMI) for neonates in intensive care units. *Journal of Obstetric, Gynecologic, and Neonatal Nursing: JOGNN/NAACOG, 44*(1), 114–126.

Scher, M. S. (2004). Automated EEG-sleep analyses and neonatal neurointensive care. *Sleep Medicine, 5*(6), 533–540.

Scher, M. S., Johnson, M. W., & Holditch-Davis, D. (2005). Cyclicity of neonatal sleep behaviors at 25 to 30 weeks' postconceptional age. *Pediatric Research, 57*(6), 879–882.

Scher, M. S., Ludington-Hoe, S., Kaffashi, F., Johnson, M. W., Holditch-Davis, D., & Loparo, K. A. (2009). Neurophysiologic assessment of brain maturation after an 8-week trial of skin-to-skin contact on preterm infants. *Clinical Neurophysiology: Official Journal of the International Federation of Clinical Neurophysiology, 120*(10), 1812–1818.

Schurr, P., & Findlater, C. K. (2012). Neonatal mythbusters: Evaluating the evidence for and against pharmacologic and nonpharmacologic management of gastroesophageal reflux. *Neonatal Network, 31*(4), 229–241.

Staples, A. D., Bates, J. E., & Petersen, I. T. (2015). Bedtime routines in early childhood: Prevalence, consistency, and associations with nighttime sleep. *Monographs of the Society for Research in Child Development, 80*(1), 141–159.

Stevenson, N. J., Palmu, K., Wikström, S., Hellström-Westas, L., & Vanhatalo, S. (2014). Measuring brain activity cycling (BAC) in long term EEG monitoring of preterm babies. *Physiological Measurement, 35*(7), 1493–1508.

Tedder, J. L. (2008). Give them the HUG: An innovative approach to helping parents understand the language of their newborn. *The Journal of Perinatal Education, 17*(2), 14–20.

Thorpe, K., Staton, S., Sawyer, E., Pattinson, C., Haden, C., & Smith, S. (2015). Napping, development and health from 0 to 5 years: A systematic review. *Archives of Disease in Childhood, 100*(7), 615–622.

Trachtenberg, F. L., Haas, E. A., Kinney, H. C., Stanley, C., & Krous, H. F. (2012). Risk factor changes for sudden infant death syndrome after initiation of back-to-sleep campaign. *Pediatrics, 129*(4), 630–638.

Tronick, E., & Beeghly, M. (2011). Infants' meaning-making and the development of mental health problems. *The American Psychologist, 66*(2), 107–119.

Vasquez, V., & Cong, X. (2014). Parenting the MICU infant: A meta-ethnographic synthesis. *International Journal of Nursing Sciences, 1*(3), 281–290.

Vásquez-Ruiz, S., Maya-Barrios, J. A., Torres-Narváez, P., Vega-Martínez, B. R., Rojas-Granados, A., Escobar, C., & Angeles-Castellanos, M. (2014). A light/dark cycle in the NICU accelerates body weight gain and shortens time to discharge in preterm infants. *Early Human Development, 90*(9), 535–540.

Voos, K. C., Terreros, A., Larimore, P., Leick-Rude, M. K., & Park, N. (2015). Implementing safe sleep practices in a neonatal intensive care unit. *The Journal of Maternal-Fetal & Neonatal Medicine: The Official Journal of the European Association of Perinatal Medicine, the Federation of Asia and Oceania Perinatal Societies, the International Society of Perinatal Obstetricians, 28*(14), 1637–1640.

Watson, B. O., & Buzsáki, G. (2015). Sleep, memory and brain rhythms. *Daedalus, 144*(1), 67–82.

Weisman, O., Magori-Cohen, R., Louzoun, Y., Eidelman, A. I., & Feldman, R. (2011). Sleep-wake transitions in premature neonates predict early development. *Pediatrics, 128*(4), 706–714.

Wigert, H., Hellström, A. L., & Berg, M. (2008). Conditions for parents' participation in the care of their child in neonatal intensive care—a field study. *BMC Pediatrics, 8*, 3.

CHAPTER 8

Guidelines for Activities of Daily Living

Your perspective on life comes from the cage you were held captive in.
　　—Shannon L. Alder

This guideline presents the latest evidence-based research, along with clinical practice recommendations and implementation strategies related to infants' activities of daily living in the neonatal intensive care unit (NICU), which encompasses positioning, feeding, and skin and mucous membrane care practices as detailed in Table 8.1.

TABLE 8.1　Attributes and Criteria of Infants' Activities of Daily Living Core Measure

Attributes	Criteria
Age-appropriate postural alignment ensures comfort, safety, physiologic stability, and supports optimal neuromotor development	1. Infants are positioned and handled to support postural alignment and spontaneous movement during caregiving and at rest 2. Infants receive therapeutic interventions to optimize neuromotor and neurobehavioral performance and outcome 3. Skin-to-skin care is the position of choice for medically stable, eligible infants
Age-appropriate feeding experiences will be pain and stress free, individualized, infant driven, and nurturing	1. Breast milk is the preferred and actively recommended diet for all hospitalized infants 2. Skin-to-skin care is aggressively encouraged and prefeeding activities at the breast are supported 3. Oral-feeding encounters are introduced no sooner than 33 weeks gestational age based on the infant's feeding readiness behaviors that direct all subsequent oral-feeding experiences
Age-appropriate skin care routines and skin protective measures preserve barrier function and tissue integrity	1. Skin and mucous membrane integrity is routinely assessed (at least daily) using a validated and reliable tool 2. Recommended bathing frequency (sponge, tub, swaddled) is no more than 3 times/week for the purpose of removing debris and general hygiene 3. Skin and mucous membranes are protected from potential secondary injury, transepidermal water losses, and alterations in surface microbiome

GUIDELINE OBJECTIVES

- To define the criteria and recommendations for best practice in positioning, feeding, and skin and mucous membrane care practices in the NICU
- To present the evidence that supports the criteria and best practice recommendations for activities of daily living in the NICU
- To present clinical practice strategies that facilitate adoption and integration of evidence-based best practices in positioning, feeding, and skin and mucous membrane care techniques in the NICU

MAJOR OUTCOMES CONSIDERED

The impact of the consistently reliable application of the activities of daily living core measure attributes and criteria on the NICU patient, family, and staff includes:

- Physiologic, psychosocial, and psychoemotional outcomes
- Patient safety and quality clinical outcomes

POSTURE AND MOBILITY

Posture is paramount to your future.
    —Cindy Ann Peterson

Interventions and Practice Considerations

- Create and maintain staff confidence and competence in supporting infant postural alignment and spontaneous movement during caregiving activities and at rest
  - Best practice considerations include competency-based training in postural alignment for existing and all new hires; consider an annual competency-based refresher training
  - Best practice considerations include integrating postural alignment knowledge into practices such as positioning the infant for sleep, swaddled weighing, skin-to-skin care infant transfers, swaddled bathing, swaddled transfer to and from transport incubator, and so forth
- Create and maintain a systematic integration of prevention-oriented therapy services into the infant's plan of care
  - Best practice considerations include ensuring that the clinical interdisciplinary team coordinates, collaborates, and communicates effectively to achieve patient- and family-focused goals
- Create and maintain an evidence-based practice guideline for the provision of skin-to-skin care
  - Best practice considerations include eligibility or exclusion criteria, competency-based training for parents and staff regarding the infant transfer

process, as well as documentation requirements to capture the dose-dependent impact of skin-to-skin care

The Evidence

Motor development, postural control, and sensorimotor integrity are critical for the short- and long-term neurodevelopmental and cognitive outcomes of NICU survivors (Dansk et al., 2012; Spittle et al., 2015). Muscle tone develops in a caudal cephalic direction and, in the fluid-filled uterus, the dance between extensor and flexor tone can proceed unencumbered by gravity (Allen & Capote, 1990; Sweeney & Gutierrez, 2002). However, the prematurely born infant, with limited muscle power, and even the critically ill term infant are significantly impacted by the forces of gravity that limit spontaneous, antigravity movement and increase infant vulnerability to compromised musculoskeletal and servomotor development (Burgin et al., 2008; Eli Kim, Nemea, Friesland, Dolphin, & Rage, 2002; Monterosso et al., 2002; Samos et al., 2002). It has been demonstrated that the use of postural supports can reduce the incidence of neuromotor abnormalities and protect musculoskeletal alignment. Vaivre-Douret et al. (2004) demonstrated that regular changes in posture, while preserving functional orientation and alignment, supported normal neuromuscular and osteoarticular function in a cohort of low-risk preterm infants. In order to achieve age-appropriate postural alignment and flexion, the use of postural supports or positioning aids have been investigated by several researchers and conclude that the use of postural supports and appropriately sized diapers improves hip and shoulder posture and has also shown to reduce infants' pain and stress behaviors during routine caregiving (Comaru & Miura, 2009; Monterosso et al., 1995; Monterosso et al., 2003). Postural supports and positioning devices that support a flexed posture and spontaneous movement stimulate recoil back to flexion following movement, and provide proprioceptive input that improve reflex and motor response symmetry in preterm infants (Madlinger-Lewis et al., 2014).

NICU nurses and neonatal therapists acknowledge that positioning plays a key role in the developmental well-being of the hospitalized infant, yet there is extreme inconsistency in what age-appropriate positioning looks like in the NICU (Coughlin et al., 2010; Jeanson, 2013; Perkins et al., 2004; Zarem et al., 2013). The effects of supine, prone, and semi-upright positions have been studied in relation to cerebral and mesenteric oxygenation, mechanical ventilation, and cardiac output with conflicting findings (Balaguer, Escribano, Roque I Figulus, & Rivas-Fernandez, 2013; Demirel et al., 2012; Eghbalian, 2014; Ma et al., 2015; Petrova & Mehta, 2015). Although prone position has been described to improve oxygen saturation in premature infants with respiratory distress syndrome (Eghbalian, 2014) and slightly improve oxygenation in infants receiving mechanical ventilation (Balaguer et al., 2013), Ma et al. (2015) documented a decrease in cardiac output and an increase in systemic vascular resistance for neonates positioned prone.

In addition to body position, the position of the head and neck in relation to the body has correlated with alterations in cerebral perfusion and cerebral venous drainage culminating in a systematic review recommending neutral head position to reduce the incidence of intraventricular hemorrhage in preterm infants (Ancora et al., 2010; Malusky & Donze, 2011; Pellicer et al., 2002). Coughlin et al. (2010) recommend that head position from midline be maintained at an angle less than or equal to 45°; this recommendation has been substantiated in the work of Liao et al. (2015), who looked at bilateral cerebral saturations in various head positions of stable preterm infants. Using near-infrared spectroscopy, the authors demonstrated that head position in midline to a head position changes of 45° to 60° left or right from midline (with the body in supine) demonstrated stable, bilateral cerebral saturation (Liao et al., 2015).

Studies of cranial deformation in preterm infants confirm the malleability of the immature skull resulting in mechanically influenced changes in cortical morphology as well as alterations in motor performance (Mewes et al., 2007; Nuysink et al., 2013). In a term cohort with and without deformational plagiocephaly (DP), infants with DP received lower scores in cognitive and motor domains of the Bayley Scales of Infant and Toddler Development-III (BSID-III) than the control group, and magnetic resonance imaging (MRI) findings revealed not only shape changes in the DP group, but the orientation of specific brain structures was also impacted (Collett et al., 2012). The functional implications of these findings require continued investigation, and although DP may not directly cause cognitive and developmental problems, it may be a marker for risk and prudent clinicians are recommended to minimize cranial deformation as much as possible (Collett et al., 2011; Collett et al., 2013).

Postdischarge early intervention programs for preterm infants have demonstrated a positive influence on cognitive and motor outcomes during infancy (Spittle, Orton, Anderson, Boyd, & Doyle, 2015). Pineda et al. (2013) described altered neurobehavioral patterns in preterm infants at term equivalent when compared with their full-term counterparts. Altered behaviors included a lower tolerance for handling, a lower capacity for self-regulation, more stress behaviors and excitability, as well as hyper- and hypotonia (Pineda et al., 2013). These behaviors are amenable to therapeutic intervention during the NICU hospitalization (Pineda et al., 2013). Neonatal therapists are positioned to minimize and mitigate developmental morbidity associated with neonatal intensive care, but this approach requires an interdisciplinary commitment to teamwork and collaboration (Dietz et al., 2014; Mahoney & Cohen, 2005; Mathisen et al., 2012; Nightlinger, 2011). An effective strategy to facilitate collaboration, clinical efficiency, and compliance with evidence-based best practices is the use of order sets for clinical decision support, which should include standing orders to initiate consults with neonatal therapists on admission (Bobb et al., 2007).

Besides prone, supine, and the semi-upright sitting position, the postural benefits of skin-to-skin care have been studied with exciting results. In addition to the myriad of benefits of skin-to-skin care (kangaroo care) described in the 2014 Cochrane review, early initiation of kangaroo care improves cerebral blood flow as well as increases electromyographic activity in the brachial biceps; these benefits in flexor tone persist over time (Diniz et al., 2013; Korraa et al., 2014; Miranda et al., 2014).

These findings present neonatal clinicians with a comprehensive, safe postural intervention with multisystem, short- and long-term benefits for the infant–family dyad and the clinical team. Transferring the infant from bed to skin-to-skin position can be destabilizing; however, when a standing parent transfer mode is used, the infant exhibits physiologic stability and parents build confidence and competence (Ludington-Hoe et al., 2003; Ludington-Hoe, 2013; Robinson, 2014).

Cost Analysis

The initiation of "earlier" interventions in the NICU aimed at reducing postural morbidities through a collaborative interdisciplinary approach to care reduces not only fiscal costs of compromised neurobehavioral and motor outcomes, but also reduces human and societal costs (Sweeney & Gutierrez, 2002). The economic implications of skin-to-skin care (kangaroo care) have been reported as it facilitates and supports breastfeeding, with substantial health benefits that span the infant's lifetime (Renfrew et al., 2009).

Recommendations for Best Practice in Postural Alignment and Mobility (Table 8.2)

TABLE 8.2   Major Practice Recommendations and Implementation Strategies—Postural Alignment and Mobility

Recommendations	Implementation Strategy
1. Develop and/or adopt a multimodal, interactive competency-based education program focused on evidence-based best practices in neonatal positioning (examples of postural assessment tools and mobile learning resources are shown in Figures 8.1–8.3; Grant & Coughlin, 2015)	a. Review your available education resources (instructor-led, eLearning, mobile resources, pamphlets) b. Collect baseline knowledge levels from staff and parents (this will allow you to measure your success) c. Introduce a competency-based education module; follow-up with a posttest to measure the impact of teaching d. Consider adding a practicum component to the teaching to allow application of the new knowledge e. Outline a plan for continuing education and integration of learning into interdisciplinary orientation f. Outline a plan to monitor knowledge translation into practice g. Audit practice, share results with staff

2. Identify practice improvement opportunities around positioning and supporting postural alignment and mobility in the clinical setting (i.e., swaddled weights, swaddled baths, standing infant transfer for skin-to-skin care, positioning for sleep) (Edraki et al., 2014; Mahoney & Cohen, 2005; Neu & Browne, 1997; van Sleuwen et al., 2007)	a. Establish a multidisciplinary task force to identify and prioritize postural practice improvement opportunities:
	  i. Less than or equal to 10 persons
	  ii. Balance the power (equal number of staff to leader presence)
	  iii. Voluntary participation
	  iv. Bias for action—do not meet to meet, you meet to change!

(continued)

TABLE 8.2   Major Practice Recommendations and Implementation Strategies—Postural Alignment
and Mobility   *(continued)*

Recommendations	Implementation Strategy

	b. Begin with the improvement opportunity that you believe will be the easiest to implement (e.g., swaddled weights)
	c. Collect baseline information if possible (maybe look at big data during standard weighing times; consider an observation of stress cues during weighing before and after the swaddled intervention; also, consider a survey of staff after the intervention regarding their perceptions of the new practice)
	d. Begin a test of change using the PDSA methodology)
	   i. How will you zero the scale with the swaddling materials?
	   ii. Discuss with the team how much variance in linen weight will be acceptable (all blankets don't weigh exactly the same)
	   iii. How does this new practice impact other caregiving routines associated with the weighing?
	   iv. Are there other unexpected implications that need to be addressed in relation to this new practice?
	e. Once you have refined your test of change evaluate the new practice with a larger group of supportive staff
	   i. Reevaluate the findings
	   ii. Revise as indicated
	f. Draft clinical practice algorithm and/or practice guideline
	g. Implement new practice, measure results
	h. Provide feedback to staff
	i. Publish and/or present results

3. Address preventable, hospital-acquired neuromotor and postural morbidities by proactively integrating neonatal therapists into the daily plan of care (Frolek Clark & Schlabach, 2013; Mahoney & Cohen, 2005; Nightlinger, 2011; Olson & Baltman, 1994)	a. Consider including an order set for neonatal therapy in the CPOE system
	   i. Discuss with the interdisciplinary team what the order set would include, when it would be initiated
	   ii. Identify how you will measure the impact of this new intervention before initiating—short-term and possibly postdischarge effect
	   iii. Consider testing this "order set" on a low-risk patient population
	b. Outline the documentation/communication expectations for the various therapeutic interventions
	   i. What will it look like in the EMR? How will this be available to other disciplines—can the access to the therapy progress notes be improved so that everyone on the team is aware of the infant's progress?
	   ii. How will family be informed of the various therapy interventions and included in the progress updates?
	c. Once you have tested and refined your strategy, develop a practice guideline, educate new staff on the practice
	d. Continually evaluate, measure and provide feedback to staff
	e. Publish and/or present your results

(continued)

TABLE 8.2   Major Practice Recommendations and Implementation Strategies—Postural Alignment and Mobility   *(continued)*

Recommendations	Implementation Strategy
4. Establish skin-to-skin as the recommended position for all infants and the standing transfer as the preferred transfer mode (Baley, 2015; Coughlin, 2015; Diniz et al., 2013; Ludington-Hoe et al., 2003)	a. Assess current infant transfer mode for kangaroo care in your unit; consider collecting big data, staff and parent surveys or other metrics as your benchmark before beginning your test of change b. Develop a competency-based learning module for staff and parents and include a simulation exercise for the standing transfer; consider giving the parents a certificate of completion following the simulation (examples are shown in Figures 8.4–8.6) c. Once staff and parents have met the competency requirements, introduce the new practice and collect data metrics for comparison d. Make eligibility for skin-to-skin care a point for discussion on rounds and change of shift e. Consider placing a kangaroo sticker on the incubator of eligible infants so everyone will know who can participate in skin-to-skin care when the parents are at the bedside, even if the infant is not their patient assignment f. Provide feedback to staff and parents g. Publish and/or present your results

CPOE, computerized physician order entry; EMR, electronic medical record, PDSA, Plan-Do-See-Act.

Clinical and Parent Resource

Examples and samples of mobile learning resources, postural assessment tools, competency-based checklists for parents and clinicians as well as a parent teaching sheet are shown in Figures 8.1 to 8.6.

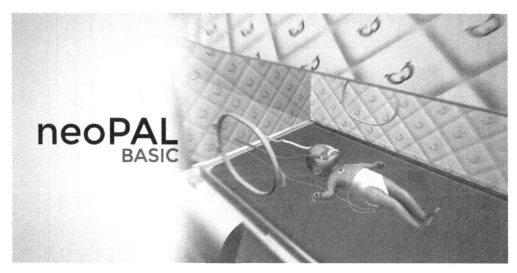

FIGURE 8.1   neoPAL BASIC—mobile learning app from Caring Essentials.

Neonatal Postural Assessment Worksheet (*neoPAW*)

Date: _____ Time: _____ Patient Identifier (bed space, or MRN): _____ GA: _____ : CGA: _____ : Prone   Supine   Side-lying

Indicator	0	1	2	Score	Comments/Limitations
Head	Lateral rotation > 45 degrees from midline L ☐ R ☐	Lateral rotation < 45 degrees from midline L ☐ R ☐	Head in a midline orientation		
Neck	Neck in extension OR Flexion Ext ☐ Flex ☐	////////	Neck in a neutral alignment		
Scapulae (shoulder blades)	Retracted L ☐ R ☐	Flat L ☐ R ☐	Softly rounded L ☐ R ☐		
Spine/torso	Mal-aligned (lateral or rotational)	////////	Aligned		
			Subtotal (page 1)		

1. Is the baby positioned in a way to support or allow for spontaneous movement? Yes ☐ No ☐

2. Did you observe spontaneous movement during your assessment? (If yes, please describe briefly.) Yes ☐ No ☐

   Describe: _____

170

Indicator	0	1	2	Score	Comments/Limitations
Hands	Not touching the body L ☐ R ☐ **Both** ☐	Touching the torso L ☐ R ☐ **Both** ☐	Touching the head/face L ☐ R ☐ **Both** ☐		
Hips	Abducted with extreme external rotation (> 45 degrees) L ☐ R ☐ **Both** ☐	Hips adducted & extended L ☐ R ☐ **Both** ☐	Hips aligned with flexion & pelvic tilt L ☐ R ☐ **Both** ☐		
Knees/ ankles	Parallel legs (knees & ankles in extension) L ☐ R ☐ **Both** ☐	Knees & ankles unsupported flexion L ☐ R ☐ **Both** ☐	Knees & ankles aligned, softly flexed and supported L ☐ R ☐ **Both** ☐		
			TOTAL Score (Subtotal + Page 2 Score)		

1. Does this baby's position need to be adjusted (If yes, please describe how and what you were able to adjust?)   Yes ☐   No ☐

   Describe: _____

FIGURE 8.2   Neonatal Postural Assessment (neoPAW) worksheet sample.

Reprinted with permission from Caring Essentials Collaborative, LLC.

Patient's name:_____ Corrected gestational age:_____

Clinician's name:_____ Date/time of assessment: _____

Indicator	0	1	2	Score
Shoulders	Shoulders retracted	Shoulders flat/in neutral	Shoulders softly rounded	
Hands	Hands away from the body	Hands touching torso	Hands touching face	
Hips	Hips abducted, externally rotated	Hips extended	Hips aligned and softly flexed	
Knees, ankles, feet	Knees extended, ankles and feet externally rotated	Knees, ankles feet extended	Knees, ankles feet are aligned and softly flexed	
Head	Rotated laterally (L or R) greater than 45° from midline	Rotated laterally (L or R) 45° from midline	Positioned midline to less than 45° from midline (L or R)	
Neck	Neck hperextended flexed	Neck neutral	Neck neutral, head slightly flexed forward 10°	
Ideal cumulative score = 10–12			**Total score**	

FIGURE 8.3   Infant position assessment tool.

Step	Action	Validation of Competence	Complete ☑
1	Completes parent education for kangaroo care in the NICU	Certificate of completion	☐
2	Reviews the unit protocol and understands the eligibility criteria for kangaroo care	Observation	☐
3	Mock-up return demonstration of the kangaroo care procedure for standing infant transfer and parent seated transfer with doll simulator	Observation	☐
4	Assess own infant's eligibility and readiness for kangaroo care	Observation	☐
5	Prepare self for kangaroo care	Observation	☐
	a. Ensure proper attire for parent		
	b. Ensure parent personal needs are attended to prior to the session		
	c. Ensure comfortable, safe seating and privacy for the session		
6	Prepare infant for kangaroo care	Observation	☐
	a. Ensure proper attire for infant		
	b. Ensure infant's personal needs are attended to prior to the session		
	c. Ensure comfortable, safe seating and privacy for the session		
6	Perform transfer in accordance with parent preference and unit protocol	Observation	☐
7	Review safety plan once settled in kangaroo position (how will the parent access a clinician, when should the parent access the clinician)	Observation	☐
10	Perform return transfer in accordance with parent preference and unit protocol	Observation	☐
11	Support your infant's transition once in the incubator with gentle containment, soothing vocalizations, etcetera.	Observation & Documentation	☐

Parent: _____
        Printed name   *Signature*   *Date*
Observer: _____
        Printed name   *Signature*   *Date*

FIGURE 8.4 Sample kangaroo care parent competency.

Step	Action	Demonstration Mode of Competence	Complete ☑
1	Complete learning module	Certificate of completion	☐
2	Mock-up return demonstration of the kangaroo care (standing transfer & seated transfer)	Observation	☐
3	Assess infant's readiness for kangaroo care	Observation	☐
4	Assess parent's readiness for kangaroo care (parent must complete parent education module and comply with parent requirements in accordance with unit practice guideline)	Observation	☐
5	Prepare infant-parent dyad for kangaroo care	Observation	☐
	a. Ensure proper attire for parent & infant		
	b. Ensure parent personal needs are attended to prior to the session		
	c. Ensure comfortable, safe seating and privacy for the session		
6	Perform transfer in accordance with unit practice guideline	Observation	☐
7	Review safety plan with parent once infant-parent dyad is in kangaroo position (how will the parent access a clinician, when should the parent access the clinician)	Observation	☐
7	Document initiation time of kangaroo care session	Documentation	☐
8	Reassess dyad every 5 minutes x 3 then every 15 minutes x 2 then every 30 minutes (or as outlined in your unit practice guideline) = record assessments	Documentation	☐
9	Document termination of kangaroo session and how the experience was tolerated by infant & parent	Documentation	☐
10	Prepare infant-parent dyad for infant transfer to incubator	Observation	☐
11	Perform return transfer in accordance with unit practice guideline	Observation	☐
12	Support infant's transition back to the incubator by monitoring/recording VS until they return to baseline	Observation & Documentation	☐

Clinician: _____ _____ _____
           Printed name   *Signature*   *Date*

Observer: _____ _____ _____
           Printed name   *Signature*   *Date*

FIGURE 8.5   Sample staff kangaroo care competency.

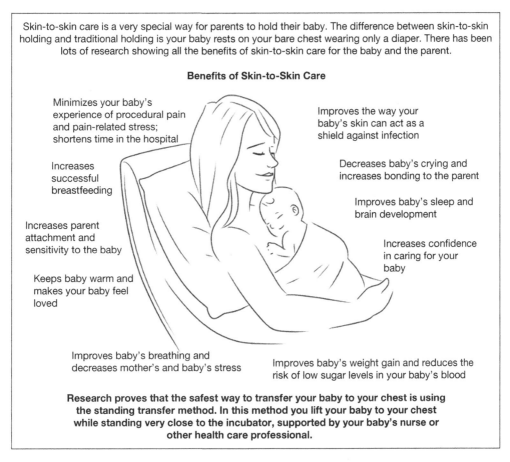

Skin-to-skin care is a very special way for parents to hold their baby. The difference between skin-to-skin holding and traditional holding is your baby rests on your bare chest wearing only a diaper. There has been lots of research showing all the benefits of skin-to-skin care for the baby and the parent.

Benefits of Skin-to-Skin Care

Minimizes your baby's experience of procedural pain and pain-related stress; shortens time in the hospital

Improves the way your baby's skin can act as a shield against infection

Increases successful breastfeeding

Decreases baby's crying and increases bonding to the parent

Improves baby's sleep and brain development

Increases parent attachment and sensitivity to the baby

Increases confidence in caring for your baby

Keeps baby warm and makes your baby feel loved

Improves baby's breathing and decreases mother's and baby's stress

Improves baby's weight gain and reduces the risk of low sugar levels in your baby's blood

Research proves that the safest way to transfer your baby to your chest is using the standing transfer method. In this method you lift your baby to your chest while standing very close to the incubator, supported by your baby's nurse or other health care professional.

FIGURE 8.6 Sample parent teaching resource for skin-to-skin (kangaroo care).

▪ FEEDING

A newborn baby has only three demands. They are warmth in the arms of his mother, food from her breasts, and security in the knowledge of her presence.
      —Grantly Dick-Read

Interventions and Practice Considerations

- Create and maintain a systematic approach to actively promote and support breast and breast-milk feeding in the NICU.
  - Best practice considerations include a comprehensive competency-based education for parents and staff on the benefits of breast milk and breast-feeding as well as effective techniques to support breast milk production

and successful breastfeeding in the NICU; include staff accountability criteria for promoting and supporting breastfeeding

- Create and maintain an evidence-based approach to prefeeding activities that promote successful breastfeeding in the NICU
  - Best practice considerations include frequent skin-to-skin care, dedicated NICU lactation support, ensuring the first oral feed is a breastfeeding, and outline staff accountability criteria for operationalizing these best practices
- Create and maintain an evidence-based approach to the initiation of oral feeding based on the infant's maturational competencies and feeding-readiness behaviors
  - Best practice considerations include educating staff and parents on feeding-readiness behaviors (include a competency-based assessment following the education); use an objective assessment tool to describe not only the infant's readiness behaviors, but also a tool that assesses the quality of the oral-feeding experience; avoid volume-based feeding plans; identify staff accountability criteria for adherence to these best practices.

The Evidence

The benefits of breastfeeding and human milk feeding impact health outcomes across an individual's life span with a dose–response benefit that includes decreased incidence of otitis media, recurrent upper respiratory tract infections, asthma, necrotizing enterocolitis, atopic dermatitis, inflammatory bowel disease, obesity, celiac disease, type I and type II diabetes, sudden infant death syndrome (SIDS), and leukemia (American Academy of Pediatrics [AAP], 2012). Challenges and barriers to breastfeeding in the NICU and the post-NICU discharge period are complex and include a lack of support for the breastfeeding mother, difficulty expressing breast milk, interference from the physical and caregiving/caregiver environments of the NICU, and maternal stress (Briere et al., 2014; Cricco-Lizza, 2011; Lucas et al., 2014; Purdy et al., 2012). In a prospective cohort study looking at maternal human milk feeding goals, more than half of mothers predelivery planned for exclusive human milk feedings; however, these goals decreased significantly during the NICU stay (Hoban et al., 2015). Frequently stated reasons for changes in breastfeeding goals include a decrease in milk supply, the need to return to work, and an inability to pump; however, when lactation support and counseling is provided, maternal anxiety decreases and there is an increase in breast-milk feeding (Hoban et al., 2015; Ikonen et al., 2015; Sisk et al., 2006).

Educational programs and "feeding care maps" aimed at increasing nurses' knowledge about infant capabilities, developmental feeding milestones, and breastfeeding have been shown to improve lactation support and breastfeeding rates (Bernaix et al., 2008; Dougherty & Luther, 2008; Pineda, Foss, Richards, & Pane, 2009; Siddell et al., 2003). Integrating the Baby-Friendly Hospital Initiative, 10 Steps for the NICU provides a clear operational framework that facilitates success (Benoit & Semenic, 2014; Nyqvist et al., 2013). Addressing parents' knowledge gaps about breastfeeding, especially fathers', plays a key role in initiating and sustaining breastfeeding (Benoit & Semenic, 2014; Maycock et al., 2013; Nyqvist et al., 2013). Mitchell-Box and Braun (2013) completed a systematic review looking at the impact of male-partner–focused breastfeeding interventions and concluded that breast-feeding education for fathers has a significant impact on increasing breastfeeding initiation and exclusive breast-milk feedings.

Summarizing the evidence on breastfeeding initiation for premature infants, Lucas & Smith (2015) concluded stable premature infants as young as 27 to 28 weeks postconceptual age (PCA) are able to maintain physiologic stability during exposure to the breast and, for some infants, breast exposure before 30 weeks PCA have resulted in exclusive breastfeeding by 33 weeks PCA. Mother–infant dyads in the NICU, who experience frequent kangaroo care sessions, receive emotional and lactation support (to include pumping support), and are encouraged to initiate early breastfeeding were most likely to sustain breastfeeding following NICU discharge (Benoit & Semenic, 2014; Lucas et al., 2014; Renfrew et al., 2009; Walker et al., 2014).

Understanding the maturational processes associated with oral feeding is critical for safe, efficient, and enjoyable feeding experiences (both breast and bottle). However, current NICU feeding practices do not reflect this understanding (Lau, 2015). Oral-feeding readiness is impacted by neurodevelopmental and neurobehavioral maturity, physiologic stability, as well as caregiver feeding style and the feeding culture in the NICU (Kish, 2013). Pickler et al. (2015) report a shorter time to full oral feedings and a shorter hospital stay when oral feedings are introduced no sooner than 34 weeks post-menstrual age (PMA) in combination with the infant exhibiting signs of physiological and behavioral readiness for feeding (see Table 8.1). These findings are corroborated in a systematic review by Watson and McGuire (2015) suggesting that responsive feeding results in a shorter transition time from enteral tube feeding to full oral feedings.

Cue-based feeding in the NICU is challenged by the existing volume-driven paradigm, which results in maladaptive feeding behaviors, patient safety concerns related to aspiration, excess energy expenditure, and future feeding aversions as well as parental anxiety (Pickler et al., 2015; Shaker, 2013a, 2013b; Stevens et al., 2014; see Table 8.3).

A multidisciplinary approach is mandatory to transform feeding culture from an emphasis on volume to a cue-based or infant-driven model for feeding (Newland et al., 2013). Comprehensive education for staff and parents, clear practice guidelines and performance expectations, order entry and documentation requirements, and objective assessment criteria facilitate adoption of this evidence-based best practice (Gelfer et al., 2015; Ludwig & Waitzman, 2007; Newland et al., 2013; Ross & Philbin, 2011).

Cost Analysis

The cost–benefit of promoting and providing human milk feedings in the NICU are calculated by a reduction in several prematurity-related morbidities, specifically

TABLE 8.3 Post-Menstrual Age and Time in Days to Full Oral Feeding and Discharge From First Oral Feeding

	Intervention Groups			
	Group 1: 32 Slow ($n = 18$)	Group 2: 32 Max ($n = 25$)	Group 3: 34 Slow ($n = 24$)	Group 4: 34 Max ($n = 19$)
Mean time in days from first oral feeding to full oral feedings (SD; min–max)	17.8 (1.9; 14.0–21.6)	17.8 (1.6; 14.6–21.0)	14.1 (1.9; 10.8–17.4)	8.8[a] (1.9; 5.1–12.4)
Mean PMA in weeks at full oral feeding (SD; min–max)	34.8 (0.286; 34.2–35.4)	34.8 (0.243; 34.3–35.3)	36.0[a] (0.253; 35.4–36.4)	35.1 (0.284; 34.6–35.7)
Mean time in days from first oral feeding to discharge (SD; min–max)	25.7 (2.2; 21.2–30.1)	24.8 (1.9; 21.1–28.6)	19.3[c] (1.9; 15.4–23.1)	15.1[b] (2.2; 10.8–19.4)
PMA in weeks at discharge (SD; min–max)	35.9 (0.337; 35.3–36.6)	35.8 (0.286; 35.3–36.4)	36.7 (0.286; 36.1–37.2)	36.0 (0.329; 35.4–36.7)

[a] Significantly different from Groups 1 and 2 at $p < 0.05$.
[b] Significantly different from Groups 1 and 2 at $p < 0.01$.
[c] Significantly different from Group 1 at $p = 0.03$.
PMA, post-menstrual age; SD, standard deviation.
Reprinted with permission from Creative Commons, Pickler et al. (2015).

necrotizing enterocolitis (NEC) and late-onset sepsis (Johnson et al., 2014). An exclusive human milk–based diet is linked to a shorter length of hospital stay and a decrease in NEC, with estimated cost savings approaching $10,000 (Ganapathy, Hay, & Kim, 2012; Herrmann & Carroll, 2014). Breast-milk feedings in the NICU not only optimize cognitive development but also reduce the need for early intervention and special education services (Vohr et al., 2006). Additionally, successful breastfeeding in the postdischarge period saves families in excess of $1,500/ yr in direct costs for feeding supplies and formula as well as the cost savings to families for fewer medical bills and fewer lost days of work (Association of Women's Health, Obstetric and Neonatal Nurses [AWHONN], 2015). Focusing on feeding behaviors and using an infant-driven feeding protocol has also been demonstrated to decrease transition time to full oral feedings and hospital stay, both of which are associated with significant cost savings (Horner et al., 2014; Sables-Baus et al., 2013).

Recommendations for Best Practices in Nurturing Feeding in the NICU (Table 8.4)

TABLE 8.4   Major Practice Recommendations and Implementation Strategies—Nurturing Feeding

Recommendations	Implementation Strategy
1. Develop a competency-based multimodal staff and parent education program on the benefits of breast milk and breastfeeding in the NICU (Alves et al., 2013; Hallowell et al., 2014; Renfrew et al., 2009) 2. Develop a competency-based multimodal staff and parent education program on effective and supportive techniques to initiate and sustain breastfeeding in the NICU (Alves et al., 2013; Hallowell et al., 2014; Renfrew et al., 2009)	a. Review your available education resources (instructor-led, eLearning, mobile resources, pamphlets) b. Collect baseline knowledge levels from staff and parents (this will allow you to measure your success) c. Review the literature to identify the latest information regarding breast milk feeding in the NICU as well as the evidence-based best practices to support, initiate, and sustain breastfeeding in the NICU d. Introduce a competency-based education module; follow-up with a posttest to measure impact of teaching e. Consider adding a practicum component to the teaching to allow application of the new knowledge f. Outline a plan for continuing education and integration of learning into interdisciplinary orientation g. Outline a plan to monitor knowledge translation into practice h. Audit practice, share results with staff
3. Ensure optimal lactation consultant staffing ratios (Mannel & Mannel, 2006; USLCA, 2010)	a. Review your current lactation consultant staff ratios b. Recommendations for tertiary care settings = 1.9 FTE/1,000 deliveries per year c. If you do not meet this recommendation, review your current breastfeeding rates, propose a test of change trialing the recommended staffing ratios d. Measure the breastfeeding rates following the staffing adjustment e. Consider quantifying your results beyond breastfeeding rates (e.g., length of stay, decrease infection rate) f. If you are operating with the correct staffing ratios, again calculate your breastfeeding rates and consider a SWOT (strengths, weaknesses, opportunities, and threats) analysis (Figure 8.7) of your existing work flow/productivity g. Address threats, explore opportunities using the PDSA model h. Evaluate interval improvements, revise and refine work flow and continual reevaluate i. Publish and/or present your results

(continued)

TABLE 8.4   Major Practice Recommendations and Implementation Strategies—Nurturing Feeding   (*continued*)

Recommendations	Implementation Strategy
4. Develop and sustain guidelines for breastfeeding support and practice expectations to include plans for prefeeding activities during skin to skin, ensuring the first oral feeding is at the breast, protecting privacy, etc. (Alves et al., 2013; Hallowell et al., 2014; Renfrew et al., 2009)	a. Review your existing practice guideline related to breastfeeding—consider integrating the Neo-BFHI 10 steps (see Tables 8.5 and 8.6) b. Establish a breastfeeding task force with clear, achievable goals and timelines c. Prioritize opportunities for improvement d. Utilize the PDSA model for improvement e. Consider an FMEA (for more information, see link under resources) f. Review your current feeding progression plan and consider a controlled test of change to facilitate transitioning from enteral tube feeding to direct breastfeeding g. Consider an algorithm to guide practice expectations; revise as necessary (Figures 8.9 and 8.10) h. Remember to capture your challenges and how they were resolved i. Refine your new practice and expand the test of change j. Make sure to identify and measure key metrics for success k. Provide feedback to staff l. Continually audit practice m. Publish and/or present your results
5. Ensure optimal communication between clinical staff and parents as well as administrative support and physician buy-in to promote and protect ongoing breast milk production (Lee et al., 2013)	a. Review your existing lines of communication among the maternity staff, NICU staff, and parents b. Are there gaps in communication and how can they be improved in relation to breastfeeding support (pumping and storing of human milk in-hospital and home)? c. What hospital resources are available to mothers expressing human milk? d. Consider collaborating with parents and administrators to identify resources that will support breast milk production in the NICU e. Draft a test of change; identify goals and success metrics f. Implement, evaluate, revise g. Measure results h. Publish and/or present results
6. Develop or obtain a staff and parent competency-based education program on feeding-readiness behaviors (Ludwig & Waitzman, 2007; Newland et al., 2013)	a. Assess current staff and parent knowledge of feeding readiness behaviors/cues b. Design (or outsource your education from an expert, clinically reliable source) a multimodel education module with a competency component (e.g., have staff and parents assess and identify readiness behaviors from video footage); include this into new hire orientation; consider it as an annual competency until the practice has become consistent and reliable (determine what that would look like) c. Assess the transfer of knowledge into practice—consider integrating feeding behavior assessment into the provider order set d. Measure and evaluate your results e. Refine or revise your education strategy based on learner feedback f. Publish and/or present your results

(*continued*)

TABLE 8.4   Major Practice Recommendations and Implementation Strategies—Nurturing Feeding   (*continued*)

Recommendations	Implementation Strategy
7. Adopt and integrate infant-driven or a responsive cue-based feeding model into your culture of care (Ludwig & Waitzman, 2007; Newland et al., 2013; Ross & Philbin, 2011; Waitzman et al., 2014; Wellington & Perlman, 2015)	a. Review your current oral-feeding strategy and collect benchmark data points (days to full oral feeds, average daily weight gain, frequency of feeding intolerance, even big data during feeds if available, etc.) b. Consider adopting the Infant-Driven Feeding® model of practice (see Figures 8.9 and 8.10), the SOFFI (see Figure 8.11) algorithm, or integrating the National Association of Neonatal Nurses Guidelines for Infant-Directed Oral Feeding for Premature and Critically Ill Hospitalized Infants (see link in resource section) c. Draft a test of change using the PDSA model (consider replicating the work of Gelfer et al., 2015) d. Implement a test on a designated patient population; evaluate results, revise/refine the plan, retest with the multidisciplinary team e. Share the project outcomes and integrate into the standard of care f. Continuously refine and improve your practice through audit and success metric trends g. Publish and/or present your results

FMEA, failure modes and effects analysis; PDSA, Plan-Do-Study-Act; SOFFI, supporting oral feeding in fragile infants; SWOT, strengths, weaknesses, opportunities, and threats.

Clinician and Parent Resources

This section presents a variety of resources you may find helpful as you transform your feeding practices. Assessing your existing strengths and weaknesses is a good place to start (Figure 8.7). Once you have a clear picture of your current reality you can then use the PDSA methodology to test change and identify the best path to your practice improvement objective. Tables 8.5 and 8.6 present the guiding principles and 10 steps in the Neonatal Baby Friendly Initiative. Various algorithms to guide infant-driven feeding and supporting oral feeding for fragile infants are outlined in Figures 8.9 and 8.10. Tables 8.7 to 8.9 are reprinted with permission from Sue Ludwig and Kara Ann Waitzman and provide information about the work they have done on feeding readiness behaviors and infant-driven feeding scales.

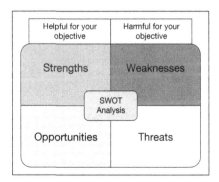

FIGURE 8.7   Sample SWOT analysis tool. In each quadrant, list the strengths, weaknesses, opportunities, and threats to your identified project objective/aim.

TABLE 8.5   Neonatal-Baby-Friendly Hospital Initiative (Neo-BFHI) Guiding Principles

1. Staff attitudes toward the mother must focus on the individual mother and her situation.
2. The facility must provide family-centered care, supported by the environment.
3. The health care system must ensure continuity of care from pregnancy to after the infant's discharge.

Source: Nyqvist et al. (2015).

TABLE 8.6   Neonatal-Baby-Friendly Hospital Initiative (Neo-BFHI)—10 Steps to Protect, Promote, and Support Breastfeeding

1. Have a written breastfeeding policy that is routinely communicated to all health care staff.
2. Educate and train all staff in the specific knowledge and skills necessary to implement this policy.
3. Inform hospitalized pregnant women at risk of preterm delivery or birth of a sick infant about the benefits of breastfeeding and the management of lactation and breastfeeding.
4. Encourage early, continuous, and prolonged mother–infant skin-to-skin contact/kangaroo mother care.
5. Show mothers how to initiate and maintain lactation and establish early breastfeeding with infant stability as the only criterion.
6. Give newborn infants no food or drink other than breast milk, unless medically indicated.
7. Enable mothers and infants to remain together 24 hours a day.
8. Encourage demand breastfeeding or, when needed, semi-demand feeding as a transitional strategy for preterm and sick infants.
9. Use alternatives to bottle feeding at least until breastfeeding is well established, and use pacifiers and nipple shields only for justifiable reasons.
10. Prepare parents for continued breastfeeding and ensure access to support services/groups after hospital discharge.

Neo-BFHI, Neonatal-Baby-Friendly Hospital Initiative.
Source: Nyqvist et al. (2015). Copyright 2015. Reprinted by permission of Kerstin Hedberg Nyqvist. http://www-conference.slu.se/neobfhi2015/Neo-BFHI_Core_document_2015_Edition.pdf

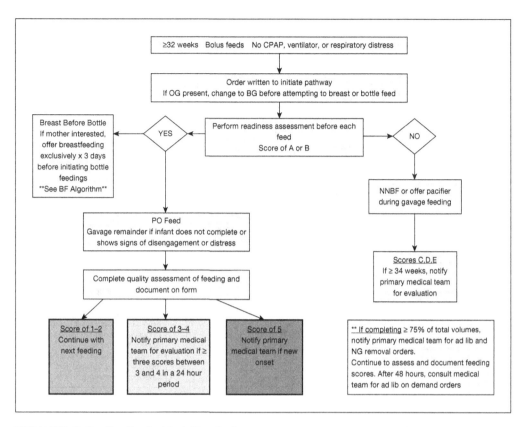

FIGURE 8.8 Algorithm for infant-driven feeding.

CPAP, continuous positive airway pressure; NG, nasogastric; NNBF, nonnutritive breastfeeding; OG, orogastric.

Reprinted with permission from Dr. Polina Gelfer.

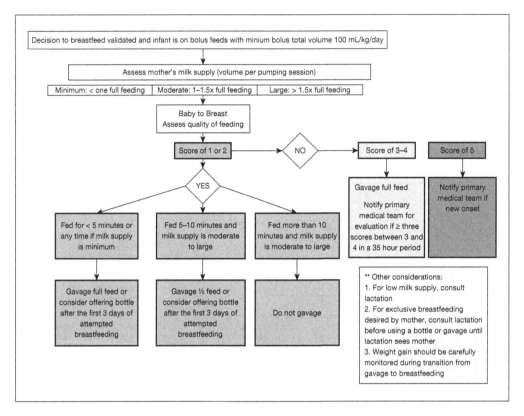

FIGURE 8.9   Algorithm for infant-driven breastfeeding.

Reprinted with permission from Dr. Polina Gelfer.

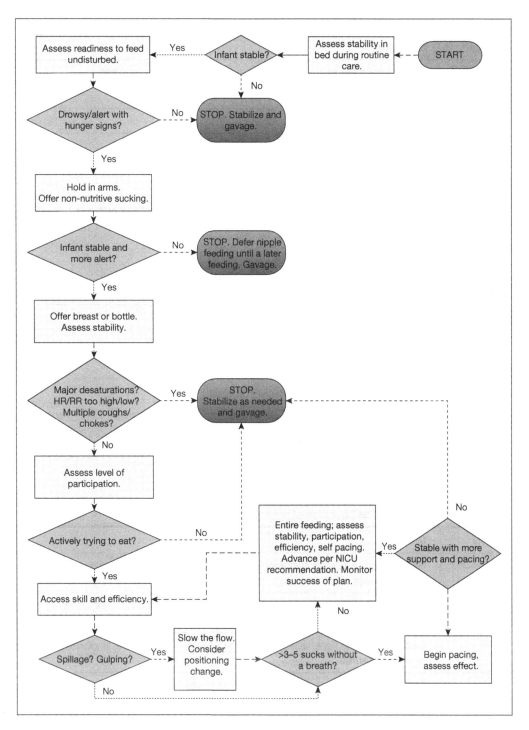

FIGURE 8.10   SOFFI (supporting oral feeding in fragile infants) method algorithm for bottle-feeding.

Source: Horner et al. (2014). Reprinted with permission from Dr. Erin Ross. Copyright © 2011. Reprinted by permission of Wolters Kluwer Health, Inc.

TABLE 8.7   Infant-Driven Feeding Scales©—Readiness

Score	Description
1	Alert or fussy before care. Rooting and/or hands-to-mouth behavior. Good tone.
2	Alert once handled. Some rooting or takes pacifier. Adequate tone.
3	Briefly alert with care. No hunger behaviors. No change in tone.
4	Sleeping throughout care. No hunger cues. No change in tone.
5	Significant change in heart rate, respiratory rate, O_2, or work of breathing outside safe parameters.

Reprinted with permission from Sue Ludwig and Kara Ann Waitzman. For permission to use Infant-Driven Feeding Scales in your hospital, please e-mail: info@infantdrivenfeeding.com

TABLE 8.8   Infant-Driven Feeding Scales©—Quality

Score	Description
1	Nipples with a strong coordinated SSB throughout feed.
2	Nipples with a strong coordinated SSB but fatigues with progression.
3	Difficulty coordinating SSB despite consistent suck.
4	Nipples with a weak/inconsistent SSB. Little to no rhythm.
5	Unable to coordinate SSB pattern. Significant change in heart rate, respiratory rate, O_2, work of breathing outside safe parameters or clinically unsafe swallow during feeding.

Reprinted with permission from Sue Ludwig and Kara Ann Waitzman. For permission to use Infant-Driven Feeding Scales in your hospital, please e-mail: info@infantdrivenfeeding.com

TABLE 8.9   Infant-Driven Feeding Scales©—Caregiver Techniques

Score	Description
A	Modified Sidelying: Position infant in inclined sidelying position with head in midline to assist with bolus management.
B	External Pacing: Tip bottle downward/break seal at breast to remove or decrease the flow of liquid to facilitate SSB pattern
C	Specialty Nipple: Use nipple other than standard for specific purpose, that is, nipple shield, slow-flow, Haberman
D	Cheek Support: Provide gentle unilateral support to improve intraoral pressure.
E	Frequent Burping: Burp infant based on behavioral cues not on time or volume completed
F	Chin Support: Provide gentle forward pressure on mandible to ensure effective latch/tongue stripping if small chin or wide jaw excursion.

SSB, suck-swallow-breath.
Reprinted with permission from Sue Ludwig and Kara Ann Waitzman. For permission to use Infant-Driven Feeding Scales in your hospital, please e-mail: info@infantdrivenfeeding.com

Infant-Driven Feeding® Model of Practice (for permission to use the IDFS in your hospital, please e-mail info@infantdrivenfeeding.com): For resources related to providing unit-wide online education on the Infant-Driven Feeding® Model of Practice, visit: www.infantdrivenfeeding.com

Additional Resources

- Neo-BFHI Core Document: www-conference.slu.se/neobfhi2015/ Neo-BFHI_Core_document_2015_Edition.pdf
- National Association of Neonatal Nurses Guidelines for Infant-Directed Oral Feeding for Premature and Critically Ill Hospitalized Infants: apps.nann .org/Default.aspx?TabID=251&productId=1416099

■ SKIN CARE

Who shall measure the subtlety of those touches which convey the quality of soul as well as body . . . ?
  —Georg Elliot

Interventions and Practice Considerations

1. Create and maintain a systematic approach to the assessment of skin and mucous membrane integrity
   - Best practice considerations include the use of a validated age-appropriate assessment tool and a clinical algorithm or practice guideline that addresses the utilization of evidence-based interventions when alterations in skin and mucous membrane integrity is identified
2. Create and maintain clear practice guidelines regarding bathing and hygiene practices in the NICU
   - Best practice considerations include outlining an individualized bathing mode and frequency for each infant, using colostrum/breast milk for oral care, educating parents on meeting the hygiene needs of their infant, and staff role-modeling best practices in infant hygiene consistently and reliably
3. Create and maintain a practice guideline for the protection of skin and mucous membranes
   - Best practice considerations include using protective skin barrier films when applying medical devices, adhering to pressure ulcer prevention recommendations, frequent repositioning of infants with limited mobility and frequently repositioning medical devices to minimize pressure points, minimizing transepidermal water losses, as well as frequent skin-to-skin care experiences to optimize infant's microbiome and positive hedonic touch

The Evidence

The skin is the largest organ of the human body and serves as a physical barrier to environmental threats, provides a resilient foundation for internal structural integrity and thermal regulation, and facilitates sensory discrimination and motivational-affective sensations (Abraira & Ginty, 2013; Morrison et al., 2010; Visscher & Narendran, 2014). The skin arises from the same ectodermal germ layer as the brain, and from a neurodevelopmental perspective, the skin is the surface of the brain participating in multiple caregiving interactions that contribute to the infant's meaning making of self and other (Gibbins et al., 2008; Tronick & Beeghly, 2011). Maintaining optimal functionality is key to survival (both physiologically and psychoemotionally) and challenging when caring for critically ill infants as their susceptibility to injury is related to not only their severity of illness and the developmental maturity of their skin, but also their vulnerability in social encounters, particularly those mediated by touch (McGlone et al., 2014; Ness et al., 2013; Visscher & Narendran, 2014). Mechanisms of skin injury for the hospitalized infant include mechanical, thermal, chemical, infectious, vascular, and/or developmental (Fox, 2011; Oranges, Dini, & Romanelli, 2015). Table 8.10 presents a general overview of the various mechanical injuries that can occur in the NICU.

Routinely assessing skin and mucous membrane integrity must be combined with a thoughtful risk assessment of the infant for infection, skin breakdown, vulnerability to the absorption of topical agents, as well as thermoregulatory failure; caregiving activities are implicated in increasing the hospitalized infant's level of these risks through individual hygiene practices and the level of clinician "presence" at the shared care interface (Boldrini et al., 2013; Gibbins et al., 2008; Oranges et al., 2015). Although the use of standardized pressure ulcer risk-assessment scales has not been linked to improved clinical outcomes, it is nonetheless considered best practice. *Take-away message*: *Choose a valid and reliable tool but don't let the tool replace clinical judgment* (Kottner & Balzer, 2010; Kottner et al., 2013; Lund et al., 2013).

Bathing as a routine care practice takes on new meaning in the NICU. Beyond aesthetics, bathing in the NICU aims to reduce infection as well as preserve skin integrity, but it is not without consequence to the hospitalized infant. Liaw et al. (2006) examined the relationship between infant distress and state behaviors during different phases of routine tub bathing and concluded that tub bathing not only disrupts infants' sleep, but increases their distress behaviors. Modifying the caregiving experience during tub bathing by providing containment and positional support decreases stress behaviors; conversely, when the caregiver is not attentive to the infant's stress behaviors, is rushed and "rough" during the care encounter, the infant's stress behaviors escalate and this wastes precious calories that are no longer available for growth and recovery (Liaw et al., 2010; Lin et al., 2014). In a randomized clinical trial comparing the effects of swaddled bathing with conventional bathing, the authors report a statistically significant decrease in crying time and stable thermoregulation in the swaddled group (Edraki et al., 2014). Loring

TABLE 8.10   Mechanical Injuries in Neonatal Skin

Mechanical Injury			
Pressure	**Abrasion and Lacerations**	**Skin Stripping (Denuding)**	**Trauma**
External, perpendicular force is applied to the skin impeding local perfusion and inducing shear to subcutaneous structures (these structures are forcibly displaced [shear] by the exerted surface pressure)—common sites of injury: • Ear lobes • Occiput • Nasal septum (CPAP induced injury) • Any interface between skin and medical device poses a threat to skin integrity	Rough or jagged surfaces/ devices exert a tangential force that abrades or pierces the skin (depth of injury will vary based on the surface/device)— common causes include: • Rough drying of the skin • Sliding the infant across a surface (as opposed to lifting) • Performing any needle or lance procedures	Mechanical interface removes the epidermal layer (with or without dermal elements) from the surface of skin—common causes include: • Tape removal • Adhesive removal	External forces applied to the skin cause various ranges of tissue injury and possibly underlying structures— common causes include: • Forceps • Vacuum extraction • Scalp electrode • Surgical incisions • Tubes and drains

Thermal Injury		Infectious Injury	
Either hot or cold devices/objects come in contact with the skin—common causes include • Burn from a transilluminator • Burn from a heated blanket or glove • Burn from humidified gas tubing • Cooling equipment • Frozen breast milk		Invasion of the skin by microorganisms— common causes include: • Infected surgical site or drain • Candidiasis • Staphylococcal scaled skin syndrome	

Chemical Injury			
Irritants		**Incontinence**	**Extravasation**
Solutions or substances that remove protective components of the stratum corneum—common causes include: • Dermatitis from soaps • Alcohol-induced hemorrhagic skin necrosis • Peri-stomal effluent from G-tube site		Diaper use macerates skin as the chemical components of urine and feces alter the protective acid mantle of the skin and activate enzymes and bile salts, which exacerbate perineal/peri-anal tissue injury—common causes include: • Diaper dermatitis • Infrequent diaper changes (Rough cleaning to the diaper area with soaps can complicate the degree of skin injury)	The chemical composition of various intravenous fluids can cause extensive damage to fragile extravascular structures up to and including necrosis—common causes include: • Extravasation of parenteral nutrition and other vesicant solutions • Infiltration of non-vesicant solutions

et al., (2012) compared body temperature in a cohort of late preterm infants before and after immersion tub bathing and sponge bathing and report significantly less body temperature variability in the infants who received the immersion tub bath. Sponge bathing preterm infants is associated with physiologic and behavioral consequences to include a decrease in vagal tone and oxygen saturation as well as increased motoric stress behaviors (Lee, 2002; Lee, Hong, Nam, Lee, & Jung, 2000; Peters, 1998).

The interval between tub bathing that has demonstrated safety with regard to skin flora and pathogen colonization is up to 4 days (Franck et al., 2000; Quinn et al., 2005). Involving families in the care of their hospitalized infants has long-lasting positive effects across physical, cognitive, and psychosocial domains; transitioning the bath from a nursing task to a parenting task validates parental role identity and increases parents' confidence and competence in caring for their hospitalized infant (Craig et al., 2015; Elser, 2013). Although best practice suggests bathing infants no more than three times per week, this does not mean that basic daily hygiene care is not necessary. Daily basic skin hygiene practices including keeping nails short and clean, gently wiping the infant's hands with either an infant wipe or washcloth with pH neutral soap (hands-to-mouth may be a vector for pathogen transmission from the infant's microenvironment), changing and washing the diaper area frequently using water and a washcloth or infant wipe, and gently washing the infant's face and neck area after feeding can be integrated into daily caregiving activities (Afsar, 2009; Coughlin et al., 2014; Landers et al., 2012; Visscher et al., 2009).

Providing oral care with mother's own milk in the NICU has been associated with several benefits to include a decrease in the rate of positive tracheal aspirates and positive blood cultures in mechanically intubated very low birth weight (VLBW) infants, increased levels of secretory immunoglobulin A and lactoferrin, a significant decrease in the incidence of sepsis, a reduced time to full enteral feedings, and an increase in weight gain (Gephart & Weller, 2014; Lee et al., 2015; Seigel et al., 2013; Thibeau & Boudreaux, 2013). Administration of mother's own milk via the oropharyngeal route has been demonstrated to be safe, feasible, and well tolerated by the most vulnerable of infants and is linked to an increase in breast-milk feeding; dosing regimen of at least once per day is a minimum recommendation with more frequent dosing of every 2 to 3 hours following each pumping session, when the mother is present and pumping at the bedside (Edwards & Spatz, 2010; Gephart & Weller., 2014; Meier et al., 2010; Rodriguez et al., 2010). In addition, applying a coating of breast milk to the infant's lips acts as a moisturizer and can prevent drying and cracking, thereby reducing the risk of infection as well as avoidable discomfort. Protecting neonatal skin and mucous membranes from medical adhesive-related skin injury (MARSI), and other hospital-acquired conditions (to include pressure ulcers and nosocomial infections) requires a collaborative, interprofessional commitment to patient quality and safety. This commitment begins with the adoption of evidence-based best practices in skin safety. The use of silicone adhesive products is recommended for the NICU patient population as these products attach quickly to the skin and can be removed easily and painlessly over hairy skin (Lund, 2014).

Most adhesive removers contain toxic chemicals that can cause topical injury but also pose a hazard via transcutaneous absorption and are not recommended for the neonatal patient population; the use of a water soaked cotton ball and slow, gently applied pressure is a safe alternative to remove adhesives until there is more neonatal testing on silicone-based removers (Lund, 2014).

Pressure ulcer prevalence rates as high as 23% have been reported in the NICU with more than 50% of pressure ulcers related to equipment and medical devices (Baharestani & Ratliff, 2007). Effective prevention strategies include the use of water, air, and gel mattresses and sheepskins as well as gel pads placed beneath pressure points (bony prominences to include the occiput) for pressure ulcer prevention in neonates less than 32 weeks gestation as well as frequent position changes for infants who are unable to reposition themselves (Baharestani & Ratliff, 2007; Lund, 1999). A frequent cause of pressure ulcer in the NICU is the use of nasal continuous positive airway pressure (CPAP)—although medically necessary, challenges with the patient interface can be a factor in this hospital-acquired condition. McCoskey (2008) describes a prevention-oriented approach to nares and nasal septal injury secondary to CPAP, which includes ensuring proper fit of the device, continuously assessing the vulnerable structures of the nares and septum, alternating between prongs and mask and positioning the infant prone for comfort and consequently minimizing the pressures variations that predispose the tissue to injury. In a prospective controlled study of 65 infants with an average gestational age of 32.6 weeks receiving nasal CPAP, the use of a hydrocolloid dressing as an interface between the infant's skin and the CPAP device demonstrated a statistically significant decrease in the incidence and severity of nasal injury (Xie, 2014).

With new, emerging evidence regarding the role of the microbiome in late-onset sepsis and necrotizing enterocolitis, interventions to minimize dysbiosis or perturbations in the fragile ecosystem of the microbiome are poised to minimize morbidity and mortality (Gritz & Bhandari, 2015). Factors that affect the infant's microbiome encompass prenatal factors such as maternal diet, antibiotics, and infections; perinatal factors that include maternal antibiotics and mode of delivery; and postnatal factors that include bathing practices, incubator versus mother care, hand hygiene practices, mechanical ventilation, indwelling feeding tubes, invasive lines, diet, the presence of an infection, and the use of antibiotics (Cacho & Neu, 2014; Cong et al., 2015; Johnson & Versalovic, 2012; Madan et al., 2012). In a randomized clinical trial, skin-to-skin contact performed twice a day for 60 minutes statistically significantly decreased methicillin-oxacillin-resistant *Staphylococcus aureus* (MRSA) and methicillin-oxacillin-resistant coagulase-negative *Staphylococcus epidermidis* (MRSE) nasal colonization after 7 days in a cohort of premature infants (Lamy Filho et al., 2015). The safety and effectiveness of this noninvasive strategy in combination with strict hygiene protocol and sterile central line care should be considered as an alternative to other, more potentially injurious strategies that compromise the fragile skin integrity of the hospitalized infant, particularly in the setting that the leading causative pathogen of neonatal late-onset sepsis is coagulase-negative staphylococci—MRSE (Dong & Speer, 2015; Gritz & Bhandari, 2015; Ponnusamy et al., 2014).

The tactile or touching dimensions of caregiving play an important role in how infants experience the world and how they make meaning about themselves in relation to other; positive, supportive interactions that respect the dignity of the developing human being at the shared surface interface influence infants' mental health development. Tronick and Beeghly (2011) argue that experiences that limit an infant's engagement with the world (e.g., when clinicians are unresponsive to an infant's behavioral stress cues, limited positive social/tactile interactions/experiences), translate into maladaptive meaning making that, when chronic, heightens the infant's vulnerability to psychological pathology.

Cost Analysis

The economic benefits gained from preserving and protecting infants' first line of defense against infection, the skin, is substantial, not to mention benefits in minimizing the associated pain, both physical and psychoemotional, with alterations in skin and mucous membrane integrity. With the average NICU cost of care associated with a bloodstream infection approaching $20,000, investments in the reliable implementation of evidence-based interventions to reduce infection by preserving skin integrity and skin ecosystems provide a substantial return on investment (Donovan et al., 2013; Gritz & Bhandari, 2015). Additionally, the preterm and hospitalized infant is at high risk for significant psychological pathology including autism spectrum disorders that not only undermine the infant's and family's quality of life, but also contributes to the societal burden of these chronic conditions (Fraley et al., 2013; Nosarti et al., 2012). Providing effective, no-cost interventions by acknowledging and interacting with the skin as a social organ may reduce individual morbidity and societal burden (McGlone et al., 2014; Morrison et al., 2010).

Recommendations for Best Practices in Skin Care of the Hospitalized Infant (Table 8.11)

TABLE 8.11   Major Practice Recommendations and Implementation Strategies—Skin Care

Recommendations	Implementation Strategy
1. Adopt an age-appropriate, validated and reliable skin assessment tool; connect assessment findings with appropriate interventions and prevention strategies	a. Review existing skin assessment and prevention strategies—do they meet the needs of the patient and the caregiver? b. Consider developing an algorithm to guide clinical practice when deviations in skin and mucous membrane integrity are assessed c. Test your algorithm d. Evaluate, revise, implement e. Measure results (number of consults for skin injury, infections, pressure ulcers, etc.) f. Provide continual feedback to staff g. Publish and/or present your results

(continued)

TABLE 8.11   Major Practice Recommendations and Implementation Strategies—Skin Care   (continued)

Recommendations	Implementation Strategy
2. Develop a competency-based education module for staff and parents on swaddled bathing; include a simulated return demonstration	a. Review your available education resources (instructor-led, eLearning, mobile resources, pamphlets) b. Collect baseline knowledge levels from staff and parents regarding bathing (this will allow you to measure your success) c. Introduce a competency-based education module; follow up with a posttest to measure impact of teaching d. Include a simulated practicum component to the teaching to allow application of the new knowledge e. Outline a plan for continuing education and integration of learning into interdisciplinary orientation f. Outline a plan to monitor knowledge translation into practice g. Audit practice, share results with staff
3. Establish swaddled bathing as a parenting task and, in partnership with parents, outline an individualized bathing routine; capture this plan in the patient's medical record and the parents' diary	a. Review your existing bathing practices, consider collecting big data during bathing events, staff/parent survey data about the bathing experiences, parent confidence, engagement, and other tools to measure parent skills, development/satisfaction before and after the new practice has been implemented, etc. b. Verify that parents have completed the required education and any gaps have been resolved (e.g., cultural concerns) c. Implement the new practice, monitor for unexpected outcomes d. Measure results and compare top baseline metrics e. Provide feedback to staff and parents f. Publish and/or present results

4. Develop a daily hygiene routine that minimizes distress to the infant while minimizing infectious risks	a. Review your current routine hygiene practices (washing hands and face, cleansing diaper area, changing bed linens)
	b. Outline a test of change to integrate these routines
	   i. Consider the use of mild infant wipes
	   ii. Maintain a container at each infant's bedside, and so forth
	c. Consider monitoring frequency of skin eruptions, bloodstream infections, diaper dermatitis, and gastrointestinal distresses before and after implementation
	d. Outline how this practice will be documented
	e. If there are additional costs for wipes, contrast this cost to outcomes (i.e., infection rates)
	f. Revise and refine practice
	g. Publish and/or present results

5. Adopt an oral immune therapy plan of care using mother's own milk; ensure that staff are competent in the proper administration	a. Review your existing oral care practice b. Educate staff and parents on the benefits of oral immune therapy c. Develop and implement a competency on oropharyngeal administration of colostrum/mother's milk for staff and parents (*do not assume everyone knows how to do it!*)

(continued)

TABLE 8.11 Major Practice Recommendations and Implementation Strategies—Skin Care   *(continued)*

Recommendations	Implementation Strategy
	d. Once everyone is competent with the proper administration technique, implement the practice (consider giving parents a certificate of achievement following their competency completion) e. Make sure the EMR is able to capture this intervention (minimum frequency is daily, but the record should be able to capture additional interventions [Gephart & Weller, 2014]) f. Consider including this practice in the admission order set (outline criteria for this standing order) g. Identify quality metrics—breastfeeding rates, incidence of NEC, feeding intolerance, late-onset sepsis, and so forth h. Outline the process for collection, storage, and delivery with parents i. Compare before and after selected metrics j. Audit and trend practice and provide continual feedback to staff and parents k. Publish and/or present results

6. Support and facilitate continuous skin-to-skin care with eligible infants	a. Review your existing skin-to-skin care practice guidelines and infant transfer method
	b. Revise the guidelines to ensure clear eligibility criteria, documentation requirements, and standardize the infant transfer method to the standing transfer
	   i. Create a competency-based learning module for staff and parents with simulation to ensure confidence and competence in the practice
	   ii. Consider start and stop times for monitoring skin-to-skin care sessions (to capture and compare dose-dependent effect)
	c. Identify success metrics and collect baseline and intervention data points
	d. Provide feedback to staff and parents
	e. Incorporate performance expectations for skin-to-skin care in the annual staff review process
	f. Publish and/or present results

7. Develop clear expectations and practice guidelines for pressure ulcer prevention and MARSIs	a. Review existing practice and revise as necessary based on the latest evidence-based recommendations (e.g., using pressure-relieving sleep surfaces, barrier films for medical device interfaces, eliminating the use of toxic adhesive remover solutions) b. Outline a test of change to address your revised practice policy i. Include a more sensitive approach to the pressure ulcer surveillance process, that is, can this be done while the parent is providing skin-to-skin, can a second clinician support the infant during the head-to-toe assessment, and so forth c. Outline success metrics and collect baseline data points for postintervention evaluation d. Outline documentation criteria e. Revise your test of change and implement

(continued)

TABLE 8.11 Major Practice Recommendations and Implementation Strategies—Skin Care *(continued)*

Recommendations	Implementation Strategy
	f. Audit practice; provide feedback to staff and parents g. Publish and/or present your results

8. Develop practice expectations for positive/social touch with each caregiving encounter (parent and professional) and other types of positive touch as therapeutic interventions, that is, M-technique, massage, tactile-kinesthetic stimulation (Badr et al., 2015; Field et al., 2010; Pepino & Mezzacappa., 2015; Smith, 2012; Smith et al., 2012)	a. Review your current practice of engaging in a caregiving encounter
	b. Identify opportunities to improve that process that are repeatable and sustainable
	  i. Provide a verbal greeting to the infant with tactile input on nonvulnerable body areas (e.g., head, back, cupping the lower extremities)
	  ii. Watch the infant's response to the greeting and proceed once the infant demonstrates engagement cues
	c. Review resources for various positive touch therapies and develop a protocol with clear eligibility criteria for the selected touch therapies
	d. Ensure practitioner competence in the selected touch therapy
	e. Identify success metrics
	f. Collect benchmark data points for postintervention comparison
	g. Provide feedback to staff and parents
	h. Revise plan as indicated
	i. Publish and/or present results

EMR, electronic medical record; MARSIs, medical adhesive-related skin injuries; NEC, necrotizing enterocolitis.

Tools and Patient Resources

NEONATAL SKIN ASSESSMENT TOOLS

- Braden Q Scale
- Glamorgan Scale
- Neonatal Skin Condition Score
- Starkid Skin Scale
- Neonatal Skin Risk Assessment Scale

SWADDLED BATHING IN THE NICU
- A protocol for swaddled bathing in the NICU: www.medscape.com/viewarticle/781129
- Tender loving baths in the NICU: www.dandlelion-webinars.com/wp-content/uploads/2013/02/Tender-Loving-Baths-in-the-NICI.pdf
- *NICU Journal*—a parent's journey: www2.aap.org/sections/perinatal/pdf/NICUTab1.pdf

■ REFERENCES

Abraira, V. E., & Ginty, D. D. (2013). The sensory neurons of touch. *Neuron, 79*(4), 618–639.

Afsar, F. S. (2009). Skin care for preterm and term neonates. *Clinical and Experimental Dermatology, 34*(8), 855–858.

Allen, M. C., & Capute, A. J. (1990). Tone and reflex development before term. *Pediatrics, 85*(3 Pt. 2), 393–399.

Alves, E., Rodrigues, C., Fraga, S., Barros, H., & Silva, S. (2013). Parents' views on factors that help or hinder breast milk supply in neonatal care units: Systematic review. *Archives of Disease in Childhood. Fetal and Neonatal Edition, 98*(6), F511–F517.

American Academy of Pediatrics (AAP). (2012). Policy statement: Breastfeeding and the use of human milk. *Pediatrics, 129*(3), e827–e841.

Ancora, G., Maranella, E., Aceti, A., Pierantoni, L., Grandi, S., Corvaglia, L., & Faldella, G. (2010). Effect of posture on brain hemodynamics in preterm newborns not mechanically ventilated. *Neonatology, 97*(3), 212–217.

Association of Women's Health, Obstetric and Neonatal Nurses (AWHONN). (2015). AWHONN position statement: Breastfeeding. *Journal of Obstetric, Gynecologic and Neonatal Nursing, 44*, 145–150.

Badr, L. K., Abdallah, B., & Kahale, L. (2015). A meta-analysis of preterm infant massage: An ancient practice with contemporary applications. *MCN. The American Journal of Maternal Child Nursing, 40*(6), 344–358.

Baharestani, M. M., & Ratliff, C. R. (2007). Pressure ulcers in neonates and children: An NPUAP white paper. *Advances in Skin & Wound Care, 20*(4), 208, 210, 212, 214, 216, 218–208, 210, 212, 214, 216, 220.

Balaguer, A., Escribano, J., Roque i. Figulus, M., & Rivas-Fernandez, M. (2013). Infant position in neonates receiving mechanical ventilation. *Cochrane Database of Systematic Reviews, 2013*(3), CD003668.

Baley, J.; Committee on Fetus and Newborn. (2015). Skin-to-skin care for term and preterm infants in the neonatal ICU. *Pediatrics, 136*(3), 596–599.

Benoit, B., & Semenic, S. (2014). Barriers and facilitators to implementing the Baby-Friendly Hospital Initiative in neonatal intensive care units. *Journal of Obstetric, Gynecologic, and Neonatal Nursing: JOGNN/NAACOG, 43*(5), 614–624.

Bernaix, L. W., Schmidt, C. A., Arrizola, M., Iovinelli, D., & Medina-Poelinez, C. (2008). Success of a lactation education program on NICU nurses' knowledge and attitudes. *Journal of Obstetric, Gynecologic, and Neonatal Nursing: JOGNN/NAACOG, 37*(4), 436–445.

Bobb, A. M., Payne, T. H., & Gross, P. A. (2007). Viewpoint: Controversies surrounding use of order sets for clinical decision support in computerized provider order entry. *Journal of the American Medical Informatics Association, 14*(1), 41–47.

Boldrini, A., Scaramuzzo, R. T., & Cuttano, A. (2013). Errors in neonatology. *Journal of Pediatric and Neonatal Individualized Medicine, 2*(2), e020231.

Briere, C. E., McGrath, J., Cong, X., & Cusson, R. (2014). An integrative review of factors that influence breastfeeding duration for premature infants after NICU hospitalization. *Journal of Obstetric, Gynecologic, and Neonatal Nursing: JOGNN/NAACOG, 43*(3), 272–281.

Bruggink, J. L., Einspieler, C., Butcher, P. R., Van Braeckel, K. N., Prechtl, H. F., & Bos, A. F. (2008). The quality of the early motor repertoire in preterm infants predicts minor neurologic dysfunction at school age. *The Journal of Pediatrics, 153*(1), 32–39.

Cacho, N., & Neu, J. (2014). Manipulation of the intestinal microbiome in newborn infants. *Advances in Nutrition, 5*(1), 114–118.

Collett, B. R., Aylward, E. H., Berg, J., Davidoff, C., Norden, J., Cunningham, M. L., & Speltz, M. L. (2012). Brain volume and shape in infants with deformational plagiocephaly. *Child's Nervous System: Official Journal of the International Society for Pediatric Neurosurgery, 28*(7), 1083–1090.

Collett, B. R., Gray, K. E., Starr, J. R., Heike, C. L., Cunningham, M. L., & Speltz, M. L. (2013). Development at age 36 months in children with deformational plagiocephaly. *Pediatrics, 131*(1), e109–e115.

Collett, B. R., Starr, J. R., Kartin, D., Heike, C. L., Berg, J., Cunningham, M. L., & Speltz, M. L. (2011). Development in toddlers with and without deformational plagiocephaly. *Archives of Pediatrics & Adolescent Medicine, 165*(7), 653–658.

Comaru, T., & Miura, E. (2009). Postural support improves distress and pain during diaper change in preterm infants. *Journal of Perinatology: Official Journal of the California Perinatal Association, 29*(7), 504–507.

Cong, X., Henderson, W. A., Graf, J., & McGrath, J. M. (2015). Early life experience and gut microbiome: The brain-gut-microbiota signaling system. *Advances in Neonatal Care: Official Journal of the National Association of Neonatal Nurses, 15*(5), 314–323; quiz E1.

Coughlin, C. C., Frieden, I. J., & Eichenfield, L. F. (2014). Clinical approaches to skin cleansing of the diaper area: Practice and challenges. *Pediatric Dermatology, 31*(Suppl. 1), 1–4.

Coughlin, M. (2015). The Sobreviver (survive) project. *Newborn and Infant Nursing Reviews, 15*(4), 169–173.

Coughlin, M., Lohman, M. B., & Gibbins, S. (2010). Reliability and effectiveness of an infant positioning assessment tool to standardize developmentally supportive positioning practices in the neonatal intensive care unit. *Newborn and Infant Nursing Reviews, 10*(2), 104–106.

Craig, J. W., Glick, C., Phillips, R., Hall, S. L., Smith, J., & Browne, J. (2015). Recommendations for involving the family in developmental care of the NICU baby. *Journal of Perinatology: Official Journal of the California Perinatal Association, 35*(Suppl. 1), S5–S8.

Cricco-Lizza, R. (2011). Everyday nursing practice values in the NICU and their reflection on breastfeeding promotion. *Qualitative Health Research, 21*(3), 399–409.

Danks, M., Maideen, M. F., Burns, Y. R., O'Callaghan, M. J., Gray, P. H., Poulsen, L., . . . Gibbons, K. (2012). The long-term predictive validity of early motor development in "apparently normal" ELBW survivors. *Early Human Development, 88*(8), 637–641.

Demirel, G., Oguz, S. S., Celik, I. H., Erdeve, O., & Dilmen, U. (2012). Cerebral and mesenteric tissue oxygenation by positional changes in very low birth weight premature infants. *Early Human Development, 88*(6), 409–411.

Dietz, A. S., Pronovost, P. J., Mendez-Tellez, P. A., Wyskiel, R., Marsteller, J. A., Thompson, D. A., & Rosen, M. A. (2014). A systematic review of teamwork in the intensive care unit: What do we know about teamwork, team tasks, and improvement strategies? *Journal of Critical Care, 29*(6), 908–914.

Diniz, K. T., Cabral-Filho, J. E., Miranda, R. M., Souza Lima, G. M., & Vasconcelos, D. d. A. (2013). Effect of the kangaroo position on the electromyographic activity of preterm children: A follow-up study. *BMC Pediatrics*, *13*, 79.

Dong, Y., & Speer, C. P. (2015). Late-onset neonatal sepsis: Recent developments. *Archives of Disease in Childhood. Fetal and Neonatal Edition*, *100*(3), F257–F263.

Donovan, E. F., Sparling, K., Lake, M. R., Narendran, V., Schibler, K., Haberman, B., . . . Meinzen-Derr, J.; Ohio Perinatal Quality Collaborative. (2013). The investment case for preventing NICU-associated infections. *American Journal of Perinatology*, *30*(3), 179–184.

Dougherty, D., & Luther, M. (2008). Birth to breast—A feeding care map for the NICU: Helping the extremely low birth weight infant navigate the course. *Neonatal Network*, *27*(6), 371–377.

Edraki, M., Paran, M., Montaseri, S., Razavi Nejad, M., & Montaseri, Z. (2014). Comparing the effects of swaddled and conventional bathing methods on body temperature and crying duration in premature infants: A randomized clinical trial. *Journal of Caring Sciences*, *3*(2), 83–91.

Edwards, T. M., & Spatz, D. L. (2010). An innovative model for achieving breast-feeding success in infants with complex surgical anomalies. *The Journal of Perinatal & Neonatal Nursing*, *24*(3), 246–253; quiz 254.

Eghbalian, F. (2014). A comparison of supine and prone positioning on improves arterial oxygenation in premature neonates. *Journal of Neonatal-Perinatal Medicine*, *7*(4), 273–277.

Eliakim, A., Nemet, D., Friedland, O., Dolfin, T., & Regev, R. H. (2002). Spontaneous activity in premature infants affects bone strength. *Journal of Perinatology: Official Journal of the California Perinatal Association*, *22*(8), 650–652.

Elser, H. E. (2013). Bathing basics: How clean should neonates be? *Advances in Neonatal Care: Official Journal of the National Association of Neonatal Nurses*, *13*(3), 188–189.

Field, T., Diego, M., & Hernandez-Reif, M. (2010). Preterm infant massage therapy research: A review. *Infant Behavior & Development*, *33*(2), 115–124.

Fraley, R. C., Roisman, G. I., & Haltigan, J. D. (2013). The legacy of early experiences in development: Formalizing alternative models of how early experiences are carried forward over time. *Developmental Psychology*, *49*(1), 109–126.

Franck, L. S., Quinn, D., & Zahr, L. (2000). Effect of less frequent bathing of preterm infants on skin flora and pathogen colonization. *Journal of Obstetric, Gynecologic, and Neonatal Nursing: JOGNN/NAACOG*, *29*(6), 584–589.

Frolek Clark, G. J., & Schlabach, T. L. (2013). Systematic review of occupational therapy interventions to improve cognitive development in children ages birth–5 years. *The American Journal of Occupational Therapy: Official Publication of the American Occupational Therapy Association*, *67*(4), 425–430.

Ganapathy, V., Hay, J. W., & Kim, J. H. (2012). Costs of necrotizing enterocolitis and cost-effectiveness of exclusively human milk-based products in feeding extremely premature infants. *Breastfeeding Medicine: The Official Journal of the Academy of Breastfeeding Medicine*, *7*(1), 29–37.

Gelfer, P., McCarthy, A., & Turnage Spruill, C. (2015). Infant driven feeding for preterm infants: Learning through experience. *Newborn and Infant Nursing Reviews*, *15*(2), 64–67.

Gephart, S. M., & Weller, M. (2014). Colostrum as oral immune therapy to promote neonatal health. *Advances in Neonatal Care: Official Journal of the National Association of Neonatal Nurses, 14*(1), 44–51.

Gibbins, S., Hoath, S. B., Coughlin, M., Gibbins, A., & Franck, L. (2008). The universe of developmental care: A new conceptual model for application in the neonatal intensive care unit. *Advances in Neonatal Care: Official Journal of the National Association of Neonatal Nurses, 8*(3), 141–147.

Grant, A., & Coughlin, M. (2015). *Effectiveness of a mobile learning application to improve postural integrity.* 5th Annual National Association of Neonatal Therapists Conference, The Wigwam, Litchfield, Arizona.

Gritz, E. C., & Bhandari, V. (2015). Corrigendum: The human neonatal gut microbiome: A brief review. *Frontiers in Pediatrics, 3*, 60.

Hallowell, S. G., Spatz, D. L., Hanlon, A. L., Rogowski, J. A., & Lake, E. T. (2014). Characteristics of the NICU work environment associated with breastfeeding support. *Advances in Neonatal Care: Official Journal of the National Association of Neonatal Nurses, 14*(4), 290–300.

Herrmann, K., & Carroll, K. (2014). An exclusively human milk diet reduces necrotizing enterocolitis. *Breastfeeding Medicine: The Official Journal of the Academy of Breastfeeding Medicine, 9*(4), 184–190.

Hoban, R., Bigger, H., Patel, A. L., Rossman, B., Fogg, L. F., & Meier, P. (2015). Goals for human milk feeding in mothers of very low birth weight infants: How do goals change and are they achieved during the NICU hospitalization? *Breastfeeding Medicine: The Official Journal of the Academy of Breastfeeding Medicine, 10*(6), 305–311.

Horner, S., Simonelli, A. M., Schmidt, H., Cichowski, K., Hancko, M., Zhang, G., & Ross, E. S. (2014). Setting the stage for successful oral feeding: The impact of implementing the SOFFI feeding program with medically fragile NICU infants. *The Journal of Perinatal & Neonatal Nursing, 28*(1), 59–68.

Ikonen, R., Paavilainen, E., & Kaunonen, M. (2015). Preterm infants' mothers' experiences with milk expression and breastfeeding: An integrative review. *Advances in Neonatal Care: Official Journal of the National Association of Neonatal Nurses, 15*(6), 394–406.

Jeanson, E. (2013). One-to-one bedside nurse education as a means to improve positioning consistency. *Newborn and Infant Nursing Reviews, 13*(1), 27–30.

Johnson, T. J., Patel, A. L., Bigger, H. R., Engstrom, J. L., & Meier, P. P. (2014). Economic benefits and costs of human milk feedings: A strategy to reduce the risk of prematurity-related morbidities in very-low-birth-weight infants. *Advances in Nutrition, 5*(2), 207–212.

Johnson, C. L., & Versalovic, J. (2012). The human microbiome and its potential importance to pediatrics. *Pediatrics, 129*(5), 950–960.

Kish, M. Z. (2013). Oral feeding readiness in preterm infants: A concept analysis. *Advances in Neonatal Care: Official Journal of the National Association of Neonatal Nurses, 13*(4), 230–237.

Korraa, A. A., El Nagger, A. A., Mohamed, R. A., & Helmy, N. M. (2014). Impact of kangaroo mother care on cerebral blood flow of preterm infants. *Italian Journal of Pediatrics, 13*(40), 83. doi:10.1186/s13052–014-0083–5

Kottner, J., & Balzer, K. (2010). Do pressure ulcer risk assessment scales improve clinical practice? *Journal of Multidisciplinary Healthcare, 3*, 103–111.

Kottner, J., Hauss, A., Schlüer, A. B., & Dassen, T. (2013). Validation and clinical impact of paediatric pressure ulcer risk assessment scales: A systematic review. *International Journal of Nursing Studies, 50*(6), 807–818.

Lamy Filho, F., de Sousa, S. H., Freitas, I. J., Lamy, Z. C., Simões, V. M., da Silva, A. A., & Barbieri, M. A. (2015). Effect of maternal skin-to-skin contact on decolonization of methicillin-oxacillin-resistant *Staphylococcus* in neonatal intensive care units: A randomized controlled trial. *BMC Pregnancy and Childbirth, 15*, 63.

Landers, T., Abusalem, S., Coty, M. B., & Bingham, J. (2012). Patient-centered hand hygiene: The next step in infection prevention. *American Journal of Infection Control, 40*(4, Suppl. 1), S11–S17.

Lau, C. (2015). Development of suck and swallow mechanisms in infants. *Annals of Nutrition & Metabolism, 66*(Suppl. 5), 7–14.

Lee, H. C., Martin-Anderson, S., Lyndon, A., & Dudley, R. A. (2013). Perspectives on promoting breastmilk feedings for premature infants during a quality improvement project. *Breastfeeding Medicine: The Official Journal of the Academy of Breastfeeding Medicine, 8*, 176–180.

Lee, H. K. (2002). Effects of sponge bathing on vagal tone and behavioural responses in premature infants. *Journal of Clinical Nursing, 11*(4), 510–519.

Lee, H. K., Hong, K. J., Nam, E. S., Lee, Y. H., & Jung, E. J. (2000). Physiologic state and behavioral response to sponge bathing in premature infants. *Child Health Nursing Research, 6*(1), 32–50.

Lee, J., Kim, H. S., Jung, Y. H., Choi, K. Y., Shin, S. H., Kim, E. K., & Choi, J. H. (2015). Oropharyngeal colostrum administration in extremely premature infants: An RCT. *Pediatrics, 135*(2), e357–e366.

Liao, S. M., Rao, R., & Mathur, A. M. (2015). Head position change is not associated with acute changes in bilateral cerebral oxygenation in stable preterm infants during the first 3 days of life. *American Journal of Perinatology, 32*(7), 645–652.

Liaw, J. J., Yang, L., Chou, H. L., Yang, M. H., & Chao, S. C. (2010). Relationships between nurse care-giving behaviours and preterm infant responses during bathing: A preliminary study. *Journal of Clinical Nursing, 19*(1–2), 89–99.

Liaw, J. J., Yang, L., Yuh, Y. S., & Yin, T. (2006). Effects of tub bathing procedures on preterm infants' behavior. *The Journal of Nursing Research, 14*(4), 297–305.

Lin, H. C., Huang, L. C., Li, T. C., Chen, C. H., Bachman, J., & Peng, N. H. (2014). Relationship between energy expenditure and stress behaviors of preterm infants in the neonatal intensive care unit. *Journal for Specialists in Pediatric Nursing, 19*(4), 331–338.

Loring, C., Gregory, K., Gargan, B., LeBlanc, V., Lundgren, D., Reilly, J., . . . Zaya, C. (2012). Tub bathing improves thermoregulation of the late preterm infant. *Journal of Obstetric, Gynecologic, & Neonatal Nursing, 41*(2), 171–179.

Lucas, R., Paquette, R., Briere, C. E., & McGrath, J. G. (2014). Furthering our understanding of the needs of mothers who are pumping breast milk for infants in the NICU: An integrative review. *Advances in Neonatal Care: Official Journal of the National Association of Neonatal Nurses, 14*(4), 241–252.

Lucas, R. F., & Smith, R. L. (2015). When is it safe to initiate breastfeeding for preterm infants? *Advances in Neonatal Care: Official Journal of the National Association of Neonatal Nurses, 15*(2), 134–141.

Ludington-Hoe, S. M. (2013). Kangaroo care as a neonatal therapy. *Newborn and infant Nursing Reviews, 13*(2), 73–75.

Ludington-Hoe, S. M., Ferreira, C., Swinth, J., & Ceccardi, J. J. (2003). Safe criteria and procedure for kangaroo care with intubated preterm infants. *Journal of Obstetric, Gynecologic, and Neonatal Nursing: JOGNN/NAACOG, 32*(5), 579–588.

Ludwig, S. M., & Waitzman, K. A. (2007). Changing feeding documentation to reflect infant-driven feeding practice. *Newborn and Infant Nursing Reviews, 7*(3), 155–160.

Lund, C. (1999). Prevention and management of infant skin breakdown. *The Nursing Clinics of North America, 34*(4), 907–920, vii.

Lund, C. (2014). Medical adhesives in the NICU. *Newborn and Infant Nursing Reviews, 14*(4), 160–165.

Lund, C. H., Brandon, D., Holden, A. C., Kuller, J., & Hill, C. M. (2013). *Neonatal skin care: Evidence-based clinical practice guideline* (3rd ed.). Washington, DC: Association of Women's Health, Obstetrics and Neonatal Nursing.

Ma, M., Noori, S., Maarek, J. M., Holschneider, D. P., Rubinstein, E. H., & Seri, I. (2015). Prone positioning decreases cardiac output and increases systemic vascular resistance in neonates. *Journal of Perinatology: Official Journal of the California Perinatal Association, 35*(6), 424–427.

Madan, J. C., Farzan, S. F., Hibberd, P. L., & Karagas, M. R. (2012). Normal neonatal microbiome variation in relation to environmental factors, infection and allergy. *Current Opinion in Pediatrics, 24*(6), 753–759.

Madlinger-Lewis, L., Reynolds, L., Zarem, C., Crapnell, T., Inder, T., & Pineda, R. (2014). The effects of alternative positioning on preterm infants in the neonatal intensive care unit: A randomized clinical trial. *Research in Developmental Disabilities, 35*(2), 490–497.

Mahoney, M. C., & Cohen, M. I. (2005). Effectiveness of developmental intervention in the neonatal intensive care unit: Implications for neonatal physical therapy. *Pediatric Physical Therapy: The Official Publication of the Section on Pediatrics of the American Physical Therapy Association, 17*(3), 194–208.

Malusky, S., & Donze, A. (2011). Neutral head positioning in premature infants for intraventricular hemorrhage prevention: An evidence-based review. *Neonatal Network, 30*(6), 381–396.

Mannel, R., & Mannel, R. S. (2006). Staffing for hospital lactation programs: Recommendations from a tertiary care teaching hospital. *Journal of Human Lactation: Official Journal of International Lactation Consultant Association, 22*(4), 409–417.

Mathisen, B. A., Carey, L. B., & O'Brien, A. (2012). Incorporating speech-language pathology within Australian neonatal intensive care units. *Journal of Paediatrics and Child Health, 48*(9), 823–827.

Maycock, B., Binns, C. W., Dhaliwal, S., Tohotoa, J., Hauck, Y., Burns, S., & Howat, P. (2013). Education and support for fathers improves breastfeeding rates: A randomized controlled trial. *Journal of Human Lactation: Official Journal of International Lactation Consultant Association, 29*(4), 484–490.

McCoskey, L. (2008). Nursing care guidelines for prevention of nasal breakdown in neonates receiving nasal CPAP. *Advances in Neonatal Care: Official Journal of the National Association of Neonatal Nurses, 8*(2), 116–124.

McGlone, F., Wessberg, J., & Olausson, H. (2014). Discriminative and affective touch: Sensing and feeling. *Neuron, 82*(4), 737–755.

Meier, P. P., Engstrom, J. L., Patel, A. L., Jegier, B. J., & Bruns, N. E. (2010). Improving the use of human milk during and after the NICU stay. *Clinics in Perinatology, 37*(1), 217–245.

Mewes, A. U., Zöllei, L., Hüppi, P. S., Als, H., McAnulty, G. B., Inder, T. E.,...Warfield, S. K. (2007). Displacement of brain regions in preterm infants with non-synostotic dolichocephaly investigated by MRI. *NeuroImage, 36*(4), 1074–1085.

Miranda, R. M., Cabral Filho, J. E., Diniz, K. T., Souza Lima, G. M., & Vasconcelos, D. d. A. (2014). Electromyographic activity of preterm newborns in the kangaroo position: A cohort study. *BMJ Open, 4*(10), e005560.

Mitchell-Box, K. M., & Braun, K. L. (2013). Impact of male-partner-focused interventions on breastfeeding initiation, exclusivity, and continuation. *Journal of Human Lactation: Official Journal of International Lactation Consultant Association, 29*(4), 473–479.

Monterosso, L., Coenen, A., Percival, P., & Evans, S. (1995). Effect of a postural support nappy on "flattened posture" of the lower extremeties in very preterm infants. *Journal of Paediatrics and Child Health, 31*(4), 350–354.

Monterosso, L., Kristjanson, L., & Cole, J. (2002). Neuromotor development and the physiologic effects of positioning in very low birth weight infants. *Journal of Obstetric, Gynecologic, and Neonatal Nursing: JOGNN/NAACOG, 31*(2), 138–146.

Monterosso, L., Kristjanson, L. J., Cole, J., & Evans, S. F. (2003). Effect of postural supports on neuromotor function in very preterm infants to term equivalent age. *Journal of Paediatrics and Child Health, 39*(3), 197–205.

Morrison, I., Löken, L. S., & Olausson, H. (2010). The skin as a social organ. *Experimental Brain Research, 204*(3), 305–314.

Ness, M. J., Davis, D. M., & Carey, W. A. (2013). Neonatal skin care: A concise review. *International Journal of Dermatology, 52*(1), 14–22.

Neu, M., & Browne, J. V. (1997). Infant physiologic and behavioral organization during swaddled versus unswaddled weighing. *Journal of Perinatology: Official Journal of the California Perinatal Association, 17*(3), 193–198.

Newland, L., L'huillier, M. W., & Petrey, B. (2013). Implementation of cue-based feeding in a level III NICU. *Neonatal Network, 32*(2), 132–137.

Nightlinger, K. (2011). Developmentally supportive care in the neonatal intensive care unit: An occupational therapist's role. *Neonatal Network, 30*(4), 243–248.

Nosarti, C., Reichenberg, A., Murray, R. M., Cnattingius, S., Lambe, M. P., Yin, L.,... Hultman, C. M. (2012). Preterm birth and psychiatric disorders in young adult life. *Archives of General Psychiatry, 69*(6), E1–E8.

Nuysink, J., Eijsermans, M. J., van Haastert, I. C., Koopman-Esseboom, C., Helders, P. J., de Vries, L. S., & van der Net, J. (2013). Clinical course of asymmetric motor performance and deformational plagiocephaly in very preterm infants. *The Journal of Pediatrics, 163*(3), 658–665.e1.

Nyqvist, K. H., Häggkvist, A. P., Hansen, M. N., Kylberg, E., Frandsen, A. L., Maastrup, R.,... Haiek, L. N.; Baby-Friendly Hospital Initiative Expert Group. (2013). Expansion of the Baby-Friendly Hospital Initiative ten steps to successful breastfeeding into neonatal intensive care: Expert group recommendations. *Journal of Human Lactation: Official Journal of International Lactation Consultant Association, 29*(3), 300–309.

Nyqvist, K. H., Maastrup, R., Hansen, M. N., Haggkvist, A. P., Hannula, L., Ezeonodo, A., . . . Haiek, L. N. (2015). *Neo-BFHI: The Baby-Friendly Hospital Initiative for neonatal wards. Core document with recommended standards and criteria.* Nordic and Quebec Working Group. Retrieved from: http://www-conference.slu.se/neobfhi2015/Neo-BFHI_Core_document_2015_Edition.pdf

Olson, J. A., & Baltman, K. (1994). Infant mental health in occupational therapy practice in the neonatal intensive care unit. *The American Journal of Occupational Therapy: Official Publication of the American Occupational Therapy Association, 48*(6), 499–505.

Oranges, T., Dini, V., & Romanelli, M. (2015). Skin physiology of the neonate and infant: Clinical implications. *Advances in Wound Care, 4*(10), 587–595.

Pellicer, A., Gayá, F., Madero, R., Quero, J., & Cabañas, F. (2002). Noninvasive continuous monitoring of the effects of head position on brain hemodynamics in ventilated infants. *Pediatrics, 109*(3), 434–440.

Pepino, V. C., & Mezzacappa, M. A. (2015). Application of tactile/kinesthetic stimulation in preterm infants: A systematic review. *Jornal de Pediatria, 91*(3), 213–233.

Perkins, E., Ginn, L., Fanning, J. K., & Bartlett, D. J. (2004). Effect of nursing education on positioning of infants in the neonatal intensive care unit. *Pediatric Physical Therapy: The Official Publication of the Section on Pediatrics of the American Physical Therapy Association, 16*(1), 2–12.

Peters, K. L. (1998). Bathing premature infants: Physiological and behavioral consequences. *American Journal of Critical Care: An Official Publication, American Association of Critical-Care Nurses, 7*(2), 90–100.

Petrova, A., & Mehta, R. (2015). Alteration in regional tissue oxygenation of preterm infants during placement in the semi-upright seating position. *Scientific Reports, 5*, 8343.

Pickler, R. H., Reyna, B. A., Wetzel, P. A., & Lewis, M. (2015). Effect of four approaches to oral feeding progression on clinical outcomes in preterm infants. *Nursing Research and Practice, 2015*, 716828.

Pineda, R. G., Foss, J., Richards, L., & Pane, C. A. (2009). Breastfeeding changes for VLBW infants in the NICU following staff education. *Neonatal Network, 28*(5), 311–319.

Pineda, R. G., Tjoeng, T. H., Vavasseur, C., Kidokoro, H., Neil, J. J., & Inder, T. (2013). Patterns of altered neurobehavior in preterm infants within the neonatal intensive care unit. *The Journal of Pediatrics, 162*(3), 470–476.e1.

Ponnusamy, V., Venkatesh, V., & Clarke, P. (2014). Skin antisepsis in the neonate: What should we use? *Current Opinion in Infectious Diseases, 27*(3), 244–250.

Purdy, I. B., Singh, N., Le, C., Bell, C., Whiteside, C., & Collins, M. (2012). Biophysiologic and social stress relationships with breast milk feeding pre- and post-discharge from the neonatal intensive care unit. *Journal of Obstetric, Gynecologic, and Neonatal Nursing: JOGNN/NAACOG, 41*(3), 347–357.

Quinn, D., Newton, N., & Piecuch, R. (2005). Effect of less frequent bathing on premature infant skin. *Journal of Obstetric, Gynecologic, and Neonatal Nursing: JOGNN/NAACOG, 34*(6), 741–746.

Renfrew, M. J., Craig, D., Dyson, L., McCormick, F., Rice, S., King, S. E., . . . Williams, A. F. (2009). Breastfeeding promotion for infants in neonatal units: A systematic review and economic analysis. *Health Technology Assessment*, *13*(40), 1–146, iii.

Robinson, M. (2014, April 11). *Kangaroo care: Standing transfer* [video file]. Retrieved from https://www.youtube.com/watch?v=lZ0nWurVpO4

Rodriguez, N. A., Meier, P. P., Groer, M. W., Zeller, J. M., Engstrom, J. L., & Fogg, L. (2010). A pilot study to determine the safety and feasibility of oropharyngeal administration of own mother's colostrum to extremely low-birth-weight infants. *Advances in Neonatal Care: Official Journal of the National Association of Neonatal Nurses*, *10*(4), 206–212.

Ross, E. S., & Philbin, M. K. (2011). Supporting oral feeding in fragile infants: An evidence-based method for quality bottle-feedings of preterm, ill, and fragile infants. *The Journal of Perinatal & Neonatal Nursing*, *25*(4), 349–357; quiz 358.

Sables-Baus, S., DeSanto, K., Henderson, S., Kunz, J. L., Morris, A. C., Shields, L., . . . McGrath, J. M. (2013). *Infant-directed oral feeding for premature and critically ill hospitalized infants: Guideline for practice*. Glenview, IL: National Association of Neonatal Nurses.

Samsom, J. F., de Groot, L., Bezemer, P. D., Lafeber, H. N., & Fetter, W. P. (2002). Muscle power development during the first year of life predicts neuromotor behaviour at 7 years in preterm born high-risk infants. *Early Human Development*, *68*(2), 103–118.

Seigel, J. K., Smith, P. B., Ashley, P. L., Cotten, C. M., Herbert, C. C., King, B. A., . . . Bidegain, M. (2013). Early administration of oropharyngeal colostrum to extremely low birth weight infants. *Breastfeeding Medicine: The Official Journal of the Academy of Breastfeeding Medicine*, *8*(6), 491–495.

Shaker, C. S. (2013a). Cue-based feeding in the NICU: Using the infant's communication as a guide. *Neonatal Network*, *32*(6), 404–408.

Shaker, C. S. (2013b). Reading the feeding. *The ASHA Leader*, *18*, 42–47.

Siddell, E., Marinelli, K., Froman, R. D., & Burke, G. (2003). Evaluation of an educational intervention on breastfeeding for NICU nurses. *Journal of Human Lactation: Official Journal of International Lactation Consultant Association*, *19*(3), 293–302.

Sisk, P. M., Lovelady, C. A., Dillard, R. G., & Gruber, K. J. (2006). Lactation counseling for mothers of very low birth weight infants: Effect on maternal anxiety and infant intake of human milk. *Pediatrics*, *117*(1), e67–e75.

Smith, J. R. (2012). Comforting touch in the very preterm hospitalized infant: An integrative review. *Advances in Neonatal Care: Official Journal of the National Association of Neonatal Nurses*, *12*(6), 349–365.

Smith, J. R., Raney, M., Conner, S., Coffelt, P., McGrath, J., Brotto, M., & Inder, T. (2012). Application of the M Technique in hospitalized very preterm infants: A feasibility study. *Advances in Neonatal Care: Official Journal of the National Association of Neonatal Nurses*, *12*(Suppl. 5), S10–S17.

Spittle, A. J., Lee, K. J., Spencer-Smith, M., Lorefice, L. E., Anderson, P. J., & Doyle, L. W. (2015). Accuracy of two motor assessments during the first year of life in preterm infants for predicting motor outcome at preschool age. *PloS One*, *10*(5), e0125854.

Spittle, A., Orton, J., Anderson, P. J., Boyd, R., & Doyle, L. W. (2015). Early developmental intervention programmes provided post hospital discharge to prevent motor and cognitive impairment in preterm infants. *Cochrane Database of Systematic Reviews*, *2015*(11), CD005495.

Stevens, E. E., Gazza, E., & Pickler, R. (2014). Parental experience learning to feed their preterm infants. *Advances in Neonatal Care: Official Journal of the National Association of Neonatal Nurses*, *14*(5), 354–361.

Sweeney, J. K., & Gutierrez, T. (2002). Musculoskeletal implications of preterm infant positioning in the NICU. *The Journal of Perinatal & Neonatal Nursing*, *16*(1), 58–70.

Thibeau, S., & Boudreaux, C. (2013). Exploring the use of mothers' own milk as oral care for mechanically ventilated very low-birth-weight preterm infants. *Advances in Neonatal Care: Official Journal of the National Association of Neonatal Nurses*, *13*(3), 190–197.

Tronick, E., & Beeghly, M. (2011). Infants' meaning-making and the development of mental health problems. *The American Psychologist*, *66*(2), 107–119.

United States Lactation Consultant Association (USLCA). (July 2010). *International Board certified lactation consultant staffing recommendations for the inpatient setting.* Washington, DC: U.S. Lactation Consultant Association.

Vaivre-Douret, L., Ennouri, K., Jrad, I., Garrec, C., & Papiernik, E. (2004). Effect of positioning on the incidence of abnormalities of muscle tone in low-risk, preterm infants. *European Journal of Paediatric Neurology: EJPN: Official Journal of the European Paediatric Neurology Society*, *8*(1), 21–34.

van Sleuwen, B. E., Engelberts, A. C., Boere-Boonekamp, M. M., Kuis, W., Schulpen, T. W., & L'Hoir, M. P. (2007). Swaddling: A systematic review. *Pediatrics*, *120*(4), e1097–e1106.

Visscher, M., & Narendran, V. (2014). The ontogeny of skin. *Advances in Wound Care*, *3*(4), 291–303.

Visscher, M., Odio, M., Taylor, T., White, T., Sargent, S., Sluder, L.,…Bondurant, P. (2009). Skin care in the NICU patient: Effects of wipes versus cloth and water on stratum corneum integrity. *Neonatology*, *96*(4), 226–234.

Vohr, B. R., Poindexter, B. B., Dusick, A. M., McKinley, L. T., Wright, L. L., Langer, J. C., & Poole, W. K.; NICHD Neonatal Research Network. (2006). Beneficial effects of breast milk in the neonatal intensive care unit on the developmental outcome of extremely low birth weight infants at 18 months of age. *Pediatrics*, *118*(1), e115–e123.

Waitzman, K. A., Ludwig, S. M., & Nelson, C. L. A. (2014). Contributing to content validity of the Infant-Driven Feeding Scales© through Delphi surveys. *Newborn and Infant Nursing Reviews*, *14*, 88–91.

Walker, T. C., Keene, S. D., & Patel, R. M. (2014). Early feeding factors associated with exclusive versus partial human milk feeding in neonates receiving intensive care. *Journal of Perinatology: Official Journal of the California Perinatal Association*, *34*(8), 606–610.

Watson, J., & McGuire, W. (2015). Responsive versus scheduled feeding for preterm infants. *Cochrane Database of Systematic Reviews*, *2015*(10), CD005255.

Wellington, A., & Perlman, J. M. (2015). Infant-driven feeding in premature infants: A quality improvement project. *Archives of Disease in Childhood. Fetal and Neonatal Edition*, *100*(6), F495–F500.

Xie, L. H. (2014). Hydrocolloid dressing in preventing nasal trauma secondary to nasal continuous positive airway pressure in preterm infants. *World Journal of Emergency Medicine*, 5(3), 218–222.

Zarem, C., Crapnell, T., Tiltges, L., Madlinger, L., Reynolds, L., Lukas, K., & Pineda, R. (2013). Neonatal nurses' and therapists' perceptions of positioning for preterm infants in the neonatal intensive care unit. *Neonatal Network*, *32*(2), 110–116.

CHAPTER 9

Guidelines for Family Collaborative Care

I sustain myself with the love of family.
　　—Maya Angelou

This guideline presents the latest evidence-based research along with clinical practice recommendations and implementation strategies related to family collaborative care in the neonatal intensive care unit (NICU; see Table 9.1).

TABLE 9. 1　Attributes and Criteria of the Family Collaborative Care Measure

Attributes	Criteria
Parents are integral to the comprehensive care of their hospitalized infant(s).	1. Parents have 24-hour unrestricted access to their infant(s). 2. Parents are invited and encouraged to be present and participate in bedside rounds. 3. Supportive spaces and resources are readily available for parents to include restrooms, comfortable seating, designated space for personal belongings, and other comfort resources that support parent presence.
Assessing and supporting the emotional well-being of parents are an expressed priority.	1. The unit has appropriate staffing ratios of licensed mental health professionals. 2. Parents are assessed/reassessed routinely for postpartum depression and acute stress disorder; all staff are competent and responsible for this assessment. 3. Appropriate, effective therapeutic interventions and additional crisis support resources are available, to include family support groups, a peer-to-peer support network, and other support resources (e.g., spiritual, financial).
Competence and confidence in parenting skills are mentored, supported, and validated over the hospital stay.	1. Competency-based education is provided to all parents across all facets of the core measures for age-appropriate care to include (but not limited to) breastfeeding skills, skin-to-skin (S2S) care, safe sleep, bathing and hygiene practices, infant communication cues, nonpharmacologic pain and stress strategies, and so on.

(continued)

TABLE 9.1   Attributes and Criteria of the Family Collaborative Care Measure   *(continued)*

Attributes	Criteria
	2. All staff are culturally competent to support the parenting needs of their unique patient demographics.
	3. Parents are empowered and supported in relationship building and role validating activities with their infant(s) such as the provision of routine infant caregiving, feeding activities, supporting their infant during painful/stressful procedures, and so on.

◼ GUIDELINE OBJECTIVES

- To define the criteria and recommendations for best practice in family collaborative care in the NICU
- To present the evidence that supports the criteria and best practice recommendations for family collaborative care in the NICU
- To present clinical practice strategies that facilitate adoption and integration of evidence-based best practices in family collaborative care in the hospital

◼ MAJOR OUTCOMES CONSIDERED

The impact of the consistently reliable adoption and integration of family collaborative care practices on the NICU patient, family, and staff includes:

- Physiologic, psycho-social, and psycho-emotional outcomes
- Patient safety and quality clinical outcomes

◼ PRESENCE AND PARTNERS

Children need your presence more than your presents.
        —Jesse Jackson

Interventions and Practice Considerations

- Establish a policy for 24-hour unrestricted access of parents to their hospitalized infant
    - Best practice considerations include establishing individualized expectations for parent/family presence and involvement in daily routine

caregiving based on each family's resources and capabilities; using extended family/friends to create a consistent social network for the infant–parent dyad, and eliminating restrictive language in the family presence ("visitation") policy

- Create and maintain a practice guideline that defines the role of the parent in the comprehensive care of their hospitalized infant(s) and staff expectations to support parent presence and participation in bedside rounds
  - Best practice considerations include educating parents on the concept and process of bedside rounds, and integrating parent(s) into the discussion on rounds for questions, input, and feedback
- Create and maintain dedicated spaces for parents/family that are welcoming, inviting, and comforting
  - Best practice considerations include single-family room design or modifications to existing space that affords comforts consistent with continuous parent presence (e.g., bathroom and shower facilities, individualized storage space, respite areas, sibling spaces)

The Evidence

Parents are not visitors in the NICU; rather, they are partners with the professional team and advocates and allies for safe and quality infant care (Griffin, 2013). Although many NICU policies indicate 24/7 "visitation," parents frequently experience limited access to their infant during certain times to include admissions, resuscitations, procedures, rounds, and nurses' change of shift; however, if parents are truly to be partners in care they must indeed have full unrestricted access to their infant (Griffin, 2013; Lee, Carter, Stevenson, & Harrison, 2014). Obeidat, Bond, and Clark Callister (2009) explored parents' experiences associated with the admission of their newborns to the NICU in a systematic review and the analysis exposed several themes to include feelings of stress and strain, separation, depression, and a lack of control over the situation, as well as vacillation between hope and hopelessness. Studies have demonstrated that when parents were involved in caregiving they transitioned from a passive to an active role and became more engaged in parenting activities, felt safer and more confident, gained a sense of control over the situation, and felt more connected to their infant (Broedsgaard & Wagner, 2005; Butler & Galvin, 2003; Heermann, Wilson, & Wilhelm, 2005; Söderström, Benzein, & Saveman , 2003). Educating the parents on and integrating them into the continuous care of their hospitalized infant improve parent mental health outcomes, enhance parent–infant attachment, reduce hospital length of stay, increase breastfeeding rates, increase infant weight gain, may reduce the risk of moderate to severe bronchopulmonary dysplasia, decrease nosocomial infection rates, and meet the basic human needs of the infant and family (Craig et al., 2015; Flacking et al., 2012; Melnyk et al., 2006; O'Brien et al., 2013; Ortenstrand et al., 2010). Involving parents in the care of their hospitalized infant, sharing information, and encouraging and supporting parent presence increase parent satisfaction and reduce hospital readmission (Bastani, Abadi, & Haghani, 2015).

Including parents in bedside rounds aligns with the core principles of patient- and family-centered care to include respect and dignity, information sharing, participation, and collaboration, and this is also endorsed by The Joint Commission, the Department of Health and Human Services, the Centers for Medicaid & Medicare Services, and the American College of Critical Care Medicine (Davidson, 2013; Davidson et al., 2007; Johnson et al., 2008; Leape et al., 2009; Figure 9.1).

Parents who participate in bedside rounds are overwhelmingly positive, reporting a decrease in their anxiety and increased confidence in the health care team (Davidson, 2013; Grzyb, Coo, Ruhland, & Dow, 2014). Abdel-Latif, Boswell, Broom, Smith, and Davis, (2015), in a randomized crossover trial, compared parental presence at the clinical bedside rounds to the standard model of neonatal rounds (no parent presence) and reported overwhelming support for parent presence at the bedside rounds from both parents and professionals. The success of parent presence on clinical bedside rounds must include a thoughtful systematic approach to mitigate concerns regarding privacy, time management, and teaching opportunities in academic settings (Abdel-Latif et al., 2015; Davidson, 2013). Davidson (2013) recommends staff education on family-centered care and family presence on rounds, introducing the family to the idea of rounds and providing options for attendance, assessing family privacy concerns and addressing these concerns as necessary, explaining the purpose and process of rounds to the family, and identifying family learning needs to optimize participation.

NICU design and the presence of supportive spaces play a key role in family-centered care (Gooding et al., 2011; White, 2011). Parents who were asked to compare their experience in an open bay NICU floor plan with a private room setting indicated the private room afforded more time with their infant, more privacy, and more space for their personal items; parents also stated they felt less overstimulated by the light and noise, experienced greater access to their infant's physician, and felt better supported by the entire team (Carter, Carter, & Bennett, 2008). The physical environment must be a supportive space for healing to occur, accommodating the needs of the patient, which include the needs of the patient's support network (e.g., family) by adopting an evidence-based design approach to the physical space, which plays an important role in patient safety, workflow, and family-centered care (Ferri, Zygun, Harrison, & Stelfox, 2015; Sakallaris, MacAllister, Voss, Smith, & Jonas, 2015; Ulrich et al., 2008).

Cost Analysis

Empowering and engaging parents in the NICU reduces length of stay as well as decreases the incidence of critical morbidities, thus decreasing hospital as well as human costs associated with NICU hospitalization (Melnyk et al., 2006;

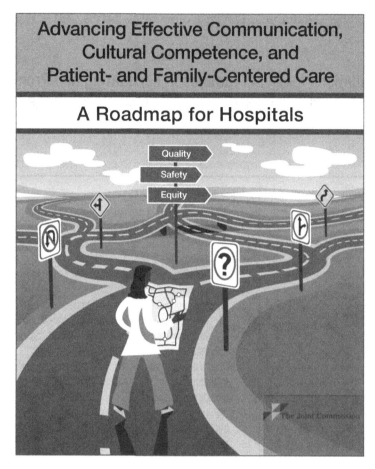

FIGURE 9.1   The Joint Commission's roadmap for patient- and family-centered care. Reprinted with permission from The Joint Commission (2010). The complete resource is available at www.jointcommission.org/assets/1/6/aroadmapforhospitalsfinalversion727.pdf

O'Brien et al., 2013; Ortenstrand et al., 2010). In a cost analysis of the Creating Opportunities for Parent Empowerment (COPE) program for parents of premature infants, the authors report a cost savings in excess of $4,500 per infant (Melnyk & Feinstein, 2009). Protecting and preserving physical and emotional closeness of the infant–parent dyad in the NICU optimize infant brain development, preserve parent psychological well-being, and enhance the parent–infant relationship; these combined benefits have a significant impact on the fiscal and societal outcomes associated with neonatal intensive care (Flacking et al., 2012). Physical and emotional closeness can be enriched by the NICU design features, and the single-family room design has been shown to be more conducive to family-centered care, enhancing infant medical progress and breastfeeding success, both of which impact short-term and long-term economic and societal variables (Domanico, Davis, Coleman, & Davis, 2011; Flacking et al., 2012).

Recommendations for Best Practices in Facilitating and Promoting Parent Presence and Partnerships with Professionals in the NICU (Table 9.2)

TABLE 9.2   Major Practice Recommendations and Implementation Strategies—Presence and Partners

Recommendations	Implementation Strategy

1. Develop an open unit policy to facilitate parents' 24-hour access to their infant (Davidson, 2013; Davidson et al., 2007; Griffin, 2013; Lee et al., 2014)	a. Review your current "visitation" policy
	  i. Is it open or restrictive?
	  ii. If it is restrictive, revisit the evidence; revise as indicated
	b. Educate all staff on the importance for parents to have 24-hour unrestricted access to their infant
	c. Consider a phased approach to an open unit policy
	  i. Collect baseline metrics to evaluate the impact of your change (parent presence, infection, breastfeeding, etc.)
	d. Draft a new unit access policy (ensure clarity to avoid misinterpretations that can lead to inconsistency and confusion); include family definition—extended family, siblings, and so on (see links for sample of wording)
	e. Implement and evaluate the effect on selected success metrics
	f. Revise as indicated and implement
	g. Revisit your policy every 3 to 6 months if you are using a phased approach to change
	h. Audit compliance, identify accountability measures
	i. Publish and/or present your results

2. Parents are invited and encouraged to participate in bedside rounds (Davidson 2013; Davidson et al., 2007; Griffin, 2013)	a. Review your current practice for bedside rounds and examine how to include and partner with parents during this daily routine
	  i. Outline a process for the rounds (bedside nurse presents the 24-hour clinical updates, parents add their observations/questions, team discusses plan for the day, parents may ask additional questions—have a plan if the discussion goes on too long to follow up with the parent at a designated time to avoid infringing on other parents' time for rounds)
	b. Develop a teaching strategy for parents
	  i. Educate parents on the purpose and process of bedside rounds, share the outline for rounds, gather parent feedback

(continued)

TABLE 9.2   Major Practice Recommendations and Implementation Strategies—Presence and Partners   *(continued)*

Recommendations	Implementation Strategy
	c. Test your process/revise and refine d. Consider collecting baseline data points (e.g., parent satisfaction, time for rounds, staff satisfaction) e. Implement f. Collect data following implementation, compare, provide feedback to parents and staff g. Revise if necessary h. Publish and/or present your results

3. Ensure that comfort and support spaces are readily accessible for parents in the NICU to include bathrooms and shower facilities, individualized storage space, respite areas, and sibling spaces	a. Review your current unit footprint
	   i. Are there opportunities for modification to your existing space?
	   ii. Is your space welcoming/inviting/comfortable for parents to spend extended periods of time with their infant?
	   iii. Consider speaking with the chief experience officer at your facility or another chief executive for support and buy-in (be prepared to present the evidence to support your changes)
	b. Brainstorm with former and current parents to identify opportunities to modify the space to meet parenting needs
	c. Prioritize ideas and begin a test-of-change
	d. Evaluate results, revise, implement
	e. Consider comparing parent and staff satisfaction before and after the modifications (in addition, look for interval changes in parental presence, S2S, breastfeeding, etc.)
	f. Publish and/or present your results

S2S, skin to skin.

See the fact sheet on Health Insurance Portability and Accountability Act of 1996 (HIPAA) Privacy and Security and Patient- and Family-Centered Care at the end of this chapter.

■ EMOTIONAL WELL-BEING

Step with care and great tact, and remember that life's a great balancing act.
      —Dr. Seuss

Interventions and Practice Considerations

- Create and maintain appropriate staffing levels of mental health professionals to meet the psycho-emotional needs of the parents and the staff in the NICU
  - Best practice considerations include a review of your existing mental health resources, existing service capabilities, and service priorities
- Create and maintain a systematic approach to parent mental health assessments during the NICU stay
  - Best practice considerations include ensuring all staff are competent in basic assessments of mental health (e.g., early signs of depression)
- Create and maintain a systematic support system for NICU parents
  - Best practice considerations include establishing unit-based family support groups and/or peer-to-peer support networks or collaborations with community or web-based support groups for the NICU parent and family

The Evidence

Parents whose infants are hospitalized in the NICU have a higher risk for mental health challenges (Candelori, Trumello, Babore, Keren, & Romanelli, 2015; Gonulal, Yalaz, Altun-Koroglu, & Kultursay, 2014; Vazquez & Cong 2014). Parents struggle with role identity and providing parenting activities in a critical care environment; the stress associated with this lived reality is correlated with clinically significant anxiety, fatigue, depression, and sleep disturbances (Busse, Stromgren, Thorngate, & Thomas, 2013; Lasiuk, Comeau, & Newburn-Cook, 2013). The prevalence of postpartum depression in mothers of premature and low birth weight infants had been reported to be as high as 40% and is associated with a perceived lack of social support, maternal distance from the hospital, and married maternal status (Alkozei, McMahon, & Lahav, 2014; Vigod, Villegas, Dennis, & Ross, 2010). Maternal stress of mothers of preterm infants correlated with symptoms of depression and an increased risk for acute stress disorder (ASD), which can negatively impact social relationships, caregiving, and parenting competencies (Alkozei et al., 2014; Jubinville, Newburn-Cook, Hegadoren, & Lacaze-Masmonteil, 2012).

Although the majority of the studies looking at postpartum depression, anxiety, and posttraumatic stress disorder (PTSD) have been done on mothers of premature infants, there is also substantial evidence that reveals fathers suffer from their infants' hospitalization as well (Candelori et al., 2015; Gonulal et al., 2014). Cheng, Kotelchuck, Gerstein, Taveras, and Poehlmann-Tynan (2016), analyzing the prevalence and impact of postnatal depression in mothers and fathers of preterm infants, discovered the incidence of postpartum depression is higher in fathers of preterm infants than fathers of term infants, especially fathers who are nonresident. In addition, paternal depression is associated with significantly lower cognitive function in the child at 2 years of age (Cheng et al., 2016). Supporting fathers in their NICU parent journey through engagement and participation in caregiving such as skin-to-skin (S2S) care is a crucial component of family-centered collaborative care with lifelong implications for the dyad (Anderzen-Carlsson, Lamy, & Eriksson, 2014; Lundqvist, Westas, & Hallstrom, 2007; Panter-Brick et al., 2014).

The trauma experienced by parents whose infant is admitted to the NICU is linked to ASD symptoms with the severity of symptoms strongly related to concerns regarding the parental role, which can be significantly altered in the NICU setting (Shaw, DeBlois, et al., 2006). In addition, there is a significant correlation between ASD symptoms in NICU parents and PTSD and depression, with fathers at even greater risk than mothers (Shaw, Bernard, et al., 2009). Parents of preterm infants are at increased risk for psychological distress at 9 months postpartum, which can compromise cognitive, behavioral, and emotional outcomes in the infant (Alkozei et al., 2014; Carson, Redshaw, Gray, & Quigley, 2015). Understanding the high levels of psychological distress associated with the trauma of NICU hospitalization, clinicians must try to prepare parents for the various psychological reactions they may experience during the NICU stay and actively validate their role and identity as parent (Shaw, Bernard, et al., 2009, Shaw, DeBlois, et al., 2006).

As parental well-being and psychological health are critical for infant long-term developmental outcomes, NICU services must include access to qualified mental health resources to mitigate and manage the trauma experience of the NICU parent. Hynan et al. (2015) outline recommendations for mental health professionals in the NICU to include appropriate staffing ratios of mental health professionals, physical accommodations for confidential discussions, scheduling of mental health assessments, the availability of layered levels of support (e.g., family support groups and peer-to-peer support resources), psychiatric referral criteria, and telemedicine supports. In a descriptive study exploring the characteristics of NICU mothers who would benefit from on-site psychiatric support services, Friedman et al. (2013) concluded that the early intervention of psychiatric services decreased mental health symptomatology, improved early parent functioning, fostered parent–infant relationships, and positively impacted the morale of the clinical team. Early interventions using trauma-focused, cognitive behavioral therapy for mothers at risk for PTSD statistically significantly decreased symptoms of trauma, anxiety, and depression and strongly suggest a transdisciplinary approach to screening parents for psychological distress (Bicking & Moore, 2012; Friedman et al., 2013; Shaw et al., 2014).

Peer support in the NICU has been identified as a crucial factor in the development of the maternal role in the NICU (Rossman, Greene, & Meier, 2015). Hall, Ryan, Beatty, and Grubbs (2015b) describe the various types of peer-to-peer support to include in-person support or telephone support, parent support groups, and Internet support groups (see Table 9.3 for details of each type). Budgetary constraints and the availability of volunteer resources are potential barriers to developing peer support resources; however, institutionalizing this resource is an integral component of family-centered collaborative care with benefits far outweighing investment challenges (Hall et al., 2015b).

TABLE 9.3   Types of NICU Peer Support Resources

Type of Support	Description
In-person or telephone support	Current NICU parent is matched with a veteran NICU parent who serves as a mentor
Parent support groups	Formal group with scheduled meetings and agendas; often run by a NICU staff member (although jointly run groups [parent and professional] show more stability)
Internet support groups	Web-based resource, usually monitored by veteran parents to include blog posts, helpful links, live chats, and FAQ resources (see parent resources in the following for a list of links to Internet parent support groups)

FAQ, frequently asked questions.

Cost Analysis

Parental mental health impacts the long-term developmental outcomes of infants across cognitive, behavioral, and emotional domains. Understanding the NICU parent's vulnerability to psychological distress, establishing transdisciplinary competency in assessing risk, and identifying symptoms of compromised mental health facilitate early effective intervention that significantly decreases long-term morbidity and the associated economic implications.

Recommendations for Best Practices in Assessing and Supporting the Emotional Well-Being of NICU Parents and Families (Table 9.4)

TABLE 9.4   Major Practice Recommendations and Implementation Strategies—Emotional Well-Being

Recommendations	Implementation Strategy
1. Ensure adequate staffing ratios for mental health professionals (social workers, psychologists, psychiatrists)	a. Review staffing recommendations from your mental health professionals' national organization (e.g., National Association of Perinatal Social Workers: www.napsw.org) b. Address gaps in staffing, workflow, and service priorities (this may require administrative support to resolve) c. Consider a test of change in staffing/workflow/priorities and measure impact across social, clinical, and economic domains in an effort to change the existing mental health resource paradigm in your NICU/organization d. Publish and/or present your work

(continued)

TABLE 9.4 Major Practice Recommendations and Implementation Strategies—Emotional
Well-Being *(continued)*

Recommendations	Implementation Strategy

2. Develop an action plan to address acute psychiatric emergencies	a. Review your current psychiatric emergency response plan
	  i. Do you have one?
	  ii. Is everyone familiar and competent in activating it?
	  iii. If one does not exist, develop one
	b. The plan may be as simple as calling for security, psychiatric support resources, and so on
	  i. Ensure, however, that the situation is handled respectfully and does not escalate the individual's psychological distress (often when security is called the individual responds in an acute defensive and possible angry manner creating an unsafe situation for everyone)
	c. Consider strategizing with psychiatric professionals to develop a psychiatric emergency response plan
	d. Draft a test of change
	e. Evaluate the new practice, revise, refine, implement
	f. Publish and/or present your results

3. Develop and sustain a competency-based staff education program on the assessment of psychological distress in the NICU; include a simulation return demonstration component	a. Collaborate with your mental health professional resources to outline an education strategy and competency on assessing parents/family on their emotional well-being
	  i. The ASD scale (Figure 9.2) and EPDS (Figure 9.3) are self-assessment tools that can be given to the parents to complete and share with staff
	  ii. If your unit does not have a standard method for sharing these assessments with parents, consider developing one OR educate staff on signs and symptoms that should prompt the clinician to have a parent complete a self-assessment
	  iii. Discuss with your mental health colleagues which tool should be administered under which conditions/when
	  iv. Is it feasible to make these self-assessments (EPDS and ASD scale) openly available for parents?
	b. Outline various scenarios to be used as the simulation component of the competency
	c. Identify metrics for success (e.g., percent of staff competent in making appropriate referrals for mental health evaluation; percent of parents referred or assessed; decreased incidence of acute psychological disturbances)
	d. Evaluate interval improvements, revise and refine education as needed; consider including this training into NICU new-hire orientation and as an annual competency
	e. Publish and/or present your results

(continued)

TABLE 9.4   Major Practice Recommendations and Implementation Strategies—Emotional
Well-Being   *(continued)*

Recommendations	Implementation Strategy
4. Develop and sustain parent support resources	a. Review your existing parent support resources b. Identify gaps in quality and availability of your existing services c. Consider a task force and include veteran parents to brainstorm on the various parent support resources available d. Enlist champion veteran parents and professionals to sustain the resources e. Ensure that all staff are knowledgeable about the resources and share this information with parents (consider including resources in parent educational materials) f. Introduce the new resources and evaluate the efficacy for parents and staff g. Identify success metrics (just having something does not mean it has value unless there is a means to evaluate it) h. Measure, revise, and adopt i. Consider a scheduled reevaluation of your parent support resources to ensure sustained quality and efficacy j. Publish and/or present your work

5. Ensure a dedicated, readily available private space for sensitive parent–professional communications	a. Review your current resources to afford private space for parent–professional conversations
	   i. Are they immediately available?
	   ii. Are you usually searching for a space to meet with parents?
	b. Discuss these needs with leadership and brainstorm on possible cost-conscious sensitive solutions
	c. Draft a test of change using the PDSA model to evaluate your idea
	d. Identify success metrics (e.g., parent and staff satisfaction)
	e. Implement a new strategy to ensure parent privacy; evaluate results, revise/refine the plan, retest with a multidisciplinary team
	f. Share the project outcomes and integrate into the standard of care
	g. Continuously refine and improve your practice through audit and success metric trends
	h. Publish and/or present your results

ASD, acute stress disorder; EPDS, Edinburgh Postnatal Depression Scale; PDSA, Plan-Do-Study-Act.

Acute Stress Disorder Scale-5*

Name: _____   Date: _____

Briefly describe your recent traumatic experience: _____

_____

_____

Please answer each of these questions about how you have felt since the event. Circle one number next to each question to indicate how you have left.

	Not at All	Mildly	Medium	Quite a Bit	Very Much
1. Do you have distressing memories of the trauma when you do not mean to?	1	2	3	4	5
2. Do you have distressing dreams about the trauma?	1	2	3	4	5
3. Do you feel as though the trauma is happening again?	1	2	3	4	5
4. Are you upset or does your body feel uptight when reminded of the trauma?	1	2	3	4	5
5. Do you have difficulty having positive emotions?	1	2	3	4	5
6. Do things seem unreal or do you feel distant from your normal self?	1	2	3	4	5
7. Are you unable to remember an important aspect of trauma not because of head injury or alcohol?	1	2	3	4	5
8. Do you try to avoid thinking about the trauma?	1	2	3	4	5
9. Do you try to avoid situations or conversations that remind you of the trauma?	1	2	3	4	5
10. Do you have trouble falling asleep or staying asleep?	1	2	3	4	5
11. Do you behave angrily or have temper outbursts?	1	2	3	4	5
12. Are you on the look out for danger?	1	2	3	4	5
13. Do you have problems with concentration?	1	2	3	4	5
14. Are you jumpy when something surprises you?	1	2	3	4	5

FIGURE 9.2   Acute Stress Disorder Scale.

EDINBURGH POSTNATAL DEPRESSION SCALE (EPDS)

The EPDS was developed for screening postpartum women in outpatient settings, home visiting settings, or at the 6–8 week postpartum examination. It has been used among numerous populations including U.S. women and Spanish-speaking women in other countries. The EPDS consists of 10 questions. The test can usually be completed in less than 5 minutes. Responses are scored 0, 1, 2, or 3 according to increased severity of the symptom. Items marked with an asterisk (*) are reverse scored (i.e., 3, 2, 1, and 0). The total score is determined by adding together the scores for each of the 10 items. Validation studies have utilized various threshold scores in determining which women were positive and in need of referral. Cutoff scores ranged from 9 to 13 points. Therefore, to err on safety's side, a woman scoring 9 or more points or indicating any suicidal ideation—that is, she scores 1 or higher on question #10—should be referred immediately for follow-up. Even if a woman scores less than 9, if the clinician feels the client is suffering from depression, an appropriate referral should be made. The EPDS is only a screening tool. It does not diagnose depression—that is done by appropriately licensed health care personnel. Users may reproduce the scale without permission providing the copyright is respected by quoting the names of the authors, title, and the source of the paper in all reproduced copies.

Instructions for Users
1. The mother is asked to underline one of four possible responses that comes the closest to how she has been feeling the previous 7 days.
2. All 10 items must be completed.
3. Care should be taken to avoid the possibility of the mother discussing her answers with others.
4. The mother should complete the scale herself, unless she has limited English or has difficulty with reading.

Name:
Date:
Address:
Baby's Age:

As you have recently had a baby, we would like to know how you are feeling. Please UNDERLINE the answer which comes closest to how you have felt IN THE PAST 7 DAYS, not just how you feel today.

Here is an example, already completed.
    I have felt happy:
        Yes, all the time
        Yes, most of the time
        No, not very often
        No, not at all
This would mean: "I have felt happy most of the time" during the past week. Please complete the other questions in the same way.

FIGURE 9.3   Edinburgh Postnatal Depression Scale. Reprinted with permission from Cox, Holden, and Sagovsky (1987).   *(continued)*

In the past 7 days:

1. I have been able to laugh and see the funny side of things
   - As much as I always could
   - Not quite so much now
   - Definitely not so much now
   - Not at all

2. I have looked forward with enjoyment to things
   - As much as I ever did
   - Rather less than I used to
   - Definitely less than I used to
   - Hardly at all

ª3. I have blamed myself unnecessarily when things went wrong
   - Yes, most of the time
   - Yes, some of the time
   - Not very often
   - No, never

4. I have been anxious or worried for no good reason
   - No, not at all
   - Hardly ever
   - Yes, sometimes
   - Yes, very often

ª5. I have felt scared or panicky for no very good reason
   - Yes, quite a lot
   - Yes, sometimes
   - No, not much
   - No, not at all

ª6. Things have been getting on top of me
   - Yes, most of the time I haven't been able to cope at all
   - Yes, sometimes I haven't been coping as well as usual
   - No, most of the time I have coped quite well
   - No, have been coping as well as ever

ª7. I have been so unhappy that I have had difficulty sleeping
   - Yes, most of the time
   - Yes, sometimes
   - Not very often
   - No, not at all

ª8. I have felt sad or miserable
   - Yes, most of the time
   - Yes, quite often
   - Not very often
   - No, not at all

ª9. I have been so unhappy that I have been crying
   - Yes, most of the time
   - Yes, quite often
   - Only occasionally
   - No, never

ª10. The thought of harming myself has occurred to me
   - Yes, quite often
   - Sometimes
   - Hardly ever
   - Never

FIGURE 9.3   *(continued)*

▪ PARENTING CONFIDENCE AND COMPETENCE

And will you succeed? Yes, you will indeed! (98 and 3/4 percent guaranteed.)
> —Dr. Seuss

Interventions and Practice Considerations

- Create and maintain a structured, competency-based parent education program
  - Best practice considerations include the use of mobile technology, web-based resources, and scheduling flexibility to ensure participation for

all parents; partnering with veteran parents to develop and present the curriculum

- Ensure annual participation in cultural competency training for all staff
  - Best practice considerations include identifying the cultural demographics of the patients and families served in your NICU and establishing sensitivity and competence in understanding and integrating the unique customs and rituals of the families into the culture of care
- Create and maintain a systematic process aimed at empowering parents to actively and consistently parent their hospitalized infant confidently and competently
  - Best practice considerations include staff education on the psychosocial needs of NICU parents, effective communication strategies, and the importance of partnerships with parents to promote parental engagement

The Evidence

Parent involvement in the care of their hospitalized infant validates role identity, decreases risk for depression, and increases parent confidence in caring for their critically ill infant (Agostini, Neri, Dellabartola, Biasini, & Monti, 2014; Cleveland, 2008; Obeidat et al., 2009). Cue-based, responsive care enhances the quality of parent–infant relationships in the NICU and requires comprehensive, culturally sensitive education and mentoring by qualified professionals (Evans, Whittingham, Sanders, Colditz, & Boyd, 2014; Hall et al., 2015a). Educating parents on the myriad of infant caregiving practices is often constrained by unit resources and parent availability.

Traditional modes of educating parents on the NICU include the use of handouts, nurse-led group classes, and "in-the-moment" education that takes place at the infant's bedside; however, these modalities, particularly related to discharge teaching, fail to meet the parents' learning needs and sense of preparedness to care for their infant at home (Sneath, 2009). *Baby Steps to Home* is a parent education resource for clinician use to guide and prepare parents for the journey to discharge and was developed by the National Association of Neonatal Nurses in collaboration with the American Academy of Pediatrics and the Preemie Parent Alliance. Including parents in the development of parent programs and parent learning resources significantly enhances parent participation, engagement, and empowerment (Dusing, Murray, & Stern, 2008; Macdonell et al., 2013). The COPE (*Creating Opportunities for Parent Empowerment)* NICU Program (www.copeforhope.com/nicu .php) trains NICU staff on how to deliver the evidence-based content aimed at building critical parenting skills. Parents learn about their baby's appearance and behaviors, how to care for their baby in the NICU, how to cultivate rapport and build a relationship with their infant, and how to take care of their infant at home. Outcomes of this program include significant decrease in length of stay, a decrease in hospital readmission, a decrease in parental psychological distress, and an increase in developmentally sensitive parent–infant interactions in the NICU (Melnyk et al., 2006).

Alternative modes of parent education are emerging although research is limited on the impact of these innovative teaching platforms. Choi and Bakken (2010) developed a web-based educational resource for low-literate parents in the NICU, which included a touchscreen interface, voice-recorded text, and visual aids (see Figure 9.4). The prototype was well received and opens the door for this type of innovation in NICU parent education.

In a systematic review looking at the effectiveness of digital delivery methods of parent training, Breitenstein, Gross, and Christophersen (2014) found that the use of technology is expanding significantly and has the potential to reduce access gaps to knowledge. The use of mobile tablets for learning has the advantage of providing information on demand that is interactive, engaging, user friendly, and responsive to the learning style and learning needs of the individual (Alegria, Boscardin, Poncelet, Mayfield, & Wamsley, 2014). In a small (n = 28) unpublished multinational evaluation of a prototype mobile learning app for NICU parents (Figure 9.5), respondents (comprising NICU parents and clinicians) were overwhelmingly favorable with the mobile platform and 100% of the survey participants expressed interest in mobile learning as a vehicle for quality parent education in the NICU (Figure 9.6).

Providing parents with evidence-based knowledge and opportunities to apply the new knowledge in a controlled, simulated setting ensures infant safety and promotes parent confidence (Coughlin, 2015; Tessier, 2010). Ensuring competence increases not only role identity but also parental presence and participation in parent-exclusive interventions that prepare parents for their infant's discharge to home (Burnham, Feeley, & Sherrard, 2013; Coughlin, 2015; Figure 9.7).

Culturally competent care honors and respects the diversity in patient values, beliefs, and behaviors and adapts care delivery to meet the sociocultural and linguistic needs of the population served (Betancourt, Green, & Carrillo, 2002). Providing culturally competent care in an intensive care setting is complicated by the acute and often life-threatening circumstances endemic to the environment; however, ignoring diversity and operating from an ethnocentric platform adversely affect

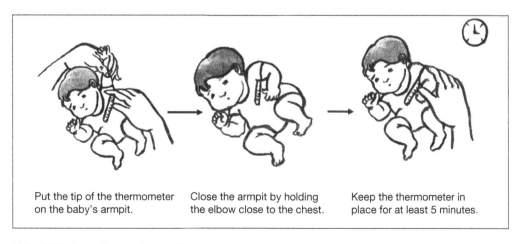

| Put the tip of the thermometer on the baby's armpit. | Close the armpit by holding the elbow close to the chest. | Keep the thermometer in place for at least 5 minutes. |

FIGURE 9.4 How to take an axillary temperature.

Source: Choi and Baken (2016). Reprinted with permission from Elsevier.

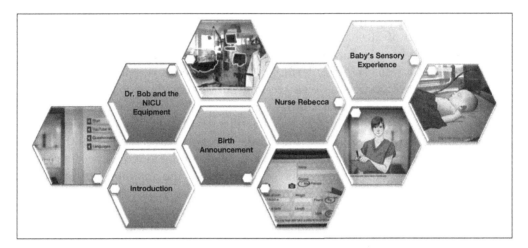

FIGURE 9.5   Sample scenes from quantum caring for parents prototype.

Reprinted with permission from Caring Essentials Collaborative, LLC.

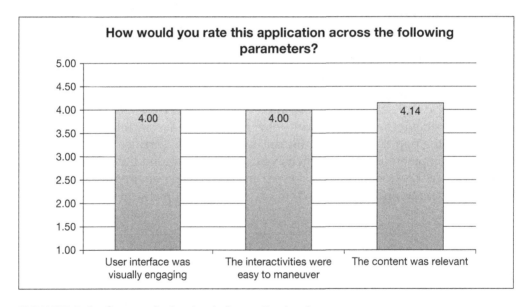

FIGURE 9.6   Survey results: 1 = strongly disagree; 5 = strongly agree.

patient outcomes and undermine patient safety (Jeffreys, 2008). An ethnographic study of a multiethnic critical care patient population revealed that the majority of conflicts arose due to a disparity in the definition of "good care" where clinicians followed a biomedical care model and families viewed good care based on a holistic life world-oriented approach (Van Keer, Deschepper, Francke, Huyghens, & Bilsen, 2015). Some critical care nurses struggle to balance their perceptions of themselves as total care providers with the family's need to participate actively in

Being a parent in the NICU is a difficult journey and each parent's journey is unique. The more time you spend with your baby—watching, touching, talking, and caring for your baby—the more you both learn about each other and begin building your lifelong relationship.

Developing a responsive relationship with your baby is an important part of becoming a parent. It begins by learning the special ways your baby communicates with you and the world around him or her. Babies communicate through their facial expressions, their movements, and their cries.

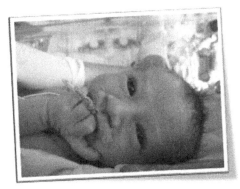

This baby is engaged and relaxed. Look at her forehead, nice and smooth without any wrinkles, her eyes are bright and she is looking at the photographer (maybe a family member is talking with her because she appears very calm). Notice her hand is at her mouth and her fingers are touching her lips (maybe she is sucking on them)—this may suggest she is a little hungry or interested in what's happening around her. Her color is smooth and pink and she does not seem agitated at all.

This little baby appears to be sleepy and possibly recovering from an event (notice the white knuckles clutching the pacifier). The baby's forehead is smooth, coloring is even, with the exception of pale shading to the nose, again it is important to know the context of what was or is happening with the baby in the moment. The baby's eyes look a little glassy which suggests he may be sleepy or overstimulated.

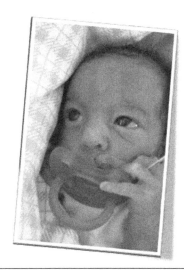

FIGURE 9.7   Parent teaching resource—infant cues.   *(continued)*

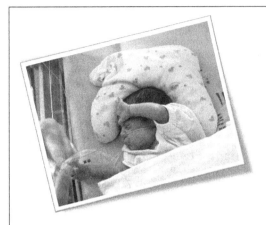

This baby appears to be overstimulated. Notice the pursed lips and both hands extended with fingers splayed. Again, it is important to understand what is happening to and around the baby when you observe these behaviors and these behaviors should then guide your interaction. Going slowly, supporting the baby during the interaction, and providing frequent timeouts let the baby know that his or her experience and feelings are important and that you are there to help him or her.

This little boy appears overstimulated. Notice how his mouth is open and his tongue is on the roof of his mouth. His eyes look like they are staring into space and his eyebrows are just a little bit raised suggesting he is trying to take everything in but it is too much for him. His hand to his face with his pinky finger hooked on his lower eye lid could suggest he may be too stimulated to release and relax his hand. He needs a quiet space and maybe even some skin-to-skin care to calm him.

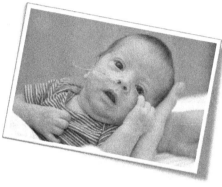

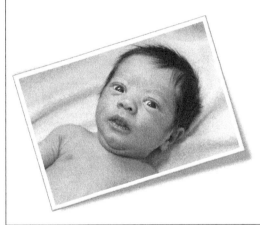

This little girl may be overstimulated. Look at her hyper alert big eyes. Her slightly protruding tongue is her response to a stressful event. Her smooth forehead and even color suggest she is trying to "hold it together" on her own, but would benefit from a break to regain a sense of calm. It's important to interpret the baby's cues or nonverbal communication in context of what is happening to him or her.

FIGURE 9.7 *(continued)*

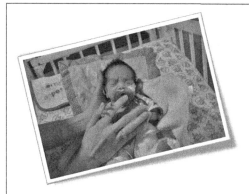

This little girl is distressed. Notice her wrinkled brow and her eyes squeezed shut. Her arms and legs are moving quite a bit as the nurse tries to comfort her with a pacifier and some gentle boundaries with her hands. The nurse offers the baby her finger to grasp to calm her. No additional cares should be done until the baby is calm. When a parent can partner with the professional during procedures and caregiving, the baby is much less likely to become distressed.

This baby does not look happy. Notice his pouty mouth and his pursed upper lip is a little blanched (whitish coloring); his eyes look tired and a little glassy. This baby needs a time-out from whatever is happening in his environment; he needs a quiet, low-lit space to recover.

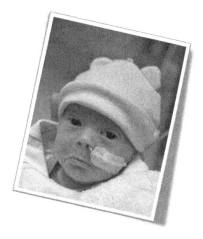

Build competence and confidence caring for your baby in the NICU; and discover your full parenting potential at www.caringessentials.org/family-use

FIGURE 9.7   *(continued)*

the care of their loved one (Hoye & Severinsson, 2010). A systematic, transformative, and seamless approach to cultural awareness and cultural sensitivity is mandatory. Schim, Doorenbos, Benkert, and Miller (2007) describe culturally congruent care as a blend of cultural realities of the client and provider (Figure 9.8) and outline a systematic approach to clinical interventions that respects and honors the personhood of provider and client.

Exploring the client level in this three-dimensional model, Wiebe and Young (2011) interviewed culturally diverse families with infants hospitalized in the NICU who indicated the primary importance of a provider–client relationship of trust and caring, respectful communication, the availability of culturally responsive social and spiritual supports, and an organizational environment that was welcoming and flexible.

Through better understanding of the family's sociocultural needs as they journey through their NICU experience, compassionate, culturally sensitive professionals can build trusting, therapeutic relationships that foster parental empowerment, parent–infant attachment, and family collaborative care (Hall et al., 2015a).

The NICU environment of care to include the physical layout and the clinical routines impact parent access to and participation in the care of their critically ill infant (Baylis et al., 2014; Flacking et al., 2012). Parents as the primary caregivers in the NICU improve short-term and long-term outcomes for the infant and family as demonstrated in the COPE program and Family-Integrated Care model (O'Brien et al., 2013; Melnyk et al., 2006). Nurses have a unique opportunity to facilitate parent engagement and promote empowerment, but this opportunity has to be cultivated in an environment that adopts a systematic, standardized approach to care (Cleveland, 2008; Coughlin, 2015). Potentially, better practices in the provision of family-centered care include the full participation of parents in the care of their hospitalized infant; this requires a global change in culture and behavior of the transdisciplinary team in relation to the truly crucial role of the parent and family (Craig et al., 2015; Davis, Mohay, & Edwards, 2003; Moore, Coker, DuBuisson, Swett, & Edwards, 2003).

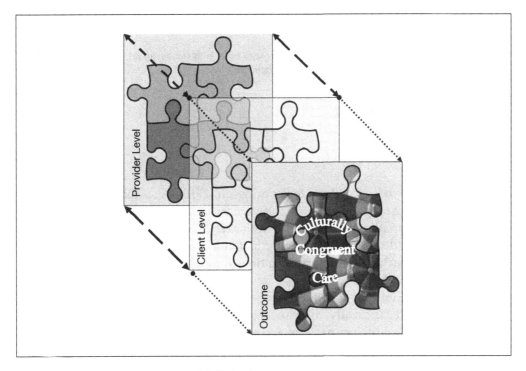

FIGURE 9.8   Three-dimensional model of cultural congruence.

Source: Schim and Doorenbos (2010). Reprinted with permission from Taylor & Francis Ltd.

Cost Analysis

As stated previously, interventions that promote parent participation, empowerment, competence, and confidence reduce the infant's length of hospital stay, improve the infant's short-term and long-term outcomes, decrease hospital readmission rates, increase parent mental well-being, and save the national health care system an excess of $2 billion per year (Melnyk & Feinstein, 2009; Melnyk et al., 2006).

Recommendations for Best Practices in Building Cultural Congruence and Promoting Parent Confidence and Competence in Caring for Their Hospitalized Infant (Table 9.5)

TABLE 9.5   Major Practice Recommendations and Implementation Strategies—Parenting Confidence and Competence

Recommendations	Implementation Strategy

1. Develop and sustain a parent education program that integrates veteran parents as content developers/reviewers, educators, mentors; include a simulation component to build confidence in the various parenting skills	a. Review your existing parent education resources in collaboration with parents (current/veteran)
	  i. Is the content current?
	  ii. What is your current delivery mode and how effective is it?
	  iii. Is there consistency in the teaching?
	  iv. Do you have parent competencies (e.g., S2S care, infant transfer, swaddled bathing, diaper change, breastfeeding, supporting their infant through procedural pain and pain-related stress—facilitated tuck, containment see sample parent competency in Figure 9.7)?
	b. Consider beginning with a competency-based approach to S2S care
	  i. Present the evidence on S2S care in the NICU to parents *and* staff
	  ii. Discuss the infant transfer method (standing transfer preferred over the seated method; Ludington-Hoe et al., 2003)
	  iii. Share your unit's updated practice policy and guideline with parents
	  iv. Take questions
	  v. Do the mock-up transfer using a doll, incubator, and whatever kangaroo care support device you use (e.g., Kangaroo Zak, Dandle Wrap, Blanket) (see Figures 9.9 and 9.10)
	  vi. Sign-off parents *and* staff in the infant transfer for both standing (preferred) and seated (see Figure 9.11)
	c. Outline your change and how you will know your change is an improvement (e.g., for S2S care, collect data on your current frequency, ask parents what they know about S2S care, how frequently have they done S2S; other clinical metrics would include breastfeeding rates, incidence of infection)

(continued)

TABLE 9.5 Major Practice Recommendations and Implementation Strategies—Parenting Confidence and Competence *(continued)*

Recommendations	Implementation Strategy
	d. Test your change using the PDSA format (see sample in the Resources section) e. Revise, refine, measure your results f. Audit practice and identify accountability metrics for staff to support the new practice g. Publish and/or present results

2. Operationalize a culturally congruent model of care	a. Review your patient demographics and, using a failure modes and effects analysis, identify opportunities for improvement in providing culturally congruent care for the families you serve (see the Standards for Culturally Competent Nursing Care in the Resources section)
	b. Your organization will have resources, guidelines that can be adapted for the unique nature of the NICU experience
	c. Consider reviewing a recent culturally sensitive patient–family case
	   i. Outline what happened
	   ii. What could have been different (failure modes and effects analysis)
	   iii. Identify opportunities for improvement
	   iv. Outline a test of change
	   v. Evaluate your test of change; revise, refine
	d. Ensure that staff participate in an annual cultural competency training
	e. Identify accountability components to the implementation of your test of change to improve cultural competence and cultural congruence
	f. Consider publishing/presenting your work

3. Develop and sustain a staff competency-based education program on the importance of parent caregiving in the NICU	a. Review current staff education on parent caregiving/family-centered care
	b. Identify opportunities to improve content, delivery mode, and competencies
	c. Prioritize opportunities and test new ideas
	   i. Describe/outline what parent caregiving looks like (staff usually resist parent caregiving when they have concerns for safety—address safety concerns)
	   ii. Consider a tiered approach to transitioning caregiving tasks from nursing to parents based on safety factors
	d. Identify success metrics for the education
	   i. Percentage of staff who are competent
	   ii. Percentage of staff who are translating the new skills into practice
	e. Revise education content as indicated, expand staff competencies in facilitating parent caregiving beyond the test parameters
	f. Publish and/or present your results

(continued)

TABLE 9.5   Major Practice Recommendations and Implementation Strategies—Parenting Confidence and Competence   *(continued)*

Recommendations	Implementation Strategy
4. Develop and sustain a care-by-parent model (O'Brien et al., 2013; Melnyk et al., 2006)	a. Review your current model of care and the parent role and consider a failure modes and effects analysis b. Identify ALWAYS EVENTS for parents (patient–family experience that should *always* occur when patients interact with health care professionals and the delivery system—see Resources section for more information) c. Prioritize these ALWAYS EVENTS and develop tests of change to implement (PDSA cycles) d. Include a parent competency-based education intervention with the ALWAYS EVENT parent caregiving activities e. Identify metrics for success; collect benchmarks f. Outline your test for change in collaboration with NICU parents using the PDSA model g. Evaluate your test, revise and refine as necessary h. Implement and draft practice guideline i. Consider publishing/presenting your work

PDSA, Plan-Do-Study-Act; S2S, skin to skin.

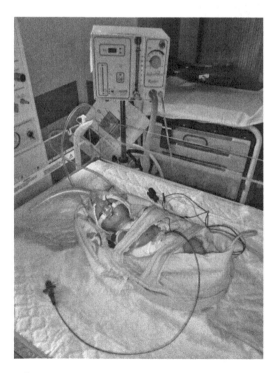

FIGURE 9.9   Mock-up of a neonatal intensive care unit infant for skin-to-skin infant transfer.

Reprinted with permission from Caring Essentials Collaborative, LLC.

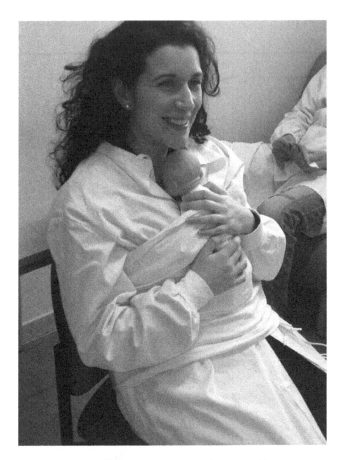

FIGURE 9.10   Successful simulated standing infant transfer for skin-to-skin care.
Reprinted with permission from Caring Essentials Collaborative, LLC.

▪ STANDARDS FOR CULTURALLY COMPETENT CARE

- **Social Justice**—advocate for the patients and families you serve with impartiality and objectivity from the standpoint of our shared humanity
- **Critical Reflection**—understand your own cultural values and beliefs as this self-awareness enables you to develop understanding and respect for other cultural values and beliefs
- **Knowledge of Cultures**—gain understanding of the impact of various cultures on attitudes, traditions, and behaviors particularity related to health and family
- **Culturally Competent Practice**—integrate cultural knowledge into a culturally congruent practice
- **Cultural Competence in Health Care Systems**—organizations must ensure they have the necessary resources to evaluate and meet the cultural and language needs of the population served

Kangaroo Care in the NICU Competency—Parent

Step	Action	Validation of Competence	Complete ✓
1	Completes parent education for kangaroo care in the NICU	Certificate of completion	☐
2	Reviews the unit protocol and understands the eligibility criteria for kangaroo care	Observation	☐
3	Mock-up return demonstration of the kangaroo care procedure for standing infant transfer and parent seated transfer with doll simulator	Observation	☐
4	Assess own infant's eligibility and readiness for kangaroo care.	Observation	☐
5	Prepare self for kangaroo care	Observation	☐
	a. Ensure proper attire for parent		
	b. Ensure parent personal needs are attended to prior to the session		
	c. Ensure comfortable, safe seating, and privacy for the session		
6	Prepare infant for kangaroo care	Observation	☐
	a. Ensure proper attire for infant		
	b. Ensure infant's personal needs are attended to prior to the session		
	c. Ensure comfortable, safe seating, and privacy for the session		
6	Perform transfer in accordance with parent preference and unit protocol	Observation	☐
7	Review safety plan with nurse once settled in kangaroo position (how will the parent access a clinician, when should the parent access the clinician)	Observation	☐
10	Perform return transfer in accordance with parent preference and unit protocol	Observation	☐
11	Support your infant's transition once in the incubator with gentle containment, soothing vocalizations, etc.	Observation & Documentation	☐

Parent: _____   _____   _____
              Printed name   *Signature*   *Date*
Observer: _____   _____   _____
              Printed name   *Signature*   *Date*

FIGURE 9.11   Sample parent kangaroo care competency.

- **Patient Advocacy and Empowerment**—recognize the harmful effects of ignorance, hate, prejudice; identify and address behaviors that compromise the patient's and family's rights to quality health care
- **Multicultural Workforce**—support your organization's efforts to increase diversity in the workplace through respectful interactions with colleagues and coworkers, role modeling culturally sensitive relationships
- **Education and Training in Culturally Competent Care**—integrate cultural care knowledge and training in cultural competence and congruence into new hire orientation and annual competency-based training for all staff
- **Cross-Cultural Communication**—ensure the use of effective, cultural competent verbal and nonverbal communication (e.g., use qualified translators and be mindful of gestures that may have different meanings within different cultures)
- **Cross-Cultural Leadership**—leadership is not hierarchical and everyone within the health care setting has a responsibility to influence individuals, groups, and systems in culturally competent care
- **Policy Development**—cultural competence requires a multilayered approach to identify, implement, and ensure accountability for culturally competent care
- **Evidence-Based Practice and Research**—evidence-based practice is a combination of best available research, clinical expertise, and patient values and must be an integral part of quality, culturally competent care

■ RESOURCES

- Institute for Patient- and Family-Centered Care free download resources: www.ipfcc.org/tools/downloads.html
- Advancing the Practice of Patient- and Family-Centered Care in Hospitals: How to Get Started: www.ipfcc.org/pdf/getting_started.pdf
- Changing Hospital "Visitation" Policies and Practices: Supporting Family Presence and Participation: www.ipfcc.org/visiting.pdf
- Parents' Involvement and Role in the NICU: www.babyfirst.com/en/parents-corner/parents-involvement-and-role.php
- National Association of Perinatal Social Workers, Standards for Social Work Services in the Newborn Intensive Care Unit: napsw.org/about/pdfs/NICU-standards.pdf
- Psychologists in the NICU: www.nationalperinatal.org/psychologists
- Internet NICU Parent Support Links
  - Graham's Foundation: grahamsfoundation.org
  - Hand to Hold: handtohold.org
  - Preemie Parent Alliance: www.preemieparentalliance.org
  - For the Love of Babies: www.suehallmd.com/links.html
  - Prematurity.org: www.prematurity.org
  - March of Dimes: www.marchofdimes.org

- Example PDSA for Competency-Based Education in the Skin-to-Skin Care Infant Transfer Method:

  Describe what you are trying to accomplish, this is your AIM
  AIM—To increase parent knowledge and confidence in providing skin-to-skin care in the NICU the frequency of skin-to-skin
  Identify Success Metrics/Outcome
  (How will you know your intervention was an improvement?)

Process Measures	Outcome Measures
• Percent of parents (mothers/fathers) who participate in the education • Percent of parents (mothers/fathers) who are competent • Percent of parents (mothers/fathers) who provide skin-to-skin care	• Increased frequency in skin-to-skin care • Increase in breast-milk feeding • Decrease in nosocomial infections • Parent and staff satisfaction

  PDSA—always include a timeline—what do you want to achieve and by when? Otherwise, nothing may really change as you will always be "in process":

  Plan—Develop a parent competency-based training module for skin-to-skin care to be completed by the end of the month (pick a date)
  Do—Parents will participate in the competency-based training module for skin-to-skin care within the first 14 days following admission to the NICU
  Study—Look at your success metrics; did you have any unexpected events? How many parents participated in the training within the designated timeline—what were the barriers or challenges to participation? What can be done to revise the plan?

  BE CREATIVE and BE COLLABORATIVE in finding solutions.

  Act—Retest your plan with your revisions and then re-evaluate.

- *Baby Steps to Home* Download: http://babystepstohome.com/nicu-discharge-module.pdf
- COPE for HOPE: www.copeforhope.com/index.php
- NICU Helping Hands Project NICU: www.nicuhelpinghands.org/programs/project-nicu
- Always Events® Toolbox: http://alwaysevents.pickerinstitute.org/?page_id=882

HIPAA Privacy and Security Rules and Joint Commission Standards Are NOT Barriers to Advancing Patient- and Family-Centered Care and Building Partnerships With Patients and Families

NOVEMBER 2013

Many hospitals and practices have questions about how to abide by HIPAA privacy and security rules while also working to advance patient- and family-centered care and partner with patients and families. In addition, many hospitals want to ensure that they adhere to Joint Commission standards.

Concerns about violating HIPAA privacy and security rules and Joint Commission standards—or an incomplete understanding of the rules and/or standards—often prevent the sharing of important information with patients and families.

It is important to note that HIPAA gives patients the right to see and receive a copy of their health information; there is no wording within the HIPAA privacy and security rules or the Joint Commission standards that prohibits health care providers from sharing information with patients and designated family members or partnering with patients and families either at the point-of-care or in governance. Furthermore, it should be noted that the Joint Commission is supportive of both patient and family engagement and of partnering with patients and families in health care redesign and improvement (e.g., patient and family advisory councils) to achieve quality and safety goals.

This document highlights frequently cited concerns and offers ways to address them.

Point-of-Care Examples

Rounds and Nursing Change of Shift Reports at the Bedside

Rounding and change of shift reports at the bedside enable patients and their designated family members to participate in discussions about the patient's health and treatment. When encouraged to actively participate, patients and family members share critical information with health care providers in these discussions.

(continued)

Concerns: *In rooms with multiple beds, does rounding or change of shift at the bedside (in earshot of other patients) violate HIPAA rules or Joint Commission standards? How do we ensure patient privacy when interacting with family members?*

▶ HIPAA allows for normal hospital and physician operations. Clinicians are freely allowed to discuss patient care for treatment purposes, and conversations may take place with patients and designated family members, unless the patient objects. Consider that, in multibed rooms, patient health information is commonly/frequently shared in ways that could be overheard by others in the course of providing care (e.g., a nurse may comment to a patient on the patient's blood pressure, or a physician may discuss discharge plans with a patient).

▶ HIPAA is intended to support greater patient control over his or her health information, and the sharing of patient information to improve care and safety. Participation in rounds or change of shift reports allows patients and family members to take greater control over their health and health information by (a) learning about the patient's condition, medications, treatments, symptoms, and problems to look out for; and (b) providing additional helpful information to providers.

▶ There is nothing in the Joint Commission standards that prohibits rounding or nurse change of shift report at the bedside. In fact, the Joint Commission has expressed explicit support for family involvement.

Additional Suggestions

▶ Design bedside change of shift reporting and rounding protocols to be sensitive to patient privacy needs. Involving patient and family advisors in designing or adapting these processes will help to ensure that patients and families are appropriately involved in their care and comfortable that their privacy is respected. Some potential strategies to consider include:

  ▶ At the beginning of a hospital stay, describe to patients and designated family members the process for rounding and change of shift report at the bedside. Be sure they understand that conversations may be overheard in shared rooms. Ask patients and families if they would like to participate in rounds and change of shift reporting at the bedside.

  ▶ Ask patients to identify designated family members and whether there are issues they would prefer to remain private if rounds or nursing shift reports are conducted with family members present.

  ▶ Ask the patient (and for a child or an incapacitated adult, the authorized parent, guardian, or designated proxy) to identify any family members who should not participate in rounds or other discussions with staff.

  ▶ Consider environmental changes to help safeguard privacy while promoting more patient- and family-centered care—for example, soundproof dividers or curtains for semiprivate rooms.

(continued)

Encouraging Family Presence

Family members are not "visitors"—they provide critical support for patients during and after a hospital stay, and are an important resource for patients' care teams. In recognition of the important role of families, many hospitals are moving away from traditional "visiting hours" and adopting policies that encourage family presence and participation.

Concerns: *If my hospital encourages "family presence" in lieu of "visiting hours," won't it be more difficult for providers to talk about sensitive medical information with patients? How can hospitals support family presence while protecting patient privacy?*

▶ Ask patients to identify the family members they would and would not like to participate in their care, and how they would like to involve them. This will ensure sensitive patient health information is shared according to their wishes.

▶ In the case of shared rooms, provide guidance to patients and their families that will help them be respectful of other patients and families who share the same patient room (i.e., keep information they might hear confidential).

▶ Engage patient and family advisors in developing guidelines for family presence that involve family members according to the patient's wishes. This work could include drafting sample language that personnel could use to deal with difficult situations, such as family members who demand access to personal health information against patient wishes.

Governance Examples

Patient and Family Advisor Participation in Governance

Involving patients and families in quality improvement workgroups, patient safety task forces, and bodies such as patient and family advisory councils (PFACs) is a key strategy for delivering patient- and family-centered care and ensuring that the end results meet the needs of patients and their families. In some case, these bodies review data on readmission rates, medical errors, or quality and safety information.

Concerns: *How can hospitals and practices make sure they are adhering to HIPAA privacy and security rules and/or Joint Commission standards while including patient and family advisors in these important discussions?*

▶ Conduct HIPAA trainings for patient and family advisors to ensure they understand the HIPAA privacy and security rules and their role in ensuring adherence to HIPAA rules.

▶ Conduct background checks on advisors who will be involved in regular ongoing task forces, committees, councils, and boards.

(continued)

▶ Create guidelines on information sharing and confidentiality that all advisors are asked to follow and require that all advisors sign a confidentiality statement. Sample wording: "As a nonemployed committee member, you may have access to protected health information. It is important that you recognize that any protected health information can only be used and disclosed as permitted by law. This information cannot be shared by written, verbal, or e-mail communication at school or home; with friends or family; or outside the hospital, clinic, or other health care facility unless specifically permitted by law."

▶ De-identify sensitive data prior to consideration by any governance bodies to comply with HIPAA's "minimum necessary" standard.

Important Steps for Success

1. Communicate clearly with clinicians, staff, patients, and families that information sharing is a priority and key to delivering high quality, safe care.

2. Implement policies and processes that encourage information sharing.

3. Provide all employees with training and guidance about how to share information in ways that adhere to HIPAA privacy and security rules and Joint Commission standards. Because of current misconceptions, it will be important to emphasize to all employees that there is no wording within the HIPAA privacy and security rules or the Joint Commission standards that prohibits health care providers from sharing information with patients and designated family members or partnering with patients and families either at the point-of-care or in governance. Engage the Risk Management Department and ask personnel to clarify any misconceptions about the HIPAA privacy and security rules.

Source: Institute for Patient- and Family-Centered Care. Retrieved from http://www.ipfcc.org/advance/topics/HIPAA-Factsheet.pdf

■ REFERENCES

Abdel-Latif, M. E., Boswell, D., Broom, M., Smith, J., & Davis, D. (2015). Parental presence on neonatal intensive care unit clinical bedside rounds: Randomised trial and focus group discussion. *Archives of Diseases in Childhood, Fetal & Neonatal Ed., 100*, F203–F209.

Agostini, F., Neri, E., Dellabartola, S., Biasini, A., & Monti, F. (2014). Early interactive behaviors in preterm infants and their mothers: Influence of maternal depressive symptomatology and neonatal birth weight. *Infant Behavior and Development, 37*(1), 86–93.

Alegria, D. A. H., Boscardin, C., Poncelet, A., Mayfield, C., & Wamsley, M. (2014). Using tablets to support self-regulated learning in the longitudinal integrated clerkship. *Medical Education Online, 19*, 10. doi:3402/meo.v19.23638

Alkozei, A., McMahon, E., & Lahav, A. (2014). Stress levels and depressive symptoms in capital and ICU mothers in the early postpartum period. *Journal of Maternal-Fetal & Neonatal Medicine, 27*(17), 1738–1743.

Anderzen-Carlsson, A., Lamy, Z. C., & Eriksson, M. (2014). Parental experiences of providing skin-to-skin care to their newborn infant—part one: A qualitative systematic review. *International Journal of Qualitative Studies on Health and Well-Being*, 9. doi:10.3402/qhw.v9.24906

Bastani, F., Abadi, T. A., & Haghani, H. (2015). Effects of family-centered care on improving parental satisfaction and reducing readmission among premature infants: a randomized controlled trial. *Journal of Clinical and Diagnostic Research, 9*(1), SC04–SC08.

Baylis, R., Ewald, U., Gradin, M., Nyqvist, K. H., Rubertsson, C., & Blomqvist, Y. T. (2014). First-time events between parents and preterm infants are affected by the designs and routines of neonatal intensive care units. *Acta Paediatrica, 103*, 1045–1052.

Betancourt, J. R., Green, A. R., & Carrillo, J. E. (2002). *Cultural competence in health care: Emerging frameworks and practical approaches*. Retrieved from http://www.commonwealthfund.org/usr_doc/betancourt_culturalcompetence_576.pdf

Bicking, C., & Moore, G. A. (2012). Maternal perinatal depression in the neonatal intensive care unit: The role of the neonatal nurse. *Neonatal Network, 31*(5), 295–304.

Breitenstein, S. M., Gross, D., & Christophersen, R. (2014). Digital delivery methods of parenting training interventions: a systematic review. *Worldviews on Evidence-Based Nursing, 11*(3), 168–176.

Broedsgaard, A., & Wagner, L. (2005). How to facilitate parents and their premature infant for the transition home. *International Nursing Review, 52*(3), 196–203.

Burnham, N., Feeley, N., & Sherrard, K. (2013). Parents perceptions regarding readiness for their infants discharged from the NICU. *Neonatal Network, 32*(5), 324–334.

Busse, M., Stromgren, K., Thorngate, L., & Thomas, K. A. (2013). Parents responses to stress in the neonatal intensive care unit. *Critical Care Nurse, 33*(4), 52–60.

Butler, C. L., & Galvin, K. (2003). Parents' perceptions of staff competency in a neonatal intensive care unit. *Journal of Clinical Nursing, 12*(5), 752–761.

Candelori, C., Trumello, C., Babore, A., Keren, M., & Romanelli, R. (2015). The experience of premature birth for fathers: The application of the Clinical Interview for Parents of High-Risk Infants (CLIP) to an Italian sample. *Frontiers in Psychology, 6,* 1444. doi:10.3389/fpsyg.2015.01444

Carson, C., Redshaw, M., Gray, R., & Quigley, M. A. (2015). Risk of psychological distress in parents of preterm children in the first year: Evidence from the UK millennium cohort study. *BMJ Open, 5*(12), e007942.

Carter, B. S., Carter, A., & Bennett, S. (2008). Families' views upon experiencing change in the neonatal intensive care unit environment: From the 'baby barn' to the private room. *Journal of Perinatology, 28*(12), 827–829.

Cheng, E. R., Kotelchuck, M., Gerstein, E. D., Taveras, E. M., & Poehlmann-Tynan, J. (2016). Postnatal depressive symptoms among mothers and fathers of infants born preterm: Prevalence and impacts on children's early cognitive function. *Journal of Developmental and Behavioral Pediatrics, 37*(1), 33–42.

Choi, J., & Bakken, S. (2010). Web-based education for low-literate parents in neonatal intensive care unit: Development of a website and heuristic evaluation and usability testing. *International Journal of Medical Informatics, 79*(8), 565–575.

Cleveland, L. M. (2008). Parenting in the neonatal intensive care unit. *Journal of Obstetric, Gynecologic, and Neonatal Nursing, 37,* 666–691.

Cox, J. L., Holden, J. M., and Sagovsky, R. (1987). Detection of postnatal depression: Development of the 10-item Edinburgh Postnatal Depression Scale. *British Journal of Psychiatry, 150,* 782–786.

Coughlin, M. (2015). The Sobreviver (Survive) Project. *Newborn & Infant Nursing Reviews, 15*(4), 169–173.

Craig, J. W., Glick, C., Phillips, R., Hall, S. L., Smith, J., and Browne, J. (2015). Recommendations for involving the family and developmental care of the NICU baby. *Journal of Perinatology, 35*(Suppl. 1), S5–S8.

Davidson, J. E. (2013). Family presence on rounds in neonatal, pediatric, and adult intensive care units. *Annals of the American Thoracic Society, 10*(2), 152–156.

Davidson, J. E., Powers, K., Hedayat, K. M., Tieszen, M., Kon, A. A., Shepard, E.,…Armstrong, D. (2007). Clinical practice guidelines for support of the family in the patient-centered intensive care unit: American College of Critical Care Medicine Task Force 2004–2005. *Critical Care Medicine, 35,* 605–622.

Davis, L., Mohay, H., & Edwards, H. (2003). Mothers' involvement in caring for their premature infants: an historical overview. *Journal of Advanced Nursing, 42*(6), 578–586.

Domanico, R., Davis, D. K., Coleman, F., & Davis, B. O. (2011). Documenting the NICU design dilemma: Comparative patient progress in open-ward and single-family room units. *Journal of Perinatology, 31*(4), 281–288.

Dusing, S. C., Murray, T., & Stern, M. (2008). Parent preferences for motor development education in the neonatal intensive care unit. *Pediatric Physical Therapy, 20*(4), 363–368.

Evans, Y., Whittingham, K., Sanders, M., Colditz, P., & Boyd, R. N. (2014). Are parenting interventions effective in improving the relationship between mothers and their preterm infants? *Infant Behavior and Development, 37,* 131–154.

Ferri, M., Zygun, D. A., Harrison, A., & Stelfox, H. T. (2015). Evidence-based design in an intensive care unit: End-user perceptions. *BMC Anesthesiology, 15,* 57. doi:10. 1186/ s12871–015-0038–4

Flacking, R., Lehtonen, L., Thomson, G., Axelin, A., Ahlqvist, S., Moran, V. H.,...Dykes, F. (2012). Closeness and separation in neonatal intensive care. *Acta Paediatrica, 101*(10), 1032–1037.

Friedman, S. H., Kessler, A., Yang, S. N., Parsons, S., Friedman, H., & Martin, R. J. (2013). Delivering perinatal psychiatric services in the neonatal intensive care unit. *Acta Paediatrica, 102*(9), e392–e397.

Gonulal, D., Yalaz, M., Altun-Koroglu, O., & Kultursay, N. (2014). Both parents of neonatal intensive care unit patients are at risk of depression. *The Turkish Journal of Pediatrics, 56,* 171–176.

Gooding, J. S., Cooper, L. G., Blaine, A. I., Franck, L. S., Howse, J. L., & Berns, S. D. (2011). Family support and family-centered care in the neonatal intensive care unit: Origins, advances, impact. *Seminars in Perinatology, 35,* 20–28.

Griffin, T. (2013). A family-centered "visitation" policy in the neonatal intensive care unit that welcomes parents as partners. *Journal of Perinatal and Neonatal Nursing, 27*(2), 160–165.

Grzyb, M. J., Coo, H., Ruhland, L., & Dow, K. (2014). Views of parents and healthcare providers regarding parental presence at bedside rounds in a neonatal intensive care unit. *Journal of Perinatology, 34*(2), 143–148.

Hall, S. L., Cross, J., Selix, N. W., Patterson, C., Segre, L., Chuffo-Siewert, R.,...Martin, M. L. (2015a). Recommendations for enhancing psychosocial support of NICU parents through staff education and support. *Journal of Perinatology, 35,* S29–S36.

Hall, S. L., Ryan, D. J., Beatty, J., & Grubbs, L. (2015b). Recommendations for peer-to-peer support for NICU parents. *Journal of Perinatology, 35,* S9–S13.

Heermann, J. A., Wilson, M. E., & Wilhelm, P. A. (2005). Mothers in the NICU: Outsider to partner. *Pediatric Nursing, 31*(3), 176–181.

Hoye, S., & Severinsson, E. (2010). Professional and cultural conflicts for intensive care nurses. *Journal of Advanced Nursing, 66*(4), 858–867.

Hynan, M. T., Steinberg, Z., Baker, L., Cicco, R., Geller, P. A., Lassen, S.,...Stuebe, A. (2015). Recommendations for mental health professionals in the NICU. *Journal of Perinatology, 35,* S14–S18.

Jeffreys, M. (2008). Dynamics of diversity: Becoming better nurses through diversity awareness. *Imprint, 55*(5), 36–41.

Johnson, B., Abraham, M., Conway, J., Simmons, L., Edgman-Levitan, S., Sodomka, P.,... Ford, D. (2008). *Partnering with patients and families to design a patient- and family-centered health care system: Recommendations and promising practices.* Bethesda, MD: Institute for Patient- and Family-Centered Care.

The Joint Commission (2010). *Advancing effective communication, cultural competence, and patient- and family-centered care: A roadmap for hospitals.* Oakbrook Terrace, IL: The Joint Commission.

Jubinville, J., Newburn-Cook, C., Hegadoren, K., & Lacaze-Masmonteil, T. (2012). Symptoms of acute stress disorder in mothers of premature infants. *Advances in Neonatal Care, 12*(4), 246–253.

Lasiuk, G. C., Comeau, T., & Newburn-Cook, C. (2013). Unexpected: An interpretive description of parental traumas associated with preterm birth. *BMC Pregnancy and Childbirth, 13*(Suppl. 1), S13.

Leape, L., Berwick, D., Clancy, C., Conway, J., Gluck, P., Guest, J.,...Isaac, T. (2009). Transforming healthcare: A safety imperative. *Quality and Safety in Health Care, 18,* 424–428.

Lee, L. A., Carter, M., Stevenson, S. B., & Harrison, H. A. (2014). Improving family-centered care practices in the NICU. *Neonatal Network, 33*(3), 125–132.

Ludington-Hoe, S. M., Ferreira, C., Swinth, J., & Ceccardi, J. J. (2003). Safe criteria and procedure for kangaroo care with intubated preterm infants. *Journal of Obstetrics, Gynecologic, & Neonatal Nursing, 32*(5), 579–588.

Lundqvist, P., Westas, L. H., & Hallstrom, I. (2007). From distance toward proximity: Fathers lived experience of caring for their preterm infants. *Journal of Pediatric Nursing, 22*(6), 490–497.

Macdonell, K., Christie, K., Robson, K., Pytlik, K., Lee, S. K., & O'Brien, K. (2013). Implementing family-integrated care in the NICU. *Advances in Neonatal Care, 13*(4), 262–269.

Melnyk, B. M., & Feinstein, N. F. (2009). Reducing hospital expenditures with the COPE (Creating Opportunities for Parent Empowerment) program for parents in premature infants: An analysis of direct healthcare neonatal intensive care unit costs and savings. *Nursing Administration Quarterly, 33*(1), 32–37.

Melnyk, B. M., Feinstein, N. F., Alpert-Gillis, L., Fairbanks, E., Crean, H. F., Sinkin, R. A.,... Gross, S. J. (2006). Reducing premature infants' length of stay and improving parents' mental health outcomes would be Creating Opportunities for Parent Empowerment (COPE) neonatal intensive care unit program: A randomized controlled trial. *Pediatrics, 118*(5), e1414–e1427.

Moore, K. A., Coker, K., DuBuisson, A. B., Swett, B., & Edwards, W. H. (2003). Implementing potentially better practices for improving family-centered care in neonatal intensive care units: Successes and challenges. *Pediatrics, 111*(4, Pt. 2) e450–e460.

Obeidat, H. M., Bond, E. A., & Clark Callister, L. (2009). The parental experience of having an infant in the newborn intensive care unit. *The Journal of Perinatal Education, 18*(3), 23–29.

O'Brien, K., Bracht, M., Macdonell, K., McBride, T., Robson, K., O'Leary, L.,...Lee, S. K. (2013). A pilot cohort analytic study of family integrated care in a Canadian neonatal intensive care unit. *BMC Pregnancy and Childbirth, 13*(Suppl. 1), S12. doi:10.1186/1471-2393-13-S1-S12.

Ortenstrand, A., Westrup, B., Brostrom, E. B., Sarman, I., Akerstrom, S., Brune, T.,... Waldenstrom, U. (2010). The Stockholm neonatal family centered care study: Effects on length of stay and infant morbidity. *Pediatrics, 125*(2), e278–e285.

Panter-Brick, C., Burgess, A., Eggerman, M., McAllister, F., Pruett, K., & Leckman, J. F. (2014). Practitioner review: Engaging fathers—recommendations for a game change in parenting interventions based on a systematic review of the global evidence. *Journal of Child Psychology and Psychiatry, and Allied Disciplines, 55*(11), 1187–1212.

Rossman, B., Greene, M. M., & Meier, P. P. (2015). The role of peer support in the development of maternal identity for "NICU moms." *Journal of Obstetric, Gynecologic and Neonatal Nursing, 44*(1), 3–16.

Sakallaris, B. R., MacAllister, L., Voss, M., Smith, K., & Jonas, W. B. (2015). Optimal healing environments. *Global Advances in Health and Medicine, 4*(3), 40–45.

Schim, S. M., Doorenbos, A., Benkert, R., & Miller, J. (2007). Culturally congruent care: Putting the puzzle together. *Journal of Transcultural Nursing, 18*(2), 103–110.

Shaw, R. J., Bernard, R. S., DeBlois, T., Ikuta, L., Ginzburg, K., & Koopman, C. (2009). The relationship between acute stress disorder and posttraumatic stress disorder in the neonatal intensive care unit. *Psychosomatics, 50,* 131–137.

Shaw, R. J., DeBlois, T., Ikuta, L., Ginzburg, K., Fleisher, B., & Koopman, C. (2006). Acute stress disorder among parents of infants in the neonatal intensive care nursery. *Psychosomatics, 47,* 206–212.

Shaw, R. J., St John, N., Lilo, E., Jo, B., Benitz, W., Stevenson, D. K., & Horwitz, S. M. (2014). Prevention of traumatic stress in mothers of pre-terms: 6-month outcomes. *Pediatrics, 134*(2), e481–e488.

Sneath, N. (2009). Discharge teaching in the NICU: Are parents prepared? An integrative review of parents' perceptions. *Neonatal Network, 28*(4), 237–246.

Söderström, I., Benzein, E., & Saveman, B. (2003). Nurses' experiences of interactions with family members in intensive care units. *Scandinavian Journal of Caring Sciences, 17*(2), 185–192.

Tessier, K. (2010). Effectiveness of hands-on education for correct child restraint use by parents. *Accident; Analysis and Prevention, 42*(4), 1041–1047.

Ulrich, R. S., Zimring, C., Zhu, X., DuBose, J., Seo, H. B., Choi, Y. S.,…Joseph, A. (2008). A review of the research literature on evidence-based healthcare design. *Health Environments Research & Design Journal, 1*(3), 61–125.

Van Keer, R. L., Deschepper, R., Francke, A. L., Huyghens, L., & Bilsen, J. (2015). Conflicts between healthcare professionals and families of a multi-ethnic patient population during critical care: An ethnographic study. *Critical Care, 19*(1), 441.

Vazquez, V., & Cong, X. (2014). Parenting the NICU infant: A meta-ethnographic synthesis. *International Journal of Nursing Sciences, 1*(3), 281–290.

Vigod, S. N., Villegas, L., Dennis, C. L., & Ross, L. E. (2010). Prevalence and risk factors for postpartum depression among women with preterm and low-birth-weight infants: A systematic review. *BJOG: An International Journal of Obstetrics and Gynaecology, 115*(5), 540–550.

White, R. D. (2011). The newborn intensive care unit environment of care: How we got here, where we're headed, and why. *Seminars in Perinatology, 35,* 2–7.

Wiebe, A., & Young, B. (2011). Parent perspectives from a neonatal intensive care unit: A missing piece of the culturally congruent care puzzle. *Journal of Transcultural Nursing, 22*(1), 77–82.

PART III

The Role of the NICU Professional
as Provider of Trauma-Informed,
Age-Appropriate Care

CHAPTER 10

Meeting the Needs of the Neonatal Clinician

Too often we underestimate the power of a touch, a smile, a kind word,
a listening ear, an honest compliment, or the smallest act of caring, all
of which have the potential to turn a life around.
        —Leo Buscaglia

■ THE WORK

Bearing witness to the suffering of others underpins the work we do as health care professionals. Whether physician, therapist, social worker, or nurse, we engage in healing relationships with our patients and their families during a time of extreme vulnerability, sadness, and fear. As their lives unfold, "our consciousness, our intentionality, our presence, makes a difference for better or for worse" (Watson, 2003). When we are unable to be present or turn away from the lived reality of our patients we fail our moral responsibility and undermine quality care and patient safety (Dill & Gumpert, 2012; Naef, 2006).

Patients depend on and trust that health care professionals will ease their suffering and provide ethically sensitive care consistently and reliably. The clinician–patient relationship is a sacred privileged trust and the cornerstone of professional clinical practice. Our trustworthiness as neonatal professionals hinges on an unequal distribution of power in a dynamic, fragile, and asymmetric patient–professional relationship (Carter 2009). This relationship defines our moral accountability and moral integrity grounded in the ethic of caring (LaSala, 2009).

Providing emotionally supportive care is an acknowledged and vital aspect of caring in the neonatal intensive care unit (NICU), but may be hindered by a knowledge deficit about effective, emotionally supportive counseling strategies for NICU parents and competing priorities in this high-tech environment (Hall et al., 2015; Jasmine, 2009; Turner, Chur-Hansen, & Winefield, 2014). Suffering is an unfortunate reality in the NICU, jeopardizing our moral accountability due to the challenges in discerning infant suffering, and placing the neonatal clinician at risk for compassion fatigue (Cavaliere, Daly, Dowling, & Montgomery, 2010; Korhonen, Haho, & Pölkki, 2013; Meadors, Lamson, Swanson, White, & Sira, 2009; Profit et al., 2014). Providing trauma-informed, age-appropriate care during neonatal intensive care recognizes the psychoemotional and physiologic vulnerabilities of the hospitalized infant–family dyad and is poised to mitigate the suffering of this extremely fragile population (Coughlin, 2014). Despite the burgeoning body of evidence to support the implementation of developmentally supportive, age-appropriate care, many clinicians miss providing this care, or if provided, lack any kind of consistency that would be beneficial in easing the suffering of the infant–family dyad (Goudarzi et al., 2015; Hall, Kronborg, Aagaard, & Ammentorp, 2010; Hendricks-Munoz et al., 2010; Valizadeh, Asadollahi, Mostafa Gharebaghi, & Gholami, 2013).

Missed care or rationed care, defined as a failure to carry out necessary tasks due to inadequate time, staffing level, and/or skill mix, has been linked to deficiencies in the work environment and is a predictor of nursing job satisfaction, patient satisfaction, and patient outcomes (Ball, Murrells, Rafferty, Morrow, & Griffiths, 2014; Kalisch, Landstrom, & Hinshaw, 2009; Papastavrou, Andreou, & Efstathiou, 2014; Papastavrou, Andreou, Tsangari, & Merkouris, 2014; Rochefort & Clarke, 2010). In a comprehensive literature review on unfinished nursing care, missed care, and implicitly rationed care, Jones, Hamilton, & Murry (2015) uncover that between 55% and 95% of international nurses in acute care hospitals report leaving at least one task undone and these errors by omission leave vulnerable patients with unmet educational, emotional, and psychological needs (see Table 10.1 for the five most frequently missed cares and least frequently missed cares).

Physicians have also described the phenomenon of care rationing at the bedside and, for many, it creates a moral dilemma (Papastavrou et al., 2014; Strech, Persad, Marckmann, & Danis, 2009). In a descriptive analysis of NICU nurses' self-reports on missed care, nurses most frequently missed rounds, oral care for ventilated infants, educating and involving parents in the care of their infant, and oral feeding opportunities for infants who exhibited feeding readiness behaviors (Tubbs-Cooley, Pickler, Younger, & Mark, 2015). Rochefort and Clarke (2010) describe care activities most frequently rationed in the NICU to include discharge planning, parental support and teaching, and infant comfort care. Missed care creates a moral conundrum for the neonatal clinician who feels forced to prioritize and rationalize what is and is not completed during any given shift, minimizing the implications of the missed care, and adding a layer of professional frustration and disappointment in abandoning moral integrity and accountability.

The work of neonatal professionals is both physically and emotionally demanding as well as morally and ethically challenging. Issues surrounding end-of-life care, futile aggressive care, patient harms, pain and suffering, depersonalization of patients,

TABLE 10.1   Categories of Care Activities Most Frequently and Least Frequently Missed

Most Frequently Missed Cares	Least Frequently Missed Cares
Emotional support	Infection control
Education	Treatments and tests
Care coordination and discharge planning	Procedures
Care planning	Nutrition
Timeliness of care	Elimination

care and cost constraints, inadequate staffing, and working with incompetent colleagues have all been associated with moral distress for nurses, physicians, and allied health professionals (Cavaliere et al., 2010; Cavinder, 2014; Hamric, & Blackhall, 2007; Kain, 2007; Mukherjee, Brashler, Savage, & Kirschner, 2009; Sannino, Giannì, Re, & Lusignani, 2015; Whitehead, Herbertson, Hamric, Epstein, & Fisher, 2015).

Moral distress is a precursor to clinician burnout, which is associated with adverse safety behaviors, medical errors, operational and clinical outcomes (Profit et al., 2014; Rushton, Batcheller, Schroeder, & Donohue, 2015). Burnout has three interrelated dimensions that include emotional exhaustion, depersonalization, and a sense of low personal accomplishment as defined by the Maslach Burnout Inventory (MBI) and is prevalent among neonatologists, neonatal nurses, and nurse practitioners as well as neonatal respiratory therapists (Bellieni et al., 2012; Maslach & Jackson, 1981; Profit et al., 2014). Compassion fatigue has been observed in professionals working in emotionally charged, challenging intensive care environments and is defined as a loss of compassion as a result of repeated exposure to suffering, often experienced by individuals with a strong empathic orientation and includes personal feelings of exhaustion, frustration, and depression (van Meadors et al., 2009; van Mol, Kompanje, Benoit, Bakker, & Nijkamp, 2015). A systematic review on the prevalence of compassion fatigue and burnout among health care professionals working in intensive care environments confirms there is an emotional price to caring for critically ill individuals including infants in the NICU (Braithwaite, 2008; van Mol et al., 2015).

At the heart of the work is caring, a desire to make a difference in the lives of others, to *be with* and bear witness to others—the authenticity of the caring relationship restores the clinician as well as the patient and must be protected, nurtured, respected, and honored at the individual and organizational level to diffuse and decrease the psychological and emotional distress associated with the complex world of neonatal intensive care (Einarsdóttir, 2012; Hogan, 2013; McDonald, Rubarth, & Miers, 2012).

■ THE ENVIRONMENT

The environment of the NICU is comprised of the physical space, the human occupants, and the organization or system culture and climate (Coughlin, Gibbins, & Hoath, 2009). The work environment plays a key role in the clinician's ability to fully operationalize his or her moral accountability and moral integrity to preserve and protect a trusting–healing relationship with the infant–family dyad as well as maintain a sense of engagement and fulfillment in service to others. In a cross-sectional survey of greater than 150,000 patients and more than 60,000 nurses in 12 countries in Europe plus the United States, Aiken et al. (2012) examined the relationship between nurse staffing patterns and hospital work environments on patient and nurse outcomes to include the levels of satisfaction and perceptions of quality and patient safety. Characteristics of the work environment were defined using the Practice Environment Scale of the Nursing Work Index (PES-NWI Revised) (see Table 10.2); optimal environments were associated with better nurse and patient outcomes (Aiken et al., 2012; Lake, 2002).

TABLE 10.2   Practice Environment Scale of the Nursing Work Index

For each item, please indicate the extent to which you agree that the item is PRESENT IN YOUR CURRENT JOB. Indicate your degree of agreement by circling the appropriate number.

Indicator	Strongly Agree	Agree	Disagree	Strongly Disagree
1. Adequate support services allow me to spend time with my patients.	4	3	2	1
2. Physician and nurses have good working relationships.	4	3	2	1
3. A supervisory staff that is supportive of the nurses.	4	3	2	1
4. Active staff development or continuing education programs for nurses.	4	3	2	1
5. Career development/clinical ladder opportunity.	4	3	2	1
6. Opportunity for staff nurses to participate in policy decisions.	4	3	2	1
7. Supervisors use mistakes as learning opportunities, not criticism.	4	3	2	1
8. Enough time and opportunity to discuss patient care problems with other nurses.	4	3	2	1
9. Enough registered nurses to provide quality patient care.	4	3	2	1
10. A nurse manager who is a good manager and leader.	4	3	2	1
11. Chief nursing officer who is highly visible and accessible to staff.	4	3	2	1
12. Enough staff to get the work done.	4	3	2	1
13. Praise and recognition for a job well done.	4	3	2	1
14. High standards of nursing care are expected by the administration.	4	3	2	1
15. A chief nurse officer equal in power and authority to other top-level hospital executives.	4	3	2	1
16. A lot of teamwork between nurses and physicians.	4	3	2	1

(continued)

TABLE 10.2   Practice Environment Scale of the Nursing Work Index   *(continued)*

Indicator	Strongly Agree	Agree	Disagree	Strongly Disagree
17. Opportunities for advancement.	4	3	2	1
18. A clear philosophy of nursing that pervades the patient care environment.	4	3	2	1
19. Working with nurses who are clinically competent.	4	3	2	1
20. A nurse manager who backs up the nursing staff in decision making, even if the conflict is with a physician.	4	3	2	1
21. Administration that listens and responds to employee concerns.	4	3	2	1
22. An active quality assurance program.	4	3	2	1
23. Staff nurses are involved in the internal governance of the hospital (e.g., practice and policy committees).	4	3	2	1
24. Collaboration (joint practice) between nurses and physicians.	4	3	2	1
25. A preceptor program for newly hired RNs.	4	3	2	1
26. Nursing care is based on a nursing, rather than a medical, model.	4	3	2	1
27. Staff nurses have the opportunity to serve on hospital and nursing committees.	4	3	2	1
28. Nursing administrators consult with staff on daily problems and procedures.	4	3	2	1
29. Written, up-to-date nursing care plans for all patients.	4	3	2	1
30. Patient care assignments that foster continuity of care, that is, the same nurse cares for the patient from one day to the next.	4	3	2	1
31. Use of nursing diagnoses.	4	3	2	1

Organizations that provide optimal work environments are perceived as safer; delivering a higher quality of care; demonstrating lower levels of burnout, depression, and anxiety; and reporting fewer instances of rationed or missed care (Aiken et al., 2012; Bronkhorst, Tummers, Steijn, & Vijverberg, 2015; Rochefort & Clarke, 2010). In a cross-sectional survey evaluating the impact of leadership walk rounds across 44 NICUs on patient safety culture and caregiver burnout, there was a statistically significant improvement on safety culture perceptions ($p < .001$) and a notable decline in burnout symptoms ($p = .07$; Sexton et al., 2014). System-level programs that recognize nursing excellence (i.e., Magnet Designation), demonstrate a statistically significant decrease in neonatal mortality and morbidity (specifically nosocomial infection and severe intraventricular hemorrhage) for very low birth weight infants when compared to hospitals that do not recognize excellence in nursing, with facilities that recognize nursing excellence also celebrating lower levels of nurse job dissatisfaction and burnout (Kelly, McHugh, & Aiken, 2011; Lake et al., 2012). Organizational climate and professionalism grounded in the ethical values of beneficence, dignity, justice, honesty, and self-discipline support the good work of caring for others, which minimizes harm for the patient *and* the clinician (Bronkhorst et al., 2015; Egener, McDonald, Rosof, & Gullen, 2012).

Attributes of the physical environment are reflective of the organizational climate and impact the patient *and* the clinician. The implications of excessive noise levels on staff encompass physiological aberrations as well as executive and emotional functioning capabilities and include tachycardia, increased blood pressure, distraction, compromised concentration and increased feelings of irritation, fatigue, and burnout (Braithwaite, 2008; Konkani & Oakley, 2012; Thomas & Martin, 2000). Intensive care unit (ICU) sound levels exceed the recommended levels established by the World Health Organization (see Table 10.3; Darbyshire & Young, 2013).

The most common sources of noise in intensive care environments include device operation noise, staff speech, alarms, and staff activity with comparable findings in the NICU (Figure 10.1; Konkani & Oakley, 2012; Krueger, Schue, & Parker, 2007; Simons et al., 2014).

Sound, light, space, and aesthetics combine to create an optimal healing environment for patient and clinician. The concept of the optimal healing environment (OHE) was originally coined in 2004 by the Samueli Institute (see Table 10.4 for the constructs and definitions of a healing environment; Sakallaris, MacAllister, Voss, Smith, & Jonas, 2015).

TABLE 10.3   Sound Level Recommendations for Hospitalized Patients' Rooms by Organizations

Shift	World Health Organization (dB)	International Noise Council (dB)	Environmental Protection Agency (dB)
Days	35	45	45
Evenings	—	40	—
Nights	30	20	35

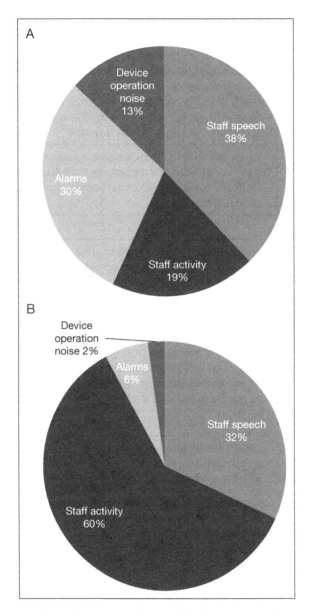

FIGURE 10.1   The contribution of each noise category in intensive care settings. (A) The acoustic energy and
(B) the number of predicted peaks in sound energy.

Source: Simons et al. (2014). Reprinted creative commons license: creativecommons.org/licenses/by/4.0

The OHE framework has been critically reviewed and has matured over the
past decade to reflect the ideals of a healing space for the healer and the patient
(Sakallaris et al., 2015).

The interpersonal construct of the OHE involves not only the patient but collegial
relationships within the environment of care. Respectful interpersonal relationships
and teamwork are fundamental for quality care, patient safety, and professional

TABLE 10.4   OHE Constructs and Definitions

Internal Environment	
Healing intention	A conscious and benevolent mental activity (thought) purposefully directed toward health, well-being, healing, or highest good for one's self or another. Healing intention is manifest in the care setting in various ways, including setting intentions, prayer, and assessing patient hopes and expectations for healing and incorporating those hopes into the plan of care.
Personal wholeness	The congruence of mind, body, and spirit, experienced through relationship with self and others, resulting in completeness and well-being. Mind–body–spirit congruence is enhanced through mind–body practices and interventions and attending to spirituality.
Interpersonal Environment	
Healing relationships	Healing relationships are the connections between persons who hold an intention for healing to occur. The attributes that distinguish a healing relationship from other positive relationships are that the connection is intentional and covenantal in nature and the connection involves positive emotional engagement and provides mutual benefit.
Healing organizations	Healing organizations are driven by a mission to promote healing and health creation. They provide appropriate structures, processes, and resources to stimulate and support healing through intention, relationships, person-centered strategic planning, and shared decision making. Healing organizations optimize the potential for well-being of their employees and the people they serve.
Behavioral Environment	
Healthy lifestyles	A healthy lifestyle involves making choices in diet, activity, relaxation, stress reduction, and sleep that create and maintain health. A healthy lifestyle is a way of life that optimizes potential for maximal healthy life years.
Integrative care	Integrative care is team-based care that is person focused and family centered and incorporates multidisciplinary care providers at their highest skill level. Integrative care blends the best of complementary therapies with conventional medicine in order to enhance self-care skills and ameliorate suffering.
External Environment	
Healing spaces	Healing spaces incorporate evidence-based design and healing principles to optimize and improve the quality of care, outcomes, and experiences of patients and staff. Healing spaces use physical design to enhance the individual's innate healing potential.
Ecological sustainability	Organizations and individuals can foster ecological sustainability by reducing their footprint and supporting the health of the planet. The chemical impact and energy use of their operations are considered. Products or practices that are resource intensive can be replaced with more ecologically friendly, less harmful, and cruelty-free alternatives.

OHE, optimal healing environment.

Reprinted with permission from Sakallaris et al. (2015).

quality of life. Organizational culture and climate set the stage for professional quality of life and patient safety influenced by managers and organizational leaders who establish or accept the norms, values, beliefs, behaviors, and assumptions that are shared by members of the organization (Stone, Hughes, & Dailey, 2008). A randomized, simulated trial evaluating the impact of mildly rude commentary on the diagnostic and procedural accuracy of a group of NICU physicians revealed that the group exposed to the rudeness were statistically and significantly less accurate than the control group (Riskin et al., 2015). The prevalence rate of workplace bullying and incivility (to include rude, dismissive, and aggressive communications) among physicians reportedly affects as many as 31% of physicians on a daily basis (Bradley et al., 2015). Anywhere from 17% to 76% of staff nurses report being bullied at one point in their career and bullying is indeed an international problem (Ariza-Montes, Muniz, Montero-Simó, & Araque-Padilla, 2013; Johnson, 2009; Vessey, Demarco, Gaffney, & Budin, 2009). Job characteristics, quality of interpersonal relationships, leadership styles, and organizational culture (to include volatility and hierarchy) have all been identified as antecedents of workplace bullying (Johnson, 2009; Hutchinson, Jackson, Wilkes, & Vickers, 2008; Trepanier, Fernet, Austin, & Boudrias, 2015). When organizational leadership turns a blind eye to bullying, this deviant disruptive behavior becomes normalized and indoctrinated into the environment of care, subverting a culture of safety and jeopardizing the patient, the professionals, and ultimately the organization (Hutchinson et al., 2008). Stone et al. (2008) developed a conceptual model looking at patient safety and quality influenced by the organizational climate. Structural characteristics enable or influence an organization's climate and is highly susceptible to the influence of senior leadership, the availability of technological resources, and communication processes and systems; organizational climate is much more malleable than organizational culture and can be a key facilitator of data-driven cultural transformation (Figure 10.2).

Organizational climate has been implicated as an underlying reason for the phenomena of missed care and implicit rationing of nursing care identifying an opportunity to improve quality and patient safety as well as professional quality of life and job satisfaction (Jones, Hamilton, Carryer, Sportsman, & Gemeinhardt, 2014; Kalisch, Tschannen, Lee, & Friese, 2011; Lake et al., 2012; Sakallaris et al., 2015).

You

The expectation that we can be immersed in suffering and loss daily
and not be touched by it is as unrealistic as expecting to be able to walk
on water without getting wet. This sort of denial is no small matter.
    —Remen, 1996, p. 52

Health care professionals have been identified as particularly susceptible to high levels of workplace stress, which has been linked to increased rates of depression, anxiety, burnout, and compassion fatigue (Rees, Breen, Cusack, & Hegney, 2015). Individual attributes have been identified as protective against these negative psychological phenomena. Psychological resilience has been described as positive

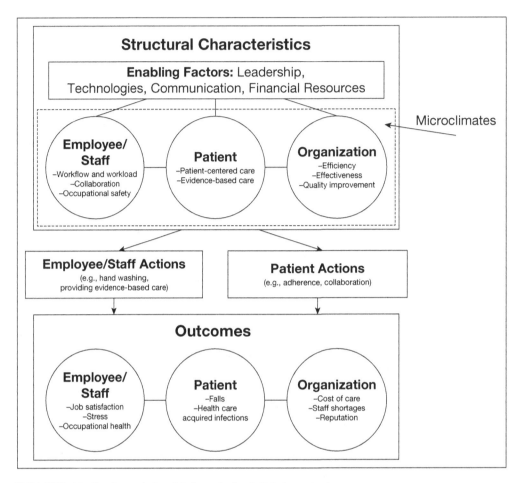

FIGURE 10.2   Conceptual model of organizational attributes and outcomes.
Adapted from Stone et al. (2008).

adaptation or recovery following a negative or emotionally distressing situation (Rees et al., 2015; Wood & Bhatnagar, 2015). The presence of resilience in ICU nurses has been reported as independently associated with a statistically significant decrease in the prevalence of posttraumatic stress disorder (PTSD) and burnout syndrome (Mealer et al., 2012). Rushton et al. (2015) confirms the relationship among precursors for burnout in nurses working in high-risk areas and identifies the modulating effects of resilience and hope in reducing vulnerability to emotional exhaustion. McCann et al. (2013) report on individual and contextual factors relating to resilience across various disciplines (Tables 10.5 and 10.6).

Work–life balance, female gender, a sense of humor, spirituality, self-reflection, and professional identity were correlated with resilience regardless of discipline (McCann et al., 2013). Although there are intrinsic neural determinants of an individual's inherent resilience or vulnerability to stress, health care professionals who participate in training interventions focused on mindfulness and self-compassion

TABLE 10.5 Factors Within an Individual That Relate to Resilience

	Factors	Nurses	Social Workers	Psychologists	Counselors	Doctors
Demographic	Age	**X**	X	X	–	–
	Gender	X	**X**	**X**	X	X
	Experience	X	X	–	–	–
	Income	X	–	X	–	–
Behavioral (personal)	Quiet leisure activities	X	–	O	X	–
	Laughter/humor	X	X	±	X	–
	Work–life balance	**X**	X	**X**	**X**	X
	Relaxation	–	X	–	–	X
	Meditation	O	–	–	X	X
	Exercise	–	±	X	–	X
	Vacations	–	–	X	O	–
	Help seeking	–	X	X	–	X̲
Behavioral (professional)	Continuing education	–	X	X	O	–
	Keeping up with literature	–	–	X	O	–
	Problem/active coping	±	±	±	–	–
Cognitive (personal)	Personal identity	–	X	–	X	–
	Self awareness	–	–	X	X	–
	Self-reflection/ insight	X	–	X	X	X
	Self-efficacy	X	–	–	O	–
	Mindfulness	–	X	–	–	X̲
	Positive self-talk/ attitude	X	–	X	O	–
	Positive reflection	–	–	O	X	–
	Hope/optimism	X	X	–	–	–
	Beliefs/spirituality	X	X	±	O	X̲
Cognitive (professional)	Professional identity	X	X	X	X	–
	Professional values	–	X	–	–	X̲
	Objectivity	–	–	O	X	–
	Commitment	±	O	O	X	–
	Challenge	±	X	X	–	–
	Control	X	X	X	O	–

X = support that this factor relates to resilience;

X = strong support that this factor relates to resilience;

± = contradicting findings regarding this factor's relationship to resilience;

X̲ = has been recommended;

O = not highly endorsed/lack of evidence;

– = has not been researched/mentioned

Source: McCann et al. (2013). Reprinted with permission.

TABLE 10.6   Contextual Factors That Relate to Resilience

	Factors	Nurses	Social Workers	Psychologists	Counselors	Doctors
Relational (personal)	Partner support	X	–	–	±	X
	Family support	X	X	X	±	–
	Friend support	X	X	X	0	–
	Therapy/ counseling	–	–	±	0	X
Relational (professional)	Validation/valued	X	–	–	–	X
	Colleague support	X	X	X	0	X
	Mentors/role models	X	X	X	–	–
	Client connection	–	X	X	–	X
	Client severity/ suicidality	–	X	X	–	X
	Making a difference	X	–	X	–	X
	Clinical supervision	**X**	X	X	0	–
	Peer supervision	–	X	X	±	–
Environmental	Low workload	–	**X**	–	X̲	–
	Job variety	–	X	–	–	X
	Skill match	–	X	–	–	X̲
	Private practice	–	–	**X**	X	–
	Culture	X̲	X	X̲	–	–

X = support for this factor has been found;
X = strong support that the factor relates to resilience;
± = contradicting findings regarding the factor's relationship to resilience;
X̲ = has been recommended;
0 = not highly endorsed/lack of evidence;
– = has not been researched/mentioned

Source: McCann et al. (2013). Reprinted with permission.

have been able to cultivate resilience and improve their coping strategies (Kemper, Mo, & Khayat, 2015; Wood & Bhatnagar, 2015).

Laura van Dernoot Lipsky coined the term and concept of *trauma stewardship*, introducing helping professionals to the realities of bearing witness to and walking with victims of trauma. Van Dernoot Lipsky describes 16 responses to trauma exposure to include:

1. Feelings of helplessness and hopelessness
2. A sense that one cannot do enough
3. Hypervigilence
4. Decreased creativity
5. An inability to grasp complexity
6. Minimizing reality
7. Chronic fatigue and/or physical ailments

8. An inability to listen and/or deliberate avoidance
9. Disconnected/dissociative moments
10. A sense of persecution
11. Feelings of guilt
12. Feelings of fear/fearfulness
13. Anger and cynicism
14. An inability to empathize/feeling numb
15. Addictions
16. A grandiose perception of self/an inflated sense of self importance related to one's work

As you review the trauma exposure responses, reflect on how many of these may apply to you, your colleagues, and your peers. What types of self-care strategies do you employ? Is your care self-intentional or do you retreat to a default setting that separates you from the lived experience of others? Cultivating compassion energy requires intention, presence, and a conscious choice to be regenerated by the good and noble work that you do (Dunn, 2009). Regenerative self-care is so much more than grabbing a glass of wine and plopping yourself on the sofa to watch another episode of your favorite sitcom at the end of a hard shift. The work, the environment, and the organizational climate affect you in measurable and meaningful ways; positively and/or negatively you are changed and you bring this new you to your personal and professional relationships (like a pebble in a pond). Acknowledging your vulnerability is key to recovering your compassion energy and developing effective self-care strategies.

Your professional quality of life incorporates the positive and negative aspects of your work experience and your work environment (Figure 10.3).

The vulnerability and susceptibility of NICU clinicians to the emotional distress associated with working with life-threatening situations and complex chronic conditions in a highly technological environment with a myriad of different personalities, priorities, personal agendas, and coping strategies contribute to an individual's professional quality of life (Figure 10.4).

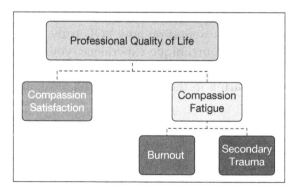

FIGURE 10.3   Diagram of professional quality of life.
Adapted from Stamm (2010). Copyright © 2010. Reprinted with permission.

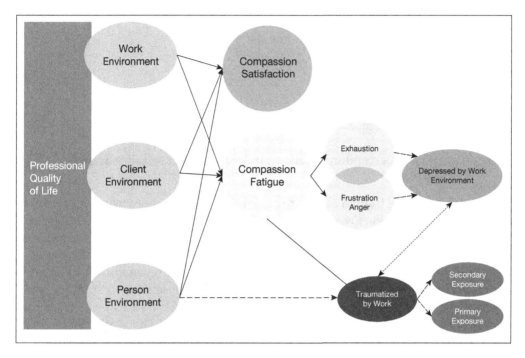

FIGURE 10.4   Theoretical path analysis.

Adapted from Stamm (2010). Copyright © 2010. Reprinted with permission.

Take a moment to complete the Professional Quality of Life (ProQOL) self-assessment that follows and then proceed to the next chapter to review evidence-based strategies to rejuvenate and reenergize your compassion energy (Figure 10.5)! To access the full ProQOL manual, visit www.proqol.org/uploads/ProQOL_Concise_2ndEd_12–2010.pdf

A word of caution on completing the ProQOL survey—do not let the results define you, but guide you. The wonderful thing about working as a health care professional is opportunity; try something new—inpatient, outpatient, home care, Starbucks barista, or ice cream parlor professional—there are many different avenues for renewal and recovery. Reflect on how YOU truly feel in the work you are pursuing and be present to your unique experience, your unique needs for rejuvenation and renewal. Cultivate your personal wholeness and return to a mind–body–spirit approach to caring in the NICU. Breathe, heal, and follow your own true path.

SECTION 8: THE ProQOL TEST AND HANDOUT
PROFESSIONAL QUALITY OF LIFE SCALE [ProQOL]

COMPASSION SATISFACTION AND COMPASSION FATIGUE
(ProQOL) VERSION 5 (2009)

When you *[help]* people you have direct contact with their lives. As you may have found, your compassion for those you *[help]* can affect you in positive and negative ways. Below are some questions about your experiences, both positive and negative, as a *[helper]*. Consider each of the following questions about you and your current work situation. Select the number that honestly reflects how frequently you experienced these things in the <u>last 30 days</u>.

| 1 = Never | 2 = Rarely | 3 = Sometimes | 4 = Often | 5 = Very Often |

1. I am happy.
2. I am preoccupied with more than one person I *[help]*.
3. I get satisfaction from being able to *[help]* people.
4. I feel connected to others.
5. I jump or am startled by unexpected sounds.
6. I feel invigorated after working with those I *[help]*.
7. I find it difficult to separate my personal life from my life as a *[helper]*.
8. I am not as productive at work because I am losing sleep over traumatic experiences of a person I *[help]*.
9. I think that I might have been affected by the traumatic stress of those I *[help]*.
10. I feel trapped by my job as a *[helper]*.
11. Because of my *[helping]*, I have felt "on edge" about various things.
12. I like my work as a *[helper]*.
13. I feel depressed because of the traumatic experiences of the people I *[help]*.
14. I feel as though I am experiencing the trauma of someone I have *[helped]*.
15. I have beliefs that sustain me.
16. I am pleased with how I am able to keep up with *[helping]* techniques and protocols.
17. I am the person I always wanted to be.
18. My work makes me feel satisfied.
19. I feel worn out because of my work as *[helper]*.
20. I have happy thoughts and feelings about those I *[help]* and how I could help them.
21. I feel overwhelmed because my case [work] load seems endless.
22. I believe I can make a difference through my work.
23. I avoid certain activities or situations because they remind me of frightening experiences of the people I *[help]*.
24. I am proud of what I can do to *[help]*.
25. As a result of my *[helping]*, I have intrusive, frightening thoughts.
26. I feel "bogged down" by the system.
27. I have thoughts that I am a "success" as a *[helper]*.
28. I can't recall important parts of my work with trauma victims.
29. I am a very caring person.
30. I am happy that I chose to do this work.

FIGURE 10.5   Professional Quality of Life (ProQOL) self-assessment.   *(continued)*

YOUR SCORES ON THE ProQOL: PROFESSIONAL QUALITY OF LIFE SCREENING

Based on your responses, place your personal scores below. If you have any concerns, you should discuss them with a physical or mental health care professional.

Compassion Satisfaction _____

Compassion satisfaction is about the pleasure you derive from being able to do your work well. For example, you may feel like it is a pleasure to help others through your work. You may feel positively about your colleagues or your ability to contribute to the work setting or even the greater good of society. Higher scores on this scale represent a greater satisfaction related to your ability to be an effective caregiver in your job.

The average score is 50 (SD 10; alpha scale reliability .88). About 25% of people score higher than 57 and about 25% of people score below 43. If you are in the higher range, you probably derive a good deal of professional satisfaction from your position. If your scores are below 40, you may either find problems with your job, or there may be some other reason—for example, you might derive your satisfaction from activities other than your job.

Burnout _____

Most people have an intuitive idea of what burnout is. From the research perspective, burnout is one of the elements of compassion fatigue (CF). It is associated with feelings of hopelessness and difficulties in dealing with work or in doing your job effectively. These negative feelings usually have a gradual onset. They can reflect the feeling that your efforts make no difference, or they can be associated with a very high workload or a non-supportive work environment. Higher scores on this scale mean that you are at higher risk for burnout.

The average score on the burnout scale is 50 (SD 10, alpha scale reliability .75). About 25% of people score above 57 and about 25% of people score below 43. If your score is below 18, this probably reflects positive feelings about your ability to be effective in your work. If you score above 57 you may wish to think about what at work makes you feel like you are not effective in your position. Your score may reflect your mood; perhaps you were having a "bad day" or are in need of some time off. If the high score persists or if it is reflective of other worries, it may be a cause for concern.

Secondary Traumatic Stress _____

The second component of compassion fatigue (CF) is secondary traumatic stress (STS). It is about your work related, secondary exposure to extremely or traumatically stressful events. Developing problems due to exposure to others' trauma is somewhat rare but does happen to many people who care for those who have experienced extremely or traumatically stressful events. For example, you may repeatedly hear stories about the traumatic things that happen to other people, commonly called vicarious traumatization. If your work puts you directly in the path of danger, for example, field work in a war or area of civil violence, this is not secondary exposure; your exposure is primary. However, if you are exposed to others' traumatic events as a result of your work, for example, as a therapist or an emergency worker, this is secondary exposure. The symptoms of STS are usually rapid in onset and associated with a particular event. They may include being afraid, having difficulty sleeping, having images of the upsetting event pop into your mind, or avoiding things that remind you of the event.

The average score on this scale is 50 (SD 10; alpha scale reliability .81). About 25% of people score below 43 and about 25% of people score above 57. If your score is above 57, you may want to take some time to think about what at work may be frightening to you or if there is some other reason for the elevated score. While higher scores do not mean that you do have a problem, they are an indication that you may want to examine how you feel about your work and your work environment. You may wish to discuss this with your supervisor, a colleague, or a health care professional.

FIGURE 10.5   *(continued)*

WHAT IS MY SCORE AND WHAT DOES IT MEAN?

In this section, you will score your test and then you can compare your score to the interpretation below.

To find your score on **each section**, total the questions listed on the left in each section and then find your score in the table on the right of the section.

Compassion Satisfaction Scale:

3. _____
6. _____
12. _____
16. _____
18. _____
20. _____
22. _____
24. _____
27. _____
30. _____
Total: _____

The Sum of My Compassion Satisfaction Questions	So My Score Equals	My Level of Compassion
22 or less	43 or less	Low
Between 23 and 41	Around 50	Average
42 or more	57 or more	High

Burnout Scale:

*1. _____ = _____
*4. _____ = _____
8. _____
10. _____
*15. _____ = _____
*17. _____ = _____
19. _____
21. _____
26. _____
*29. _____ = _____
Reverse the scores for those that are starred.
0=0, 1=5, 2=4, 3=3, 4=2, 5= 1
Total: _____

The Sum of My Burnout Questions	So My Score Equals	My Level of Burnout
22 or less	43 or less	Low
Between 23 and 41	Around 50	Average
42 or more	57 or more	High

Secondary Trauma Scale:

2. _____
5. _____
7. _____
9. _____
11. _____
13. _____
14. _____
23. _____
25. _____
28. _____
Total: _____

The Sum of My Secondary Traumatic Stress Questions	So My Score Equals	My Level of Secondary Traumatic Stress
22 or less	43 or less	Low
Between 23 and 41	Around 50	Average
42 or more	57 or more	High

FIGURE 10.5 *(continued)*

REFERENCES

Aiken, L. H., Sermeus, W., Van den Heede, K., Sloane, D. M., Busse, R., McKee, M., ... Kutney-Lee, A. (2012). Patient safety, satisfaction, and quality of hospital care: cross-sectional surveys of nurses and patients in 12 countries in Europe and the United States. *British Medical Journal (Clinical Research ed.), 344,* e1717.

Ariza-Montes, A., Muniz, N. M., Montero-Simó, M. J., & Araque-Padilla, R. A. (2013). Workplace bullying among healthcare workers. *International Journal of Environmental Research and Public Health, 10*(8), 3121–3139.

Ball, J. E., Murrells, T., Rafferty, A. M., Morrow, E., & Griffiths, P. (2014). "Care left undone" during nursing shifts: Associations with workload and perceived quality of care. *British Medical Journal Quality & Safety, 23*(2), 116–125.

Bellieni, C. V., Righetti, P., Ciampa, R., Iacoponi, F., Coviello, C., & Buonocore, G. (2012). Assessing burnout among neonatologists. *The Journal of Maternal-Fetal & Neonatal Medicine: The Official Journal of the European Association of Perinatal Medicine, the Federation of Asia and Oceania Perinatal Societies, the International Society of Perinatal Obstetricians, 25*(10), 2130–2134.

Bradley, V., Liddle, S., Shaw, R., Savage, E., Rabbitts, R., Trim, C., ... Whitelaw, B. C. (2015). Sticks and stones: Investigating rude, dismissive and aggressive communication between doctors. *Clinical Medicine (London, England), 15*(6), 541–545.

Braithwaite, M. (2008). Nurse burnout and stress in the NICU. *Advances in Neonatal Care: Official Journal of the National Association of Neonatal Nurses, 8*(6), 343–347.

Bronkhorst, B., Tummers, L., Steijn, B., & Vijverberg, D. (2015). Organizational climate and employee mental health outcomes: A systematic review of studies in health care organizations. *Health Care Management Review, 40*(3), 254–271.

Carter, M. A. (2009). Trust, power, and vulnerability: A discourse on helping in nursing. *Nursing Clinics of North America, 44,* 393–405.

Cavaliere, T. A., Daly, B., Dowling, D., & Montgomery, K. (2010). Moral distress in neonatal intensive care unit RNs. *Advances in Neonatal Care: Official Journal of the National Association of Neonatal Nurses, 10*(3), 145–156.

Cavinder, C. (2014). The relationship between providing neonatal palliative care and nurses' moral distress: An integrative review. *Advances in Neonatal Care: Official Journal of the National Association of Neonatal Nurses, 14*(5), 322–328.

Coughlin, M. (2014). *Transformative nursing in the NICU: Trauma-informed, age-appropriate care.* New York, NY: Springer Publishing.

Coughlin, M., Gibbins, S., & Hoath, S. (2009). Core measures for developmentally supportive care in neonatal intensive care units: Theory, precedence and practice. *Journal of Advanced Nursing, 65*(10), 2239–2248.

Darbyshire, J. L., & Young, J. D. (2013). An investigation of sound levels on intensive care units with reference to the WHO guidelines. *Critical Care, 17*(5), R187.

Dill, D., & Gumpert, P. (2012). What is the heart of healthcare? Advocating for and defining the clinical relationship in patient-centered care. *Journal of Participatory Medicine, 4,* e10. Retrieved from http://www.jopm.org/evidence/reviews/2012/04/25/what-is-the -heart-of-health-care-advocating-for-and-defining-the-clinical-relationship-in-patient -centered-care

Dunn, D. J. (2009). The intentionality of compassion energy. *Holistic Nursing Practice, 23*(4), 222–229.

Egener, B., McDonald, W., Rosof, B., & Gullen, D. (2012). Perspective: Organizational professionalism: Relevant competencies and behaviors. *Academic Medicine: Journal of the Association of American Medical Colleges, 87*(5), 668–674.

Einarsdóttir, J. (2012). Happiness in the neonatal intensive care unit: Merits of ethnographic fieldwork. *International Journal of Qualitative Studies on Health and Well-Being, 7*, 1–9.

Goudarzi, Z., Rahimi, O., Khalessi, N., Soleimani, F., Mohammadi, N., & Shamshiri, A. (2015). The rate of developmental care delivery in neonatal intensive care unit. *Iranian Journal of Critical Care Nursing, 8*(2), 117–124.

Hall, S. L., Cross, J., Selix, N. W., Patterson, C., Segre, L., Chuffo-Siewert, R., . . . Martin, M. L. (2015). Recommendations for enhancing psychosocial support of NICU parents through staff education and support. *Journal of Perinatology: Official Journal of the California Perinatal Association, 35*(Suppl. 1), S29–S36.

Hall, E. O., Kronborg, H., Aagaard, H., & Ammentorp, J. (2010). Walking the line between the possible and the ideal: Lived experiences of neonatal nurses. *Intensive & Critical Care Nursing: The Official Journal of the British Association of Critical Care Nurses, 26*(6), 307–313.

Hamric, A. B., & Blackhall, L. J. (2007). Nurse-physician perspectives on the care of dying patients in intensive care units: Collaboration, moral distress, and ethical climate. *Critical Care Medicine, 35*(2), 422–429.

Hendricks-Muñoz, K. D., Louie, M., Li, Y., Chhun, N., Prendergast, C. C., & Ankola, P. (2010). Factors that influence neonatal nursing perceptions of family-centered care and developmental care practices. *American Journal of Perinatology, 27*(3), 193–200.

Hogan, B. K. (2013). Carrying is a scripted discourse versus caring as an expression of an authentic relationship between self and other. *Issues in Mental Health Nursing, 34*, 375–379.

Hutchinson, M., Jackson, D., Wilkes, L., & Vickers, M. H. (2008). A new model of bullying in the nursing workplace: Organizational characteristics as critical antecedents. *Advances in Nursing Science, 31*(2), E60–E71.

Jasmine, T. (2009). Art, science, or both? Keeping the care in nursing. *The Nursing Clinics of North America, 44*(4), 415–421.

Johnson, S. L. (2009). International perspectives on workplace bullying among nurses: A review. *International Nursing Review, 56*(1), 34–40.

Jones, T., Hamilton, P., Carryer, J., Sportsman, S., & Gemeinhardt, G. (2014). International network for the study of rationalized nursing care—An overview, 2nd Annual Worldwide Nursing Conference, Singapore, June 24, 2014. doi:10.5176/2315-4330_WNC14.92

Jones, T. L., Hamilton, P., & Murry, N. (2015). Unfinished nursing care, missed care, and implicitly rationed care: State of the science review. *International Journal of Nursing Studies, 52*(6), 1121–1137.

Kain, V. J. (2007). Moral distress and providing care to dying babies in neonatal nursing. *International Journal of Palliative Nursing, 13*(5), 243–248.

Kalisch, B. J., Landstrom, G. L., & Hinshaw, A. S. (2009). Missed nursing care: A concept analysis. *Journal of Advanced Nursing, 65*(7), 1509–1517.

Kalisch, B. J., Tschannen, D., Lee, H., & Friese, C. R. (2011). Hospital variation in Mystic nursing care. *American Journal of Medical Quality, 26*(4), 291–299.

Kelly, L. A., McHugh, M. D., & Aiken, L. H. (2011). Nurse outcomes in Magnet® and non-Magnet hospitals. *The Journal of Nursing Administration, 41*(10), 428–433.

Kemper, K. J., Mo, X., & Khayat, R. (2015). Are mindfulness and self-compassion associated with sleep and resilience in health professionals? *Journal of Alternative and Complementary Medicine, 21*(8), 496–503.

Konkani, A., & Oakley, B. (2012). Noise in hospital intensive care units—A critical review of a critical topic. *Journal of Critical Care, 27*(5), 522.e1–522.e9.

Korhonen, A., Haho, A., & Pölkki, T. (2013). Nurses' perspectives on the suffering of preterm infants. *Nursing Ethics, 20*(7), 798–807.

Krueger, C., Schue, S., & Parker, L. (2007). Neonatal intensive care unit sound levels before and after structural reconstruction. *MCN. The American Journal of Maternal Child Nursing, 32*(6), 358–362.

Lake, E. T. (2002). Development of the practice environment scale of the Nursing Work Index. *Research in Nursing & Health, 25*(3), 176–188.

Lake, E. T., Staiger, D., Horbar, J., Cheung, R., Kenny, M. J., Patrick, T., & Rogowski, J. A. (2012). Association between hospital recognition for nursing excellence and outcomes of very low-birth-weight infants. *Journal of the American Medical Association, 307*(16), 1709–1716.

LaSala, C. A. (2009). Moral accountability and integrity in nursing. *Nursing Clinics of North America, 44*(4), 423–434.

Maslach, C., & Jackson, S. (1981). The measurement of experienced burnout. *Journal of Organizational Behavior, 2*(2), 99–113.

McCann, C. M., Beddoe, E., McCormick, K., Huggard, P., Kedge, S., Adamson, C., & Huggard, J. (2013). Resilience in the health professions: A review of recent literature. *International Journal of Wellbeing, 3*(1), 60–81.

McDonald, K., Rubarth, L. B., & Miers, L. J. (2012). Job satisfaction of neonatal intensive care nurses. *Advances in Neonatal Care: Official Journal of the National Association of Neonatal Nurses, 12*(4), E1–E8.

Meadors, P., Lamson, A., Swanson, M., White, M., & Sira, N. (2009). Secondary traumatization in pediatric healthcare providers: Compassion fatigue, burnout, and secondary traumatic stress. *Omega, 60*(2), 103–128.

Mealer, M., Jones, J., Newman, J., McFann, K. K., Rothbaum, B., & Moss, M. (2012). The presence of resilience is associated with a healthier psychological profile in intensive care unit (ICU) nurses: Results of a national survey. *International Journal of Nursing Studies, 49*(3), 292–299.

Mukherjee, D., Brashler, R., Savage, T. A., & Kirschner, K. L. (2009). Moral distress in rehabilitation professionals: Results from a hospital ethics survey. *PM & R: The Journal of Injury, Function, and Rehabilitation, 1*(5), 450–458.

Naef, R. (2006). Bearing witness: A moral way of engaging in the nurse–person relationship. *Nursing Philosophy: An International Journal for Healthcare Professionals, 7*(3), 146–156.

Papastavrou, E., Andreou, P., & Efstathiou, G. (2014). Rationing of nursing care and nurse-patient outcomes: A systematic review of quantitative studies. *The International Journal of Health Planning and Management, 29*(1), 3–25.

Papastavrou, E., Andreou, P., Tsangari, H., & Merkouris, A. (2014). Linking patient satisfaction with nursing care: The case of care rationing—A correlational study. *BMC Nursing, 13*, 26. Retrieved from http://bmcnurs.biomedcentral.com/articles/10.1186/1472-6955-13-26

Profit, J., Sharek, P. J., Amspoker, A. B., Kowalkowski, M. A., Nisbet, C. C., Thomas, E. J.,… Sexton, J. B. (2014). Burnout in the NICU setting and its relation to safety culture. *British Medical Journal Quality & Safety, 23*(10), 806–813.

Rees, C. S., Breen, L. J., Cusack, L., & Hegney, D. (2015). Understanding individual resilience in the workplace: The international collaboration of workforce resilience model. *Frontiers in Psychology, 6*, 73.

Remen, N. R. (1996). *Kitchen table wisdom: Stories that heal.* New York, NY: Riverhead Books.

Riskin, A., Erez, A., Foulk, T. A., Kugelman, A., Gover, A., Shoris, I.,… Bamberger, P. A. (2015). The impact of rudeness on medical team performance: A randomized trial. *Pediatrics, 136*(3), 487–495.

Rochefort, C. M., & Clarke, S. P. (2010). Nurses' work environments, care rationing, job outcomes, and quality of care on neonatal units. *Journal of Advanced Nursing, 66*(10), 2213–2224.

Rushton, C. H., Batcheller, J., Schroeder, K., & Donohue, P. (2015). Burnout and resilience among nurses practicing in high-intensity settings. *American Journal of Critical Care: An Official Publication, American Association of Critical-Care Nurses, 24*(5), 412–420.

Sakallaris, B. R., MacAllister, L., Voss, M., Smith, K., & Jonas, W. B. (2015). Optimal healing environments. *Global Advances in Health and Medicine: Improving Healthcare Outcomes Worldwide, 4*(3), 40–45.

Sannino, P., Giannì, M. L., Re, L. G., & Lusignani, M. (2015). Moral distress in the neonatal intensive care unit: An Italian study. *Journal of Perinatology: Official Journal of the California Perinatal Association, 35*(3), 214–217.

Sexton, J. B., Sharek, P. J., Thomas, E. J., Gould, J. B., Nisbet, C. C., Amspoker, A. B.,… Profit, J. (2014). Exposure to leadership walk rounds in neonatal intensive care units is associated with better patient safety culture and less caregiver burnout. *British Medical Journal Quality & Safety, 23*(10), 814–822.

Simons, K. S., Park, M., Kohlrausch, A., van den Boogaard, M., Pickkers, P., de Bruijn, W., & de Jager, C. P. (2014). Noise pollution in the ICU: Time to look into the mirror. *Critical Care, 18*(4), 493.

Stamm, B. H. (2010). *The concise ProQOL manual* (2nd ed.). Pocatello, ID: ProQOL.org.

Strech, D., Persad, G., Marckmann, G., & Danis, M. (2009). Are physicians willing to ration health care? Conflicting findings in a systematic review of survey research. *Health Policy, 90*(2–3), 113–124.

Stone, P. W., Hughes, R., & Dailey, M. (2008). Creating a safe and high-quality healthcare environment. In R. G. Hughes (Ed.), *Patient safety and quality: An evidence-based handbook for nurses* (pp. 57–71). Rockville, MD: Agency for Healthcare Research and Quality.

Thomas, K. A., & Martin, P. A. (2000). NICU sound environment and the potential problems for caregivers. *Journal of Perinatology: Official Journal of the California Perinatal Association, 20*(8 Pt. 2), S94–S99.

Tubbs-Cooley, H. L., Pickler, R. H., Younger, J. B., & Mark, B. A. (2015). A descriptive study of nurse-reported missed care in neonatal intensive care units. *Journal of Advanced Nursing, 71*(4), 813–824.

Trepanier, S.-G., Fernet, C., Austin, S., & Boudrias, V. (2016). Work environment antecedents of bullying: A review and integrative model applied to registered nurses. *International Journal of Nursing Studies, 55,* 85–97.

Turner, M., Chur-Hansen, A., & Winefield, H. (2014). The neonatal nurses' view of their role in emotional support of parents and its complexities. *Journal of Clinical Nursing, 23*(21–22), 3156–3165.

Valizadeh, L., Asadollahi, M., Mostafa Gharebaghi, M., & Gholami, F. (2013). The congruence of nurses' performance with developmental care standards in neonatal intensive care units. *Journal of Caring Sciences, 2*(1), 61–71.

Van Dernoot Lipsky, L., & Burk, C. (2009). *Trauma stewardship: An everyday guide to caring for self while caring for others.* San Francisco, CA: Barrett-Koehler Publishers.

van Mol, M. M., Kompanje, E. J., Benoit, D. D., Bakker, J., & Nijkamp, M. D. (2015). The prevalence of compassion fatigue and burnout among healthcare professionals in intensive care units: A systematic review. *PloS One, 10*(8), e0136955.

Vessey, J. A., Demarco, R. F., Gaffney, D. A., & Budin, W. C. (2009). Bullying of staff registered nurses in the workplace: A preliminary study for developing personal and organizational strategies for the transformation of hostile to healthy workplace environments. *Journal of Professional Nursing: Official Journal of the American Association of Colleges of Nursing, 25*(5), 299–306.

Watson, J. (2003). Love and caring. Ethics of face and hand—An invitation to return to the heart and soul of nursing and our deep humanity. *Nursing Administration Quarterly, 27*(3), 197–202.

Whitehead, P. B., Herbertson, R. K., Hamric, A. B., Epstein, E. G., & Fisher, J. M. (2015). Moral distress among healthcare professionals: Report of an institution-wide survey. *Journal of Nursing Scholarship: An Official Publication of Sigma Theta Tau International Honor Society of Nursing/Sigma Theta Tau, 47*(2), 117–125.

Wood, S. K., & Bhatnagar, S. (2015). Resilience to the effects of social stress: Evidence from clinical and preclinical studies on the role of coping strategies. *Neurobiology of Stress, 1,* 164–173.

CHAPTER 11

Self-Care Guidelines for the Neonatal Clinician

When you recover or discover something that nourishes your soul and brings joy, care enough about yourself to make room for it in your life.
      —Jean Shinoda Bolen

This guideline presents the latest evidence-based research, along with clinical practice recommendations and implementation strategies, related to self-care for the professional in the neonatal intensive care unit (NICU); self-care actions and behaviors apply to both the personal and the professional domains.

■ GUIDELINE OBJECTIVES

- To define the concept of self-care
- To present the evidence that supports this definition
- To present evidence-based recommendations

■ MAJOR OUTCOMES CONSIDERED

The impact of the self-care practices on the NICU patient, family, and staff includes:

- Physiologic, psychosocial, and psychoemotional outcomes
- Patient safety and quality clinical outcomes

Interventions and Practice Considerations

- Create and maintain an optimal healing environment (OHE) that supports healing intention, healing relationships, healthy lifestyles, and healing spaces
  - Best practice considerations include cultivating and supporting professional autonomy, acknowledging transdisciplinary excellence, and ensuring a work environment designed to minimize auditory overstimulation and reflect a healing intention.
- Create and maintain self-care routines encompassing home and work strategies that protect and preserve compassion energy, health, and well-being

- Best practice considerations include optimizing sleep patterns/routines, limit working more than three 12-hour shifts consecutively with a minimum of 2 rest days in between, optimize diet and exercise rituals, and cultivate self-compassion

The Evidence

Self-care practices are those self-initiated routines and rituals aimed at restoring and rebalancing one's self off-duty and on-duty. On-duty self-care practices include developing professional autonomy, acknowledging colleagues, collaborating with the interprofessional team, and making sure you take your coffee and meal breaks. OHEs in the NICU "make healing as important as curing" and support professional self-care practices across internal, interpersonal, behavioral, and external domains (Figure 11.1).

Autonomy, collaboration, and teamwork are core competencies for high-reliability organizations and high-performance work environments that result in improved communication, job satisfaction, heightened situational awareness, job fulfillment, retention, care quality, and patient safety (Brodsky et al., 2013; Weinberg, Avgar, Sugrue, & Cooney-Miner, 2013). Building high-reliability teams is a continuous journey and cultural intervention that hinges on leadership support and employee engagement across the organization driven by success metrics for quality, safety, and professional satisfaction (Salas & Rosen, 2013).

Programs that recognize nursing excellence, such as the Magnet® designation, have a powerful influence on the quality of care delivered; patient safety; and staff satisfaction, retention, and recruitment, but this nurse-focused honor does not happen in a vacuum, it takes a village—the multidisciplinary team—to achieve excellence across the board and gain compassion energy and professional fulfillment (Smith, 2006). The Daisy Award, a recognition program created to celebrate

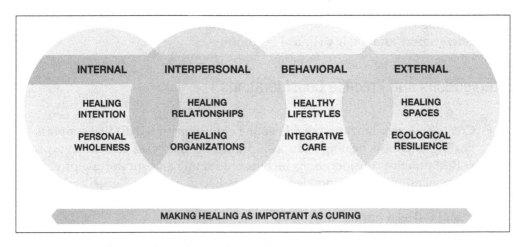

FIGURE 11.1 Optimal healing environment framework.

Reprinted with Permission from Samueli Institute.

"the super-human work nurses do" (daisyfoundation.org/daisy-award), inspires, enhances morale, and develops nursing role models.

Leadership qualities are strongly correlated with burnout and satisfaction scores (Shanafelt et al., 2015). The concept of servant leadership is a unique way of managing professionals that employs respect and honesty to empower and inspire. Operationalizing this concept through authentic praise enhances staff satisfaction and empowers bedside clinicians to adopt professional self-care strategies (Sveinsdottir, Ragnarsdottir, & Blondal, 2016). Environments that support and promote autonomy report decreased staff turnover, improved satisfaction, and enhanced quality of care and patient safety outcomes (Mark, Lindley, & Jones, 2009; Mrayyan, 2004). Recognizing excellence does not need to be a formal program per se, but the recognition should be a formalized, transdisciplinary process that validates and honors the work of the interprofessional team.

Self-care strategies in the work environment include responsible volume control over professional and personal conversations in the care area as well as promptly responding to infant cries and infant device alarms. Behavioral modifications to reduce sound levels in the NICU are effective when there is a shared sense of urgency, ownership for outcomes, a process for the continuous measurement of performance indicators, and a perceived benefit (Swathi et al., 2014). Attention to aesthetics and employing evidence-based design principles for hospital environments increases Press Ganey parent satisfaction surveys and decreases hospital staff turnover rates while improving staff satisfaction (Ferri, Zygun, Harrison, & Stelfox, 2015; Kotzer, Zacharakis, Raynolds, & Buenning, 2011).

Personal self-care strategies encompass sleep, diet, and exercise, as well as self-compassion interventions (e.g., yoga, mindfulness meditation). Sleep duration, continuity, timing, alertness versus sleepiness, and satisfaction and/or quality represent the five dimensions most relevant to define and measure sleep health, which is inescapably influenced by genetic, epigenetic, molecular, and physiologic processes (e.g., inflammatory, hormonal-, and hypothalamic–pituitary–adrenal [HPA]-mediated activity) that mediate health, disease, and function (Buysse, 2014). For health care professionals, sleep and fatigue play a critical role in clinical performance, safety, vulnerability to psychological distress and burnout as well as increasing susceptibility to altered health outcomes (i.e., hypertension, coronary heart disease, metabolic syndrome, obesity, motor vehicle accidents; Barker & Nussbaum, 2011; Buysse, 2014; Smith-Miller, Shaw-Kokot, Curro, & Jones, 2014). In light of the expansive evidence linking fatigue with compromised quality and safety in patient care delivery, the National Association of Neonatal Nurses (NANN) recommends nurses not work more than 12 hours per day or 48 hours per week, take a minimum of 20 minute meal or rest breaks when working for 6 hours or more, take a minimum of 10- to 15-minute breaks every 4 hours, limit the number of consecutive 12-hour shifts to three per week, and consider having a minimum of 2 rest days in between shifts worked (Samra & Smith, 2015). The accumulated sleep debt that builds as a result of shift work places the worker at risk for fatigue and sleepiness and can be reduced when at least 24 hours are scheduled off after each shift worked (Fischer et al., 2016). Rotating night shifts compared with permanent night duty was associated with more adverse psychological and physiological effects, with shifts longer than 12 hours associated with lower quality and safety as well as an increase in missed care (Griffiths et al., 2014; Muecke, 2005).

The challenges in keeping staff safe and well rested contrasted with the realities of staffing the NICU require creative collaboration that respects the individual professionals' need for healthy sleep.

Nurses working the night shift (permanent or rotating) have demonstrated increases in body mass index (BMI), obesity, and an increased risk for type 2 diabetes, metabolic syndrome, and ischemic heart disease (Griep et al., 2014; Pan et al., 2011; Peplonska et al., 2014; Peplonska, Bukowska, & Sobala, 2015; Szosland, 2010). Motivation plays a key role in an individual's diet and exercise routines and requires a sense of self-determination and commitment to fully realize the associated health benefits (Teixeira, Carraça, Markland, Silva, & Ryan, 2012). Self-care, intentionally identifying and incorporating health-promoting behaviors into one's daily routine, is significantly lacking among health care professionals despite the fact that this same group routinely prescribes self-care for others (Bickley, 1998; Sanchez-Reilly et al., 2013; Wells-Federman, 1996). Mindfulness, which develops self-awareness and influences self-regulation, has proven to be an effective intervention for general stress reduction (Vago & Silbersweig, 2012). Self-compassion—comprised of self-kindness, an acknowledgment of our shared humanity, and mindfulness—is associated with promoting positive health behaviors (Sirois, 2015). Self-compassion and mindfulness are both skills that can be learned (Germer & Neff, 2013). In a randomized controlled trial of the Mindful Self-Compassion (MSC) program, participants in the intervention group reported a significant increase in self-compassion, mindfulness, and well-being that was maintained up through the first-year postprogram (Neff & Germer, 2013). Resilience training through a mindfulness-based program, which integrated elements of nutrition and exercise along with mindfulness meditation, statistically significantly reduced depression, stress, and trait anxiety as well as increased staff productivity yielding a significant return on investment for the facility (Johnson, Emmons, Rivard, Griffin, & Dusek, 2015). Mindfulness-Based Stress Reduction (MBSR) programs have been implemented and evaluated since 1979 and have consistently yielded positive results for health care professionals suggesting that this intervention is a viable tool in promoting self-care and well-being (Raab, 2014).

Alternative strategies to restore work–life balance include self-help resources recommending individuals manage their time, learn to say no, leave work at work, minimize interruptions, and shorten commitments. These strategies may be difficult to implement as a first-pass solution and some colleagues turn to professional coaching as a way to navigate back from burnout. Gazelle et al. (2015) describe the effectiveness of a coaching intervention using the "wheel of life" exercise (e.g., www.mindtools.com/pages/article/newHTE_93.htm) to help the client identify work–life imbalances and develop creative and individualized meaningful strategies to regain balance and reduce emotional distress. Recognizing your vulnerability and consciously choosing to care for yourself is a critical first step in cultivating self-kindness, reestablishing work–life balance, and regaining your sense of joy and self-fulfillment in doing the good work of neonatal intensive care.

Cost Analysis

The cost–benefits associated with adopting professional and personal self-care strategies include excellence in patient care delivery defined as a decrease in missed care and other errors of both omission and commission; improved staff recruitment and retention; and a healthier health care team resulting in fewer health care dollars spent treating modifiable lifestyle-associated diseases.

Recommendations for Best Practices in Self-Care (Table 11.1)

TABLE 11.1   Major Self-Care Recommendations and Implementation—Strategies

Recommendations	Implementation Strategy
1. Build a collaborative interprofessional team–based model of care	a. Collect baseline information about current staff attitudes and perceptions of teamwork in your facility b. Establish a multidisciplinary committee to lead the initiative c. Identify opportunities for improvement based on staff feedback/survey responses; draft a vision of what this new model will look like in practice d. Create competency-based education to introduce evidence about teamwork and effective teamwork skills/behaviors/attitudes e. Introduce the new model using PDSA methodology, review, revise, and then adopt f. Resurvey staff following implementation of the new team-based model g. Trend impact of the model across key performance indicators (nosocomial infections, parent/staff satisfaction, communication challenges, etc.) h. Publish and/or present outcomes

2. Establish an excellence recognition program	a. Do you currently have some type of recognition program in your unit/hospital?
	  i. How is it perceived?
	  ii. Is it for all disciplines?
	  iii. Is it effective?
	  iv. What does it recognize (how is excellence defined)?
	  v. Who identifies the recipients of excellence?
	    – Informal praise from manager/colleague?
	    – Formal process based on specific criteria?
	  vi. Identify markers of excellence
	  vii. Identify barriers to recognizing excellence
	    – Identify what is meaningful recognition
	b. Do not be afraid to be creative
	c. Using a PDSA approach, draft a test of change for a recognition program (formal or informal)
	d. Identify performance and/or behavior metrics that you feel may be impacted and collect benchmark data points
	e. Test your idea, evaluate, refine, implement
	f. Monitor and measure the impact of this strategy on staff satisfaction, performance, and so forth
	  i. If it does not make a difference, reevaluate
	  ii. For the recognition to have meaning, it must be authentic

(continued)

TABLE 11.1   Major Self-Care Recommendations and Implementation—Strategies   (*continued*)

Recommendations	Implementation Strategy
3. Align leadership competencies with organizational objectives (i.e., high-performance organization)	a. Examine how individuals advance to leadership positions b. Does your organization identify leadership competencies that are tied to organizational priorities? c. Is there a process for talent management and succession planning that retains individuals with leadership potential? d. Is there a clinical and leadership ladder? e. If your organization does not adopt best practices in leadership development and talent management, consider exploring this opportunity—*Transformational Leadership and Evidence-Based Management, in Keeping Patients Safe: Transforming the Work Environment of Nurses* (retrieved from www.ncbi.nlm.nih.gov/books/NBK216194) f. This recommendation requires organizational commitment for transformation

4. Empower staff to create an optimal healing environment	a. Identify and prioritize opportunities to align with the OHE framework in the workplace using a PDSA approach to change (refer Chapter 5)
	b. Internal environment—personal
	  i. Evaluate how individuals are oriented to your unit, what are the performance expectations around healing intention and personal wholeness?
	  ii. Is the work about checking off boxes and completing tasks, or is healing as important as curing?
	  iii. How are staff accountable to personal wholeness (mind-body-spirit)?
	c. Interpersonal environment—relationships
	  i. Do you have a collaborative interprofessional team–based model of care or is it predominantly hierarchical?
	  ii. Are there issues with bullying? Is there a process in place to address disruptive behavior in the work place? (See the Resources section for The Joint Commission [TJC] sentinel event alert with suggested actions.)
	    – TJC Leadership Standards:
	      • EP 4: The hospital/organization has a code of conduct that defines acceptable and disruptive and inappropriate behaviors
	      • EP 5: Leaders create and implement a process for managing disruptive and inappropriate behaviors
	d. Behavioral environment—lifestyles
	  i. Does your organization provide resources to support a healthy lifestyle (gym access or memberships; nutrition counseling—nutritious healthy options in hospital; mindfulness-based training programs; other types of programs and resources to support staff health)?
	e. External environment—healing spaces
	  i. Are there enough chairs for staff at each bedside?
	  ii. Is the lighting balanced and adjustable to meet patient and staff needs within the recommended range?
	  iii. How are noise levels monitored, managed, and maintained within the recommended range?
	  iv. Is there a quiet, dedicated, aesthetically appealing space for staff to refresh and refuel during break periods?

(*continued*)

TABLE 11.1   Major Self-Care Recommendations and Implementation—Strategies   *(continued)*

Recommendations	Implementation Strategy
5. Keep a sleep diary and identify opportunities to improve your sleep health	a. Do you get "enough" sleep? i. Complete the sleep quality assessment at http://www.opapc.com/uploads/documents/PSQI.pdf b. Consider keeping a sleep diary (see the Resources section) to identify opportunities to improve your sleep quality (see Figure 11.2) c. How does your current work schedule impact your sleep health? d. Identify opportunities to improve your work schedule to improve your sleep health

6. Adopt NANN staffing recommendations to minimize shift-related fatigue	a. Does your unit adopt the NANN staffing recommendations to reduce shift-related fatigue?
	b. Identify a multidisciplinary team to review current staff scheduling patterns
	c. Are there opportunities for improvement?
	   i. Overtime limits
	   ii. Doubling back shifts
	   iii. The use of float staff or travel staff to alleviate staff shortages
	d. Select an improvement opportunity, test, revise, implement
	e. Make sure to identify metrics for success, benchmark and quantify interval improvement
	f. Publish and/or present your results

7. Develop a personal self-care strategy that is realistic, achievable, and meaningful	a. How do you care for yourself?
	   i. Complete the self-care assessment in the Resources section (see Table 11.2)
	   ii. Complete the work–life balance quiz (see Table 11.3)
	b. Based on your results, identify opportunities for self-care
	c. Ask yourself how would you like your life to be, what would balance and self-care look like?
	d. What is important to you?
	e. Who is in your support network, how can they help you?
	f. What is your biggest obstacle?
	g. Commit to resolving it—outline baby steps and a timeline to resolve it, check in on your progress daily!
	h. List one thing you will do differently tomorrow
	i. List two things you will do differently the day after that
	j. "Be the change you want to see"—Mahatma Gandhi

NANN, National Association of Neonatal Nurses; PDSA, Plan-Do-Study-Act.

Resources

- *The Joint Commission Sentinel Event Alert: Behaviors That Undermine a Culture of Safety*: www.jointcommission.org/assets/1/18/sea_40.pdf
- *Dietary Guidelines for Americans 2015–2020*: www.choosemyplate.gov
- *Mindfulness-Based Stress Reduction Activities Workbook*: tulane.edu/health/wellness/upload/MBSR-Workbook.pdf

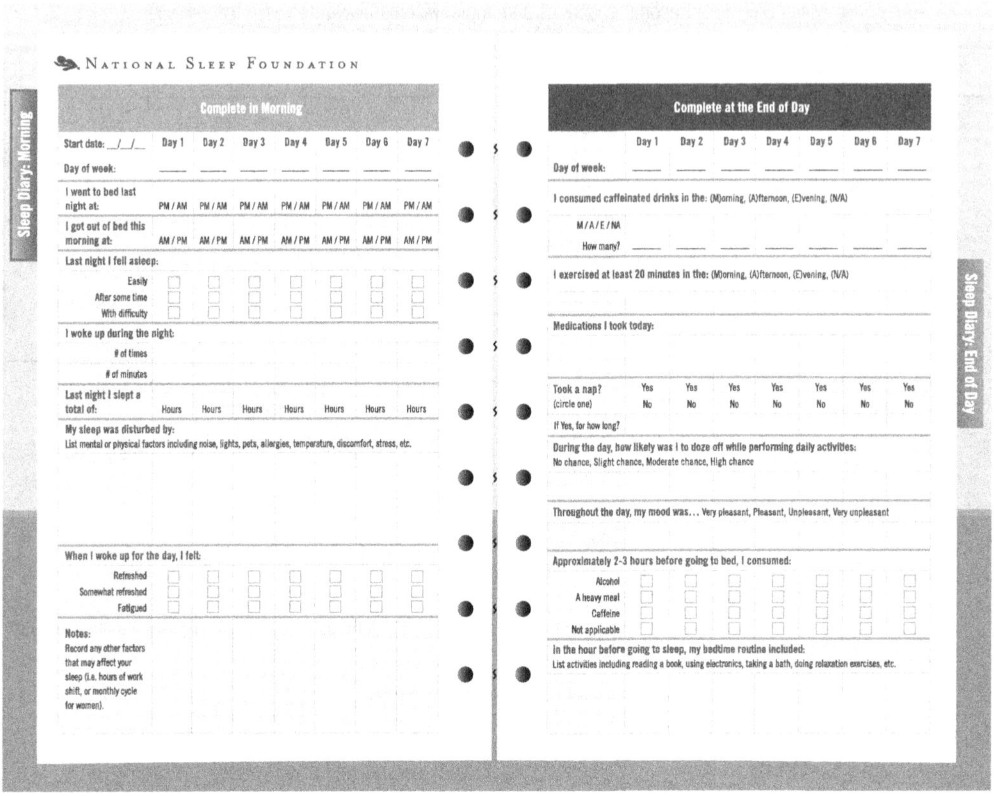

NATIONAL SLEEP FOUNDATION

Sleep Diary: Morning

Complete in Morning

Start date: __/__/__	Day 1	Day 2	Day 3	Day 4	Day 5	Day 6	Day 7
Day of week:	___	___	___	___	___	___	___
I went to bed last night at:	PM / AM	PM / AM	PM / AM	PM / AM	PM / AM	PM / AM	PM / AM
I got out of bed this morning at:	AM / PM	AM / PM	AM / PM	AM / PM	AM / PM	AM / PM	AM / PM
Last night I fell asleep:							
Easily	☐	☐	☐	☐	☐	☐	☐
After some time	☐	☐	☐	☐	☐	☐	☐
With difficulty	☐	☐	☐	☐	☐	☐	☐
I woke up during the night:							
# of times							
# of minutes							
Last night I slept a total of:	Hours	Hours	Hours	Hours	Hours	Hours	Hours
My sleep was disturbed by: List mental or physical factors including noise, lights, pets, allergies, temperature, discomfort, stress, etc.							
When I woke up for the day, I felt:							
Refreshed	☐	☐	☐	☐	☐	☐	☐
Somewhat refreshed	☐	☐	☐	☐	☐	☐	☐
Fatigued	☐	☐	☐	☐	☐	☐	☐
Notes: Record any other factors that may affect your sleep (i.e. hours of work shift, or monthly cycle for women).							

Complete at the End of Day

Sleep Diary: End of Day

	Day 1	Day 2	Day 3	Day 4	Day 5	Day 6	Day 7
Day of week:	___	___	___	___	___	___	___
I consumed caffeinated drinks in the: (M)orning, (A)fternoon, (E)vening, (N/A)							
M / A / E / NA							
How many?	___	___	___	___	___	___	___
I exercised at least 20 minutes in the: (M)orning, (A)fternoon, (E)vening, (N/A)							
Medications I took today:							
Took a nap? (circle one)	Yes No	Yes No	Yes No	Yes No	Yes No	Yes No	Yes No
If Yes, for how long?							
During the day, how likely was I to doze off while performing daily activities: No chance, Slight chance, Moderate chance, High chance							
Throughout the day, my mood was... Very pleasant, Pleasant, Unpleasant, Very unpleasant							
Approximately 2-3 hours before going to bed, I consumed:							
Alcohol	☐	☐	☐	☐	☐	☐	☐
A heavy meal	☐	☐	☐	☐	☐	☐	☐
Caffeine	☐	☐	☐	☐	☐	☐	☐
Not applicable	☐	☐	☐	☐	☐	☐	☐
In the hour before going to sleep, my bedtime routine included: List activities including reading a book, using electronics, taking a bath, doing relaxation exercises, etc.							

FIGURE 11.2 National Sleep Foundation sleep diary.

Source: National Sleep Foundation (2016).

TABLE 11.2 Self-Care Assessment Worksheet

Rate the following areas according to how frequently you do the following where 3 = frequently; 2 = occasionally; 1 = barely or rarely; 0 = never; ? = never occurred to me					
Physical Self-Care	3	2	1	0	?
1. Eat regularly (breakfast, lunch, dinner)					
2. Get regular medical check-ups					
3. Get medical care when I need it					
4. Take time off when I am sick					
5. Wear clothes I like					
6. Do fun physical activities					
7. Think positive thoughts about my body					
8. Exercise					
9. Eat healthy					

(*continued*)

TABLE 11.2   Self-Care Assessment Worksheet   (*continued*)

Physical Self-Care	3	2	1	0	?
10. Get a massage					
11. Take vacations					
12. Get enough sleep					
13. Do some fun artistic activity					
14. Other (add a self-care activity that is relevant for you)					
Psychological Self-Care	3	2	1	0	?
1. Take day trips or minivacations					
2. Have my own personal psychotherapy					
3. Make time from technology/Internet					
4. Read something unrelated to work					
5. Notice my thoughts, beliefs, feelings, attitudes					
6. Engage my intelligence in a new way					
7. Make time for self-reflection					
8. Write in a journal					
9. Minimize stress in my life					
10. Be curious					
11. Say no to extra responsibilities/work, etc.					
12. Leave work at work					
13. Other:					
Emotional Self-Care	3	2	1	0	?
1. Spend time with people I enjoy					
2. Stay in touch with important people in my life					
3. Reread favorite books or rewatch favorite movies					
4. Express my outrage in social situations					
5. Love myself					
6. Let myself cry					
7. Affirm or praise myself					
8. Find things that make me laugh					
9. Other:					

(*continued*)

TABLE 11.2   Self-Care Assessment Worksheet   (*continued*)

Spiritual Self-Care	3	2	1	0	?
1. Make time for reflection					
2. Find a spiritual or community connection					
3. Take stock in the nonmaterial aspects of life					
4. Try not to always be the expert or boss					
5. Identify what is meaningful to me					
6. Seek out nourishing or reenergizing experiences					
7. Contribute to causes I believe in					
8. Read or listen to something inspirational					
9. Spend time in nature					
10. Cherish my optimism and hope					
11. Meditate					
12. Find time for prayer or praise					
13. Have experiences of awe					
14. Other:					
Relationship Self-Care	3	2	1	0	?
1. Schedule regular dates with my partner					
2. Call, check in, or visit my relatives					
3. Share a fear, hope, dream, or secret with someone I trust					
4. Stay in contact with faraway friends					
5. Make time for personal correspondence					
6. Allow others to do things for me					
7. Make time to be with friends					
8. Ask for help when I need it					
9. Communicate with my family					
10. Enlarge my social circle					
11. Spend time with animals					
12. Other:					

(*continued*)

TABLE 11.2   Self-Care Assessment Worksheet   (*continued*)

Workplace/Professional Self-Care	3	2	1	0	?
1. Take time to chat with coworkers					
2. Identify projects and tasks that are exciting					
3. Balance my load so that nothing is too much					
4. Arrange workspace to be comfortable					
5. Get regular supervision or consultation					
6. May quiet time to work					
7. Negotiate an advocate for my needs at work					
8. Take a break during the day					
9. Set limits with my boss and peers					
10. Have a peer-support group					
11. Identify rewarding tasks					
12. Other:					
Overall Balance	3	2	1	0	?
1. Strive for balance within my work–life and work day					
2. Strive for balance among my family, friends, and relationships					
3. Strive for balance between play and rest					
4. Strive for balance between work and personal time					
5. Strive for balance and looking forward and acknowledging the moment					
Areas of Self-Care Relevant to You	3	2	1	0	?
1.					
2.					
3.					

Note: This worksheet suggests various self-care strategies. Please enter strategies that are relevant for you and, as you review the results, look for patterns and opportunities. Listen to your internal responses in the dialogue you have with yourself and take note of anything that you would like to prioritize moving forward.

Adapted from Saakvitne, Pearlman, and The Staff of the Trauma Stress Institute/Center for Adult & Adolescent Psychotherapy (1996).

TABLE 11.3   Sample Work–Life Balance Quiz

Question	True	False
1. I find myself spending more and more time thinking about work.		
2. I often feel I do not have any time for myself, my family, and my friends.		
3. No matter what I do, it seems that often every minute of every day is always scheduled for something.		
4. Sometimes I feel as though I have lost sight of who I am and why I chose this profession.		
5. I cannot remember the last time I was able to find the time to take a day off to do something fun just for me.		
6. I feel stressed out most of the time.		
7. I cannot even remember the last time I used all my allotted vacation and/or personal days.		
8. It sometimes feels as though I never even have a chance to catch my breath before I have to move on to the next project/crisis.		
9. I cannot remember the last time I read—and finished—a book that I was reading purely for pleasure.		
10. I wish I had more time for some outside interests and hobbies, but I simply do not.		
11. I often feel exhausted.		
12. I cannot remember the last time I went to the movies or visited a museum or attended some other cultural event.		
13. I do what I do because so many people depend on me for support.		
14. I have missed many of my family's important events because of work.		
15. I almost always bring work home with me.		
Count up how many times you checked the "true" column.		
If you scored:		
<3: Your life is pretty well balanced, good job!		
3–5: Your work–life balance is in jeopardy; look for opportunities to make some changes.		
>5: Your life is out of balance and you need to critically examine how you can regain balance.		

■ REFERENCES

Barker, L. M., & Nussbaum, M. A. (2011). Fatigue, performance and the work environment: A survey of registered nurses. *Journal of Advanced Nursing*, *67*(6), 1370–1382.

Bickley, J. B. (1998). Care for the caregiver: The art of self-care. *Seminars in Perioperative Nursing*, *7*(2), 114–121.

Brodsky, D., Gupta, M., Quinn, M., Smallcomb, J., Mao, W., Koyama, N.,...Pursley, D. M. (2013). Building collaborative teams in neonatal intensive care. *BMJ Quality & Safety*, *22*(5), 374–382.

Buysse, D. J. (2014). Sleep health: Can we define it? Does it matter? *Sleep*, *37*(1), 9–17.

Ferri, M., Zygun, D. A., Harrison, A., & Stelfox, H. T. (2015). Evidence-based design in an intensive care unit: End-user perceptions. *BMC Anesthesiology*, *15*, 57.

Fischer, D., Vetter, C., Oberlinner, C., Wegener, S., & Roenneberg, T. (2016). A unique, fast-forward rotating schedule with 12-hour long shifts prevents chronic sleep debt. *Chronobiology International*, *33*(1), 98–107.

Gazelle, G., Liebschutz, J. M., & Riess, H. (2015). Physician burnout: Coaching a way out. *Journal of General Internal Medicine*, *30*(4), 508–513.

Germer, C. K., & Neff, K. D. (2013). Self-compassion in clinical practice. *Journal of Clinical Psychology*, *69*(8), 856–867.

Griep, R. H., Bastos, L. S., Fonseca, M. d. e. J., Silva-Costa, A., Portela, L. F., Toivanen, S., & Rotenberg, L. (2014). Years worked at night and body mass index among registered nurses from eighteen public hospitals in Rio de Janeiro, Brazil. *BMC Health Services Research*, *14*, 603.

Griffiths, P., Dall'Ora, C., Simon, M., Ball, J., Lindqvist, R., Rafferty, A. M.,...Aiken, L. H.; RN4CAST Consortium. (2014). Nurses' shift length and overtime working in 12 European countries: The association with perceived quality of care and patient safety. *Medical Care*, *52*(11), 975–981.

Johnson, J. R., Emmons, H. C., Rivard, R. L., Griffin, K. H., & Dusek, J. A. (2015). Resilience training: A pilot study of a mindfulness-based program with depressed healthcare professionals. *Explore*, *11*(6), 433–444.

Kotzer, A. M., Zacharakis, S. K., Raynolds, M., & Buenning, F. (2011). Evaluation of the built environment: Staff and family satisfaction pre- and post-occupancy of the Children's Hospital. *HERD*, *4*(4), 60–78.

Mark, B. A., Lindley, L., & Jones, C. B. (2009). Nurse working conditions and nursing unit costs. *Policy, Politics & Nursing Practice*, *10*(2), 120–128.

Mrayyan, M. T. (2004). Nurses' autonomy: Influence of nurse managers' actions. *Journal of Advanced Nursing*, *45*(3), 326–336.

Muecke, S. (2005). Effects of rotating night shifts: Literature review. *Journal of Advanced Nursing*, *50*(4), 433–439.

National Sleep Foundation. (2016). *Sleep diary*. Washington, DC: National Sleep Foundation. Retrieved from http://www.sleepfoundation.org/sleep-diary/SleepDiaryv6.pdf

Neff, K. D., & Germer, C. K. (2013). A pilot study and randomized controlled trial of the mindful self-compassion program. *Journal of Clinical Psychology*, *69*(1), 28–44.

Pan, A., Schernhammer, E. S., Sun, Q., & Hu, F. B. (2011). Rotating night shift work and risk of type 2 diabetes: Two prospective cohort studies in women. *PLoS Medicine*, *8*(12), e1001141.

Peplonska, B., Bukowska, A., & Sobala, W. (2015). Association of rotating night shift work with BMI and abdominal obesity among nurses and midwives. *PloS One*, *10*(7), e0133761.

Peplonska, B., Burdelak, W., Krysicka, J., Bukowska, A., Marcinkiewicz, A., Sobala, W.,... Rybacki, M. (2014). Night shift work and modifiable lifestyle factors. *International Journal of Occupational Medicine and Environmental Health*, *27*(5), 693–706.

Raab, K. (2014). Mindfulness, self-compassion, and empathy among health care professionals: A review of the literature. *Journal of Health Care Chaplaincy*, *20*(3), 95–108.

Saakvitne, K. W., Pearlman, L. A.; The Staff of the Trauma Stress Institute/Center for Adult & Adolescent Psychotherapy. (1996). *Transforming the pain: A workbook on vicarious traumatization.* New York, NY: W. W. Norton [Adapted by Lisa D. Butler, PhD].

Salas, E., & Rosen, M. A. (2013). Building high reliability teams: Progress and some reflections on teamwork training. *BMJ Quality & Safety, 22*(5), 369–373.

Samra, H. A., & Smith, B. A. (2015). *The effect of staff nurses' shift length and fatigue on patient safety and nurses' health: Position statements #3066.* Chicago, IL: National Association of Neonatal Nurses.

Sanchez-Reilly, S., Morrison, L. J., Carey, E., Bernacki, R., O'Neill, L., Kapo, J.,... Thomas, J. deLima. (2013). Caring for oneself to care for others: Physicians and their self-care. *The Journal of Supportive Oncology, 11*(2), 75–81.

Shanafelt, T. D., Gorringe, G., Menaker, R., Storz, K. A., Reeves, D., Buskirk, S. J.,... Swensen, S. J. (2015). Impact of organizational leadership on physician burnout and satisfaction. *Mayo Clinic Proceedings, 90*(4), 432–440.

Sirois, F. M. (2015). A self-regulation resource model of self-compassion and health behavior intentions in emerging adults. *Preventive Medicine Reports, 2,* 218–222.

Smith, A. P. (2006). Paving and resurfacing the road to Magnet: The perspective and wisdom of Magnet-designated coordinators–part I. *Nursing Economics, 24*(2), 112–115.

Smith-Miller, C. A., Shaw-Kokot, J., Curro, B., & Jones, C. B. (2014). An integrative review: Fatigue among nurses in acute care settings. *The Journal of Nursing Administration, 44*(9), 487–494.

Sveinsdottir, H., Ragnarsdottir, E. D., & Blondal, K. (2016). Praise matters: The influence of nurse unit managers praise on nurses practice, work environment and job satisfaction: A questionnaire study. *Journal of Advanced Nursing, 72*(3), 558–568.

Swathi, S., Ramesh, A., Nagapoornima, M., Fernandes, L. M., Jisina, C., Rao, P. N., & Swarnarekha, A. (2014). Sustaining "culture of silence" in the neonatal intensive care unit during nonemergency situations: A grounded theory on ensuring adherence to behavioral modification to reduce noise levels. *International Journal of Qualitative Studies on Health and Well-Being, 18*(9), 22523. doi:10.3402/qhw.v9.22523

Szosland, D. (2010). Shift work and metabolic syndrome, diabetes mellitus and ischaemic heart disease. *International Journal of Occupational Medicine and Environmental Health, 23*(3), 287–291.

Teixeira, P. J., Carraça, E. V., Markland, D., Silva, M. N., & Ryan, R. M. (2012). Exercise, physical activity, and self-determination theory: A systematic review. *The International Journal of Behavioral Nutrition and Physical Activity, 9,* 78.

Vago, D. R., & Silbersweig, D. A. (2012). Self-awareness, self-regulation, and self-transcendence (S-ART): A framework for understanding the neurobiological mechanisms of mindfulness. *Frontiers in Human Neuroscience, 6,* 296.

Weinberg, D. B., Avgar, A. C., Sugrue, N. M., & Cooney-Miner, D. (2013). The importance of a high-performance work environment in hospitals. *Health Services Research, 48*(1), 319–332.

Wells-Federman, C. L. (1996). Awakening the nurse healer within. *Holistic Nursing Practice, 10*(2), 13–29.

Epilogue: Conclusion and a Call to Action

A hospital-acquired condition (HAC) is an undesirable situation or condition that is a result of the patient's hospitalization. Standard HACs identified by the Centers for Medicare & Medicaid Services (CMS) include such things as retained foreign objects after surgery, air embolism, blood incompatibility errors, Stage III and IV pressure ulcers, patient falls, poor glycemic control in the hospital, catheter-associated urinary tract infections, vascular catheter-associated infections, surgical site infections, and iatrogenic pneumothorax with venous catheterization.

CMS defines HACs as those complications or situations that incur additional costs and payments and could have reasonably been prevented through the application of evidence-based guidelines. In light of the evolving evidence validating the deleterious effects of toxic stress and allostatic load on the developing individual (Figure E.1) combined with our understanding of the effectiveness of various evidence-based practices that mitigate early-life adversity, one may conclude that, to some extent, the early-life adversity endured by individuals hospitalized in the neonatal intensive care unit (NICU) is a HAC and may be prevented or at the very least reduced, through the adoption and integration of evidence-based guidelines.

Grounded by the work of Ganzel, Morris, and Wethington (2010); McEwen and Gianaros (2011); Montirosso and Provenzi (2015); and Moore, Berger, and Wilson (2014), there is clearly more than enough evidence to compel neonatal clinicians to consistently and reliably integrate and implement the evidence-based practice guidelines presented in this text. Core emotional regions of the brain (cortical limbic structures) play a key role in interpreting and responding to external stressors, cultivating resilience or susceptibility to trauma, and can be modulated by authentic healing intention, presence, and relationship-based encounters (Bogdan, Pagliaccio, Baranger, & Hariri, 2016; Ganzel et al., 2010; Ganzel & Morris, 2011; Karatsoreos & McEwen 2011).

It takes a village to raise a child.
    —African proverb

Clinically relevant, transdisciplinary, evidence-based practice guidelines with effective implementation strategies create a solid foundation on which to improve and standardize the experience of care for the hospitalized infant and family. With prevention-oriented focus on quality and patient safety, the consistently reliable provision of trauma-informed, age-appropriate care in the NICU has lifelong implications for the infant–family dyad, the professional, and society at large.

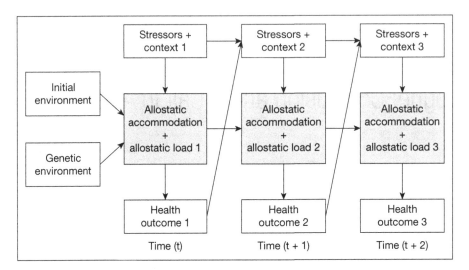

FIGURE E.1 Allostatic model across development.

Source: Ganzel, Morris, and Wethington (2010). Copyright © 2010 by the American Psychological Association. Reproduced with permission. The use of American Psychiatric Association (APA) information does not imply endorsement by APA.

This is not easy; there are competing priorities, personality challenges, and organizational barriers to change and transformation; however, these cannot get in the way of doing the right thing: *First, do no harm!*

This work requires persistence, creativity, and an unwavering commitment to excellence in service to other. It is my hope that you have found this book helpful and I invite you to visit the companion webpage (www.caringessentials.org/b2) for additional resources, guidance, and inspiration.

I would like to leave you with a few quotes to inspire you on your journey and honor the path that you have chosen!

Reach out and touch another human being not just with your hands
but with your heart.
      —Tahereh Mafi

Love and compassion are necessities, not luxuries, without them
humanity cannot survive.
      —Dalai Lama XIV

Courage. Kindness. Friendship. Character. These are the qualities that
define us as human beings, and propel us, on occasion, to greatness.
      —R. J. Palacio

Take care and care well.
      —Mary Coughlin

■ REFERENCES

Bogdan, R., Pagliaccio, D., Baranger, D. A., & Hariri, A. R. (2016). Genetic moderation of stress effects on corticolimbic circuitry. *Neuropsychopharmacology, 41*(1), 275–296.

Ganzel, B. L., & Morris, P. A. (2011). Allostasis and the developing human brain: Explicit consideration of implicit models. *Development and Psychopathology, 23*(4), 955–974.

Ganzel, B. L., Morris, P. A., & Wethington, E. (2010). Allostasis and the human brain: Integrating models of stress from the social and life sciences. *Psychological Review, 117*(1), 134–174.

Karatsoreos, I. N., & McEwen, B. S. (2011). Psychobiological allostasis: Resistance, resilience and vulnerability. *Trends in Cognitive Sciences, 15*(12), 576–584.

McEwen, B. S., & Gianaros, P. J. (2011). Stress- and allostasis-induced brain plasticity. *Annual Review of Medicine, 62*, 431–445.

Montirosso, R., & Provenzi, L. (2015). Implications of epigenetics and stress regulation on research and developmental care of preterm infants. *Journal of Obstetric, Gynecologic, and Neonatal Nursing, 44*(2), 174–182.

Moore, T. A., Berger, A. M., & Wilson, M. E. (2014). A new way of thinking about complications of prematurity. *Biological Research for Nursing, 16*(1), 72–82.

Index